Your *Clinics* subs

MW01181706

You can now access the FULL TEXT of this publication online at no additional cost! Activate your online subscription today and receive...

- Full text of all issues from 2002 to the present
- Photographs, tables, illustrations, and references
- Comprehensive search capabilities
- Links to MEDLINE and Elsevier journals

Activate Your Online Access Today!

Plus, you can also sign up for E-alerts of upcoming issues or articles that interest you, and take advantage of exclusive access to bonus features!

To activate your individual online subscription:

1. Visit our website at **www.TheClinics.com**.

2. Click on "Register" at the top of the page, and follow the instructions.

3. To activate your account, you will need your subscriber account number, which you can find on your mailing label (note: the number of digits in your subscriber account number varies from six to ten digits). See the sample below where the subscriber account number has been circled.

This is your subscriber account number

```
**********************************************3-DIGIT 001
FEB00   J0167   C7   (123456-89)  10/00   Q: 1

J.H. DOE, MD
531 MAIN ST
CENTER CITY, NY  10001-001
```

4. That's it! Your online access to the most trusted source for clinical reviews is now available.

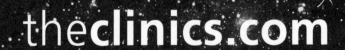

W.B. SAUNDERS COMPANY
A Division of Elsevier Inc.

The Curtis Center • Independence Square West • Philadelphia, PA 19106–3399

http://www.theclinics.com

THE OTOLARYNGOLOGIC CLINICS
OF NORTH AMERICA
April 2005
Editor: Molly Jay

Volume 38, Number 2
ISSN 0030–6665
ISBN 1-4160-2861-7

Reprints. For copies of 100 or more, of articles in this publication, please contact the Commercial Reprints Department, Elsevier Inc., 360 Park Avenue South, New York, New York 10010-1710. Tel. (212) 633-3813 Fax: (212) 462-1935 email: reprints@elsevier.com

The ideas and opinions expressed in *The Otolaryngologic Clinics of North America* do not necessarily reflect those of the Publisher. The Publisher does not assume any responsibility for any injury and/or damage to persons or property arising out of or related to any use of the material contained in this periodical. The reader is advised to check the appropriate medical literature and the product information currently provided by the manufacturer of each drug to be administered to verify the dosage, the method and duration of administration, or contraindications. It is the responsibility of the treating physician or other health care professional, relying on independent experience and knowledge of the patient, to determine drug dosages and the best treatment for the patient. Mention of any product in this issue should not be construed as endorsement by the contributors, editors, or the Publisher of the product or manufacturers' claims.

The Otolaryngologic Clinics of North America (ISSN 0030–6665) is published bimonthly by W.B. Saunders Company. Corporate and editorial offices: 1600 JFK Boulevard, Suite 1800, Philadelphia, PA 19103-2822. Accounting and circulation offices: 6277 Sea Harbor Drive, Orlando, FL 32887–4800. Periodicals postage paid at Orlando, FL 32862, and additional mailing offices. Subscription price is $199.00 per year (US individuals), $350.00 per year (US institutions), $100.00 per year (US student/resident), $269.00 per year (Canadian individuals), $430.00 per year (Canadian institutions), $280.00 per year (international individuals), $430.00 per year (international institutions), $140.00 per year (international & Canadian student/resident). Foreign air speed delivery is included in all *Clinics'* subscription prices. All prices are subject to change without notice. POSTMASTER: Send address changes to *The Otolaryngologic Clinics of North America*, W.B. Saunders Company, Periodicals Fulfillment, Orlando, FL 32887–4800. **Customer Service: 1-800-654-2452 (US). From outside the US, call 407-345-4000.**

The Otolaryngologic Clinics of North America is also published in Spanish by McGraw-Hill Interamericana Editores S.A., P.O. Box 5-237, 06500 Mexico D.F., Mexico.

The Otolaryngologic Clinics of North America is covered in *Index Medicus, Current Contents/Clinical Medicine, Excerpta Medica, BIOSIS, Science Citation Index,* and *ISI/BIOMED.*

Printed in the United States of America.

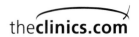

OTOLARYNGOLOGIC CLINICS OF NORTH AMERICA

Bioengineering in Otolaryngology

GUEST EDITOR
Arlen D. Meyers, MD, MBA

April 2005 • Volume 38 • Number 2

SAUNDERS

An Imprint of Elsevier, Inc.
PHILADELPHIA   LONDON   TORONTO   MONTREAL   SYDNEY   TOKYO

GUEST EDITOR

ARLEN D. MEYERS, MD, MBA, Professor, Department of Otolaryngology, University of Colorado Health Sciences Center, Denver, Colorado

CONTRIBUTORS

KRISTI S. ANSETH, PhD, Department of Chemical and Biological Engineering, University of Colorado; and Howard Hughes Medical Institute, University of Colorado, Boulder, Colorado

JEFFREY A. ARTHUR, BS, Department of Chemical and Biological Engineering, University of Colorado, Boulder, Colorado

MASOUD ASADI-ZEYDABADI, PhD, University of Colorado, Denver, Colorado

THOMAS CARROLL, MD, Department of Otolaryngology, University of Colorado Health Sciences Center, Denver, Colorado

MEISONG DING, PhD, Assistant Professor, Department of Radiation Oncology, University of Colorado Health Science Center, Aurora, Colorado

BRENNAN T. DODSON, MD, Department of Otolaryngology–Head and Neck Surgery, University of Colorado Health Sciences Center, Denver, Colorado

STEPHEN T. FLOCK, PhD, Rocky Mountain Biosystems, Golden, Colorado

G. LOUIS HORNYAK, PhD, Assistant Research Professor, Department of Physics and Astronomy, University of Denver, Denver Colorado; and Executive Director, Colorado Nanotechnology Initiative, Inc., Lakewood, Colorado

FARZIN IMANI, MD, PhD, University of Colorado Health Sciences Center, UCHSC at Fitzsimons, Aurora, Colorado

KRISTEN JAAX, MD, PhD, Advanced Bionics Corp., Valencia, California

TERRY R. KNAPP, MD, President, OrthoNetx, Inc., Superior, Colorado

DAWN BURTON KOCH, PhD, Advanced Bionics Corp., Valencia, California

KEITH LADNER, BS, Department of Otolaryngology, University of Colorado Health Sciences Center, Denver, Colorado

KEVIN S. MARCHITTO, PhD, Rocky Mountain Biosystems, Golden, Colorado

ELIZABETH MARTIN, MA, Advanced Bionics Corp., Valencia, California

KENNETH J. MCCABE, MD, Neuroradiology Fellow, Mallinkrodt Institute of Radiology, St. Louis, Missouri

ARLEN D. MEYERS, MD, MBA, Professor, Department of Otolaryngology, University of Colorado Health Sciences Center, Denver, Colorado

SILVIA MIOC, PhD, MBA, President, Colorado Photonics Industry Association, Longmont, Colorado; and Physicist, General Electric Healthcare Technologies, Louisville, Colorado

MARY-ANN MYCEK, PhD, Associate Professor, Applied Physics Program, Department of Biomedical Engineering, College of Engineering, University of Michigan; and Comprehensive Cancer Center, University of Michigan, Ann Arbor, Michigan

FRANCIS NEWMAN, MS, Assistant Professor, Department of Radiation Oncology, University of Colorado Health Science Center, Aurora, Colorado

JONATHAN M. OWENS, MD, Department of Otolaryngology–Head and Neck Surgery, University of Colorado Health Sciences Center, Denver, Colorado

DAVID RABEN, MD, Associate Professor, Department of Radiation Oncology, University of Colorado Health Science Center, Aurora, Colorado

MARK A. RICE, BS, Department of Chemical and Biological Engineering, University of Colorado, Boulder, Colorado

RANDOLPH C. ROBINSON, MD, DDS, Private Practice, Oral and Maxillofacial Surgery, Lone Tree, Colorado; and Medical Director, OrthoNetx, Inc., Superior, Colorado

DAVID RUBINSTEIN, MD, Associate Professor, Department of Radiology, University of Colorado Health Sciences Center, Denver, Colorado

RAHMAT A. SHOURESHI, PhD, Dean, School of Engineering and Computer Science, University of Denver, Denver, Colorado

STEVE STALLER, PhD, Advanced Bionics Corp., Valencia, California

RANDALL TAGG, PhD, University of Colorado, Denver, Colorado

CONTRIBUTORS

CONTENTS

The seal would be physiologically and mechanically seamless, be fluid- and air-tight, and have a tensile strength and degree of elasticity suited to the tissue. Additionally, the seal would be aesthetically acceptable, inexpensive to achieve, and easy to apply even in minimally invasive surgeries. This paper reviews tissue fusion devices and techniques that may one day provide us with such biologically invisible wound closures.

ways to mix radionuclides for enhanced radiobiologic effects, and different fractionation schemes that have grown in clinical importance. Intensity-modulated radiotherapy has become a mainstay in head and neck cancer treatment, and the authors discuss several popular and emerging approaches. Patient immobilization and imaging are also discussed.

Although the steel blade and monopolar electrocautery remain widely used and are often preferred by practicing otolaryngologists, newer, emerging technologies have been shown to improve surgical time, decrease postoperative pain, and reduce collateral tissue damage and unwanted side effects for select procedures. This article presents four alternative surgical dissection techniques including the ultrasonically activated scalpel, bipolar electrosurgical scissors, coblation, and temperature-controlled radiofrequency ablation, describes how the instruments work, and discusses the advantages and disadvantages of each technique, its application in otolaryngology, and complications and controversies surrounding its use.

FORTHCOMING ISSUES

The Clinics are now available online!

Access your subscription at
www.theclinics.com

ELSEVIER
SAUNDERS

Otolaryngol Clin N Am
38 (2005) xi–xiii

OTOLARYNGOLOGIC
CLINICS
OF NORTH AMERICA

Preface

Bioengineering in Otolaryngology

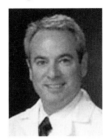

Arlen D. Meyers, MD, MBA
Guest Editor

This issue of the *Otolaryngology Clinics of North America* reflects three basic trends in biomedical technology research, development, and transfer and, more specifically, their application to otolaryngology-head and neck surgery.

First, in the life sciences, interdisciplinary collaboration in discovery and development has become the norm. Interactions between scientists and engineers in the fields of biology, chemistry, physics, photonics, computer science, aerospace engineering, nanotechnology, and materials science have spawned a new generation of smart materials, microelectronics, and intelligent biomedical clothing. All of these inventions have emerging applications in otolaryngology.

In an effort to facilitate and coordinate bioengineering research, The National Institute of Biomedical Imaging and Bioengineering was formed a few years ago as the newest addition to the National Institutes of Health. The mission of the National Institute of Biomedical Imaging and Bioengineering is to improve health by promoting fundamental discoveries, design and development, and translation and assessment of technologic capabilities in biomedical imaging and bioengineering, enabled by relevant areas of information science, physics, chemistry, mathematics, materials science, and computer sciences. In addition, the National Institutes of Health has highlighted interdisciplinary collaboration as a key component of its new strategic plan, placing cross-disciplinary partnerships at the top of its funding priorities. An Alliance for Nanotechnology at the National

0030-6665/05/$ - see front matter © 2005 Elsevier Inc. All rights reserved.
doi:10.1016/j.otc.2004.10.002

Cancer Institute has been formed, and the National Science Foundation is sponsoring the formation of Nanocenters of Excellence around the United States.

The acceleration of technology transfer is a second theme. Universities and colleges are increasingly realizing the value of intellectual property invented by their faculties. A 2002 report from the Association of University Technology Mangers noted that

- Running royalties on product sales were $1.005 billion, an 18.9% increaser over fiscal year 2001.
- In fiscal year 2002, 450 new companies were established for a total of 4320 since 1980.
- At the end of fiscal year 2002, 2741 of those start-ups were still operating.

Millions of dollars in revenue are being realized by commercializing ideas that otherwise would have sat on the shelf. This push to the marketplace has benefited patients and providers and has fueled the impressive growth of medical device companies, biotechnology start-ups, and the necessary service providers that are essential to their formation. The devices and innovations described in this volume are but a few of the applications in otolaryngology.

In addition to interdisciplinary collaboration and technology transfer, this book also reflects the third major trend—increasing academic–industry collaboration. A new generation of bioentrepreneurs and faculty inventors are working together to invent, commercialize, and finance exciting new ventures. As a result of the emergence of national and international bioclusters, workforce development and training in pharmaceutical bio-technology and bioengineering has rapidly moved to the top of the economic development agenda in numerous states and countries that are eager to take advantage of well-paying jobs, clean industries, and tax revenues. Several of the authors in this book are bioentrepreneurs, having started life science companies from discoveries made at universities.

I would like to thank the authors and industry colleagues who have contributed to this issue of the *Otolaryngology Clinics of North America*. In addition, I would like to congratulate the editors at Elsevier for recognizing the emerging importance of bioengineering and for publishing this ground-breaking book. I hope that future publications will describe bioengineering advances in specialties other than otolaryngology.

Despite the naysayers who whine about how the health care sky is falling, this is an exciting time in the history of science and health care innovation. New health care products and services will continue to emerge at an accelerating pace, forcing us to debate the important social, economic, and ethical issues they will present. The authors and I, representatives from both academia and industry, hope you enjoy this issue, a brief glimpse into the future of bioengineering in otolaryngology.

Arlen D. Meyers, MD, MBA
Professor, Department of Otolaryngology
University of Colorado Health Sciences Center
4200 East Ninth Avenue, B 205
Denver, CO 80262, USA

E-mail address: Arlen.Meyers@UCHSC.edu

ELSEVIER
SAUNDERS

Otolaryngol Clin N Am
38 (2005) 185–197

OTOLARYNGOLOGIC
CLINICS
OF NORTH AMERICA

Introduction to Bioengineering: Melding of Engineering and Biological Sciences

Rahmat A. Shoureshi, PhD

Dean, School of Engineering and Computer Science, University of Denver, East Boettcher Center 2050 East Iliff Avenue, 227, Denver, Colorado 80208, USA

Bioengineering uses engineering principles and techniques in the analysis and solution of problems in medicine and biology. Engineering disciplines rely on the principles of analysis and synthesis; through the integration of these principles, quantitative design principles that demonstrate the role of component properties in the overall system behavior are derived.

Engineering disciplines use measurement systems, mathematical and experimental modeling, and actuators to manipulate systems based on mathematics, physics, and chemistry. Recently, engineering has found biology to be another scientific area that is accessible and amenable. Therefore, a new discipline of bioengineering has emerged and is aimed at analysis of biological systems. These systems could be the building blocks for synthesis of technologies that would benefit, modify, and control living systems.

What is bioengineering?

The second half of the twentieth century experienced a revolution in the biological sciences. The March 10, 1997, issue of *Business Week* stated that biology will define scientific progress in the twenty-first century and called this century "the biotech century."

Engineering has traditionally been focused on the outward extension of biological organisms, namely external extensions such as transportation systems (eg, high-rise buildings, entertainment systems). In contrast, bioengineering is concerned with processes inside the biological organism. Unlike other engineering disciplines, there is no particular subject matter or set of techniques that belongs exclusively to bioengineering. Bioengineering applies the techniques of all the traditional engineering disciplines to

E-mail address: rshoures@du.edu

problems encountered in living systems. These challenges presented by living systems do not exist for physical systems.

Therefore, the bioengineering discipline is focused on educating engineers who can analyze a problem from both engineering and biologic perspectives. Bioengineers design medical devices such as imaging machines (eg, MRI machines), artificial organs, cardiac pacemakers, and hip and knee implants, among other devices. They also develop biologically compatible materials and design instrumentation and measurement techniques for drug delivery, bioprosthetic devices, information processing in the brain, control of heart function, artificial retinas, and advanced hearing systems.

As the field of bioengineering matures, its findings and developments will blur the distinction between inward and outward processes. Design of machines that draw inspiration from biologic processes (eg, biomimetics) and biomachines that intimately integrate a biologic organism and a machine are examples of this blurring of the inward and outward thrusts of bioengineering with respect to biologic organisms. The schematic diagram shown in Fig. 1 depicts this concept.

As stated by Bugliavello [1], the goal of physics as a science is to understand nature and universe. The goal of biology is to understand

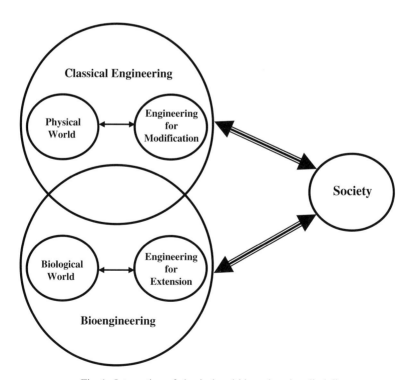

Fig. 1. Interaction of classical and bioengineering disciplines.

biologic nature. The goal of engineering, however, is to modify nature and extend the life of living systems. The domain of physics is universal; the domain of biology is limited to the biologic organisms; the goal of medicine is limited to humans and animals. The domain of engineering is limitless. It ranges from machines and alterations of nature (eg, nanomachines moving through the body) to macroenvironmental machines or processes. The key instruments of both physics and biology are theory. Those of medicine are diagnosis and therapy. The key instruments of engineering are design and synthesis. Thus, bioengineers deal with design of machines, instruments, processes, and technologies that will extend the life of living systems.

Arthur Johnson [2] attempts to define bioengineering in terms of attributes of a discipline. He states that there are two generally accepted characteristics associated with a discipline: (1) a distinct body of knowledge, and (2) distinct methods. Without these two characteristics, a new discipline is just an extension of prior disciplines. Within engineering, there are two categories of disciplines: application-based engineering and science-based engineering. The first category defines the discipline by those served (eg, petroleum engineering). The second category defines the discipline by its scientific foundations (eg, mechanical engineering, which is based on physics, and chemical engineering, which is based on chemistry).

The field of bioengineering is peculiar in that it can be categorized as application based or as science based (ie, based on biology). This dual categorization arises partly because a body of knowledge has not been defined and partly because unique methods have not been identified for bioengineering. This duality can be observed in the subdisciplines within bioengineering.

The Bioengineering Consortium within the National Institutes of Health has given the following definition for bioengineering:

> Bioengineering integrates physical, chemical, or mathematical sciences and engineering principles for the study of biology, medicine, behavior, or health. It advances fundamental concepts, creates knowledge for the molecular to organ systems levels, and develops innovative biologics, materials, processes, implants, devices, and informatics approaches for the prevention, diagnosis, and treatment of disease, for patient rehabilitation, and for improving health.

Subdisciplines of bioengineering

Some regard the work of Watson and Crick, which revealed the double-helix structure of DNA, as the formation of biological sciences and bioinformatics [3]. Also, the introduction of this field is referenced to the advent of cell culture in the work of Leff [3] that made it possible to grow living cells in the research laboratory. In the late 1980s bioengineering products began to appear in the marketplace, and the field has experience exponential growth during last 20 years.

The Whitaker Foundation became an important catalyst in the formation of biomedical engineering departments at many universities across the nation. The multimillion-dollar estate left to the Foundation has made a profound impact on the progress in research and education of bio-engineering. Research in the field can range from using computers to map DNA strands to designing artificial limbs and organs to enhancing rehabilitative therapy with cell and tissue regeneration.

Through research and educational programs, both nationally and internationally, the subdisciplines of bioengineering discussed in the following sections have been introduced. This list is not all inclusive; rather, it defines the most common disciplines identified and described by institutions such as John Hopkins University, the Massachusetts Institute of Technology, Duke University, the University of Denver, and others.

Cell and tissue engineering

Tissue engineering, one of the most rapidly growing areas in biomedical engineering, offers great potential for changing traditional approaches to meeting many critical health care needs. In the years to come, many tissues or organs, including bone, cartilage, liver, pancreas, skin, blood vessel, and peripheral nerve, may be strong candidates for engineering reconstruction.

Cardiovascular systems

As the country's primary cause of death, cardiovascular disease poses a major health problem for thousands of individuals. In response to national concern, researchers from across the disciplines of physiology, biophysics, biomechanics, mathematics, system identification, and computer modeling have come together to work collaboratively on a number of cardiovascular research projects.

Biomedical imaging science

Technological advances now allow imaging of the human body at scales ranging from a single molecule to the whole body. Researchers are linking the anatomic data, collected with emerging imaging technologies, to computer simulations to form truly functional images of individual patients. These images will allow physicians to see what a patient's organs look like and also how they are functioning, even at the smallest dimensions. A major challenge is how to store, analyze, distribute, understand, and use the enormous amount of data associated with every one of these thousands of images.

Systems neuroscience

The brain, perhaps the greatest and most complicated learning system, exercises control over virtually every aspect of human behavior. Systems neuroscience is dedicated to understanding the brain's architecture and how it learns and controls a variety of functions. Dramatic advances in experimental methods for studying neural systems have occurred during the past decade. Investigators in this area are working to produce quantitative models of information coding and processing in neural systems.

Molecular and cellular engineering physiology

The human body is comprised of some 100 trillion cells, each of which is capable of performing most of the fundamental functions of life. A central biologic problem is understanding how molecules interact to produce observable cell functions. This staggering challenge holds the keys to understanding human biology at its most basic level and to designing potential treatments for disease. Training in molecular and cellular systems equips researchers to navigate one of the most critical interfaces of modern scientific research: the intersection of molecular and cellular biology with the disciplines of engineering and mathematics.

Computational biology and bioinformatics

Vast amounts of genetic and biochemical information are becoming rapidly available. Every day, researchers in biomedical engineering draw on these data as they combine the knowledge of the human genome with the massive power of modern computers to construct simulations of human organs. These simulations or models will be so realistic that they can be used to design and test novel therapeutics, including medical devices, pharmaceuticals, and clinical procedures.

Neuroscience and neuroengineering

Engineering, computational, and mathematical approaches to solving problems in basic and clinical neurosciences form the foundation of neuroengineering. Researchers are developing novel and advanced sensors, instrumentation, micro- and nanotechnologies, and signal-processing algorithms for neurosciences. Close association with researchers in clinical neuroscience (ie, in neurology, neurosurgery, and psychiatry) enables neuro-engineers to focus on problems with important clinical applications, for example the design of diagnostic monitors for detecting brain injury in the operating room and neurologic ICU.

Biomechanics

Biomechanics focuses on the human musculoskeletal system and its intricacies such as joint movement and orthopedics. Biomaterials, joint motion analysis, three-dimensional modeling of implants, in vivo and in vitro measurements of joints and implant dynamics, design of smart implants, and the impact of loading on musculoskeletal systems are some of the topics addressed by the discipline of biomechanics.

Rehabilitation engineering

Rehabilitation engineering addresses the development of new rehabilitation techniques and the design of new assistive devices. Bioinstrumentation, biocontrol, man–machine interactions, mobility of disabled persons, and devices and techniques for cognitively and physically impaired persons are covered under the disciplines of rehabilitation and assistive technology.

Nanoscale engineering of biological sciences

Nanoscale bioengineering focuses on the development of a fundamental understanding of nanobiostructures and processes, nanobiotechnology, and techniques for a broad range of applications in biomaterials, biosystem-based electronics, agriculture, and health. This discipline provides understanding of the relationships among chemical composition, single-molecule behavior, and physical shape at the nanoscale level of biologic functioning. Design of molecular motors, construction of nanoprobes, and synthesis of nanoscale materials based on the principles of biologic self-assembly are concepts covered in this discipline.

Sample projects in bioengineering

This section provides two examples of the bioengineering projects that are being performed under the author's supervision.

Portable brain functional imaging using near-infrared light

There are a variety of functional brain imaging techniques, but these devices are not portable, many of them do not allow movement, and measurement collection can be cumbersome. New to the field is the use of near-infrared spectroscopy (NIRS) [4–9]. NIRS is possible because biologic tissue is relatively transparent to light in the near-infrared range between 700 and 1000 nm. Water absorption and hemoglobin absorption are relatively small within this wavelength region. NIRS, therefore, allows the noninvasive recording of cortical activity. Four types of activity-related signals can be recorded noninvasively: (1) changes in hemoglobin oxygenation, (2) changes in blood volume, (3) changes in CO_2 oxidation, and (4) fast optical signals presumably related to changes in light scattering. Thus, the author's research has focused on investigating the feasibility of NIRS for imaging brain functioning.

The key instrument of the author's research in functional brain imaging is a cognoscope. The cognoscope provides light sources and detectors on a band worn around the head. Consisting of four light-emitting diode (LED) sources and 10 Opto 101 photodiode detectors, this multichannel device can make an entire sampling pass in 200 milliseconds. The LEDs provide two different wavelengths of near-infrared light, which easily passes through biologic tissues and is highly scattered. The penetration depth is roughly 7 cm, depending upon the skull thickness. This depth allows visualization of the cerebral cortex. Literature reviews have shown that different groups have used this near-infrared technique for a variety of studies including prefrontal cortex research that examines thought processes, monitoring of the visual cortex during stimulation, and even some basic monitoring of the motor cortex during simple finger movements. This research is the first major step toward tracking brain activation and patterns associated with specific activities and large-motor movements. Fig. 2 shows the sources and detectors of the device mounted on a headband.

The selected unit for near-infrared imaging is the LEDI system (Near Infrared Monitoring, Inc., Philadelphia, PA), shown in Fig. 2. This sensor has been applied in a broad variety of areas of clinical research including research in cognitive function, breast cancer imaging, and muscle function. Additionally, when compared with previous generations of near-infrared imaging systems, the LEDI system provides a notable increase in the number of channels available, a decrease in power consumption per channel, and an increase in system reliability and robustness with respect to probe design and signal integrity. Moreover, the LEDI system includes a number of options that facilitate the capturing, storage, and analysis of data.

Fig. 3 demonstrates one of many analysis options provided with the LEDI system. An interface allows the operator to analyze the data with a number of features. Fig. 3 shows a plot of the relative blood oxygen and blood volume levels with respect to the individual channels.

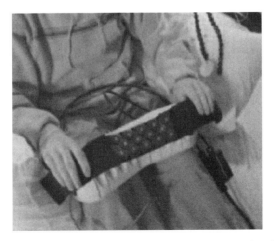

Fig. 2. The cognoscope with the sensors and detectors turned up for display.

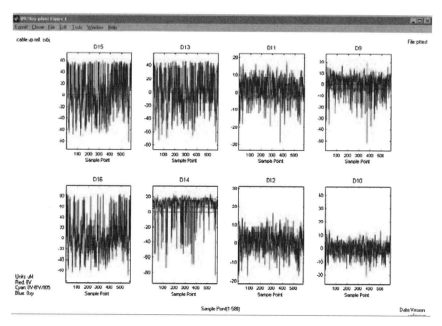

Fig. 3. Blood oxygenation and blood volume levels for each channel.

To assess the accuracy and performance of the cognoscope, the author and his colleagues are using the output of a magnetoencephalography (MEG) brain-imaging device as the benchmark. MEG was first reported in the late 1960s when a researcher at MIT saw evidence of an alpha-frequency magnetic field emanating from the heads of human subjects. MEG is based on the principle that all electric currents generate magnetic fields. The main source of the extracranial magnetic fields that are detected with the MEG instruments is current flow in the long apical dendrites of the cortical pyramidal cells. A distal excitatory synapse will induce a dipolar dendritic current toward the soma of the pyramidal cell; the electricity is flowing in one direction along the entire length of the dendrite, which therefore may be considered an electric dipole. Pyramidal neurons constitute nearly 70% of neocortical neurons, and the cells are oriented with their long apical dendrites perpendicular to the brain cortex. Fig. 4 shows the cognoscope on the head of a researcher who is seated in an MEG machine.

There are more than 100,000 of these cells per square millimeter of cortex. Dipolar currents flowing in these dendrites induce time-varying magnetic fields perpendicular to the dendrite direction. Therefore only cells oriented parallel to the skull surface produce magnetic fields that extend extracranially. The pattern of these external magnetic fields can be used to determine the location, orientation, and strength of the source electric dipoles.

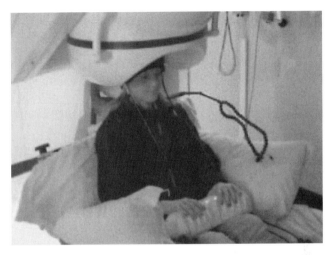

Fig. 4. A researcher sits with her head partially inserted into the MEG device and the cognoscope wrapped around the prefrontal cortex.

This research is in progress and has the potential for developing devices that can be directly controlled by the human brain. This project illustrates how the integration of electrical engineering, anatomy, and biology can result in a unique process and device for portable brain imaging.

Shoe insole for prevention of neuropathy in diabetic patients

Another project is aimed at developing a shoe insole equipped with a wireless temperature monitoring system that provides feedback to the patient about a pattern of activities that may lead to ulceration. This insole could have the potential for reducing amputation in diabetic patients. Several hypotheses are being investigated within this bioengineering project. The author and colleagues are investigating whether subjects using an insole temperature monitoring device and prescriptive self-care will have

- A significantly decreased risk over time of foot ulceration, Charcot fractures, and amputations, significantly better health-related quality of life, and changes in self-efficacy scale and subscale scores
- Fewer infections and cases of osteomyelitis
- Shorter ulcer-related length of stay for those hospitalized with foot ulcers or Charcot fractures
- Decreased healing time for foot ulcers or Charcot fractures when compared with the usual-care group

Diabetic foot wounds are the most common underlying cause of lower-extremity amputation in the United States. Amputations have a tremendous physical, emotional, and financial impact on patients and their families.

Once a person with diabetes has an amputation, the risk of developing a foot ulcer or requiring a second amputation increases dramatically [10–12]. Five percent to 19% of amputees die during their hospitalization, and as many as 50% die within the 5-year period after the amputation. Besides death, amputation of the contralateral limb and disability are frequent sequelae of a diabetic limb amputation. It is generally assumed that diabetes-related lower-extremity amputations have a significantly deleterious impact on quality of life [13–16].

Over the last 3 decades, several authors have suggested that skin temperature monitoring may be a valuable tool to detect sites at risk of potential breakdown in patients who are insensate. As early as 1971 Goller reported an association between increased local temperature and localized pressure leading to tissue injury. In 1972 Sandrow and coworkers subsequently used thermometry as a tool to diagnose occult neuropathic fractures in patients with diabetes.

Stess et al described the use of infrared thermography to assess skin temperatures in persons with diabetes, persons with diabetes with neuropathic fractures, persons with diabetes with ulcers, patients with leprosy, and controls. They found that neuropathic foot ulcers frequently had increased skin temperatures surrounding a central necrotic area and suggested that infrared thermometry may be a useful technique to identify patients at risk for ulceration. Benbow and coworkers took this work a step further and evaluated foot temperatures as a means of identifying persons with diabetes who were at risk of foot ulceration. They suggested that thermographic patterns could be used to screen high-risk patients.

In this project, the author of this article and his colleagues have designed shoe insole prototypes that are instrumented with thermistors. These prototypes have been used in a clinical study performed at the Denver VA Medical Center. The first part of the project focused on creating a durable prototype that selected the Fenwal 192-103LEV-A01 sensor (Honeywell, Minneapolis, MN) for use in the insoles. Bench testing was preformed on the prototypes for durability and efficacy in temperature reading. The Fenwal thermistor collected the most accurate temperature readings, when compared with a digital thermometer exposed to identical conditions, and had the smoothest first-order response to a step change in temperature. The Fenwal thermistor has a maximum outer diameter of 2.4 mm or 0.095 inches. The operating range of this thermistor is $0°$ to $70°C$ with a tolerance of $±0.5°C$. The Fenwal 192-103LEV-A01 has a maximum time constant of 15 seconds, but the nominal response is much faster. These thermistors do not require individual resistance-temperature calibration. Once the prototypes were considered appropriate for use in clinical trials, a 60-patient pilot study was initiated. The prototypes used were PW Minor extra-depth shoes (PW Minor, Golden, CO), and each patient was provided with an identical pair of sturdy, acrylic/nylon socks. Institutional review board approval was granted by the Colorado Multiple Institutional Review Board. The pilot study used 20 patients in each of the following groups: control diabetic, control neuropathic, and diabetic/neuropathic patients.

Each prototype insole was instrumented with seven thermistors located at the hallux, the five metatarsal heads, and the heel. The data were collected using instruNet data acquisition boards, read into LabVIEW, and then stored into patient files. The sampling rate was 0.1 Hz (once every 10 seconds). Every patient had three temperature-testing visits, each lasting approximately 45 minutes each; both sitting and walking data were collected at each visit.

The goal of this study was to establish temperature ranges for presymptomatic patients, examine differences between in-shoe temperature values for each of the three patient groups, and begin some basic procedures for correctly classifying patients into the appropriate health groups (control, diabetic without neuropathy, or diabetic/neuropathic).

The first statistical tests performed were one-way ANOVAs to search for differences in mean temperatures between the groups at specified locations in time. The investigators then analyzed resting temperatures, active temperatures, and the change in temperature between resting and active (ΔT). The last 30 seconds of sitting data were examined at each sensor location, and F tests were preformed for significance at the $\alpha = 0.05$ and $\alpha = 0.01$ level. These tests showed that the mean temperature differed among the three groups at all locations except the fourth metatarsal head on the right foot. Tukey's test for simultaneous contrasts was used to determine whether the temperature differences among the groups of subjects were statistically significant for each foot location. The results are presented in Table 1.

Many clinicians use the contralateral foot as a control. Some researchers have even given quantitative suggestions as to when a patient should be more thoroughly examined based on a predetermined temperature difference between the same location in the right foot and the left foot. Because some difference in temperature between feet is expected even in healthy patients, it seemed inappropriate to test the null hypothesis that the

Table 1
Tukey test results for the last 30 seconds of sitting temperature data

| | Sensor Locations | | | | | | | | | | | | | |
Comparisons	RHa	LHa	R1	L1	R2	L2	R3	L3	R4	L4	R5	L5	RHe	Lhe
Control–Diabetic	1.42	1.37	1.03	1.04	0.95	1.04	0.77	1.0	1.27	0.94	0.5	0.56	0.35	0.63
Control–Neuropathic	2.63[a]	2.6[a]	2.2[a]	2.1[a]	2.23[a]	2.1[a]	2.11[a]	1.91[b]	1.32	1.98[b]	1.96[a]	1.84[b]	1.73[a]	1.58[b]
Diabetic–Neuropathic	1.21	1.23	1.17	1.05	1.28	1.05	1.34	0.9	0.05	1.04	1.46	1.28	1.38	0.93

[a] Significant at the 0.01 level.
[b] Significant at the 0.05 level.

temperatures in the right foot and the left foot are identical. Therefore, histograms were constructed to suggest an upper boundary for the temperature differences in our three test groups.

This quantitative and graphic examination of left versus right foot temperatures used histograms to plot maximum differences noticed between the feet. The last 5 minutes of sitting data were selected for each patient, and temperature differences were determined for each trial (allowing 180 [60 × 3] data sets to be included). The maximum absolute temperature differences over time for each of the seven sensor locations were then plotted on histograms. The same procedure was employed for the last 5 minutes of walking as well. A sample of rearfoot, midfoot, and forefoot was used to create the graphs. Therefore the heel, third metatarsal head, and the hallux data were selected. Fig. 5 shows a sample of these histograms for the hallux.

Examination of the histograms shows that members of the control group commonly experience differences of up to 2°C during sitting. These histograms have been shown as approximate probability density functions of the right versus left temperature data. The diabetic group has somewhat larger differences, and the neuropathic group commonly shows differences as high as 3° to 3.5°C. There seems to be a tendency towards increased temperature differences during walking.

Results from the first phase of this project have demonstrated that a temperature-registering shoe insole might allow early detection of ulcer formation. Therefore, the research is continuing toward the development of a wireless insole capable of performing pattern recognition and generating feedback signals for both the patient and the physician.

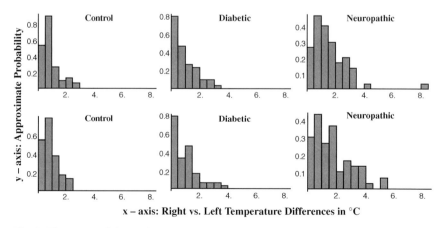

Fig. 5. Histograms of the maximum temperature differences (in °C) noted at the hallux during the last 5 minutes of sitting data collection (*top row*) and the last 5 minutes of walking data collection (*bottom row*).

References

[1] Bugliavello G. The experiences and challenges of science and ethics. Washington (DC): National Academic Press; 2003.

[2] Johnson AT. Bioengineering in the US: the rush is on. College Park (MD): University of Maryland, Department of Bioengineering.

[3] Nerem R. The emergence of bioengineering. National Academy of Engineering. The Bridge Archives 1997;27(4).

[4] Bluestone AH, Abdoulaev G, Schmitz CH, et al. Three-dimensional optical tomography of hemodynamics in the human head. Optics Express 2001;9(6):272–86.

[5] Sutton J. Brain-imaging cap [press release]. National Space Biomedical Research Institute (NSBRI), May 8, 2002.

[6] Chance B, Nioka S, Chen Y. Shining new light on brain function. SPIE's OE Magazine 2003.

[7] Chance B, Nioka S, Zhou S, Hong L, et al. A novel method for fast imaging of brain function, non-invasively, with light. Opt Express 1998;2(10):411–23.

[8] The deceit detector. Technol Rev 2003.

[9] Luo Q, Zeng S, Chance B, et al. Monitoring of brain activity with near-infrared spectroscopy. In: Tuchin VV, editor. Handbook of optical biomedical diagnostics. Society of Photo-Optical Instrumentation Engineers; 2002. p. 455–86.

[10] Pecoraro RE, Reiber GE, Burgess EM. Pathways to diabetic limb amputation: basis for prevention. Diabetes Care 1990;13:513–21.

[11] Lavery LA, Armstrong DG, Vela SA, et al. Practical criteria for screening patients at high risk for diabetic foot ulceration. Arch Intern Med 1998;158:158–62.

[12] Goldner MG. The fate of the second leg in the diabetic amputee. Diabetes 1960;9:100–3.

[13] Lavery LA, van Houtum WH, Armstrong DG. Institutionalization following diabetes-related lower extremity amputation. Am J Med 1997;103(5):383–8.

[14] Cameron HC, Lennar-Jones LE, Robinson MD. Amputations in diabetics: outcomes and survival. Lancet 1964;2:605–7.

[15] Armstrong DG, Lavery LA, van Houtum WH, et al. Amputation and reamputation of the diabetic foot. J Am Podiatr Med Assoc 1997; in press.

[16] Childs MR, Peters EJG, Armstrong DG, et al. What is the effect of amputations on the quality of life in diabetic patients? Diabetologia 1998;47(Suppl 1):A279.

ELSEVIER
SAUNDERS

Otolaryngol Clin N Am
38 (2005) 199–214

OTOLARYNGOLOGIC
CLINICS
OF NORTH AMERICA

Cell-based Therapies and Tissue Engineering

Mark A. Rice, BS[a], Brennan T. Dodson, MD[b],
Jeffrey A. Arthur, BS[a], Kristi S. Anseth, PhD[a,c],*

[a]*Department of Chemical and Biological Engineering, University of Colorado,
Boulder, CO 80309, USA*
[b]*Department of Otolaryngology–Head and Neck Surgery, University of Colorado Health
Sciences Center, Denver, CO 80262, USA*
[c]*Howard Hughes Medical Institute, University of Colorado,
Boulder, CO 80309-0424, USA*

Tissue engineering involves the restoration of tissue structure or function through the use of living cells [1]. The specific applications may include direct injection of cells, combination of cells with a biomaterial scaffold in vitro or in situ, or implantation of a biomaterial scaffold alone that can induce surrounding cells into tissue restoration. The basic concept of tissue engineering is summarized in Fig. 1. This general process consists of cell isolation and expansion followed by a reimplantation procedure that may include cells and a scaffold material or, more likely, a combination of the two.

From an otolaryngologic perspective, most head and neck applications would probably involve chondrocytes (cartilage cells) and osteoblasts (bone-producing cells) along with some type of scaffold material because of the importance of initial shape and support. At first glance, tissue engineering seems to be a simple concept, but a number of major challenges must be addressed before it will become a widely approved and accepted method for tissue replacement. A basic summary and classification of some of the major challenges are presented in Table 1. Some of these challenges are cellular; they range from identifying an appropriate cell source to devising ways to expand the cells and make sure that they function appropriately once they are being depended on to produce new tissue. Many engineering challenges

* Corresponding author. Department of Chemical and Biological Engineering, ECCH 111, Campus Box 424, University of Colorado, Boulder, CO 80309.
E-mail address: Kristi.Anseth@colorado.edu (K.S. Anseth).

doi:10.1016/j.otc.2004.10.010

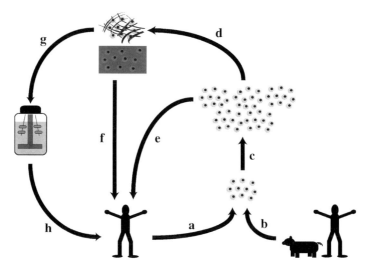

Fig. 1. Tissue engineering concept. Cells are harvested from an autologous (a), allogenic (b), or xenogenic source. These cells can be expanded (c) to a number more effective for treatment. The expanded cells can be seeded (d) onto a polymer mesh or encapsulated in a natural or synthetic hydrogel, or they can be reinjected (e) to the patient with or without an in situ–forming scaffold material. Cell-laden constructs can be implanted (f) or cultured (g) in a bioreactor and implanted (h) later.

also exist. For example, the properties of the scaffold material can have a major impact on the viability of cells and the quality of tissue created. In addition, engineered neotissues must overcome clinical challenges, including adhesion and integration into defect sites that may be poorly vascularized.

Basic cellular aspects

The choice of cell source can have a major effect on a particular tissue-engineering application. Sources can be autologous cells (from the patient in whom they will be used), allogenic cells (from another human donor), or xenogenic cells (from another species). Clearly, allogenic and xenogenic sources will face problems with immune rejection by the patient. Autologous cells would seem to be the best choice, but a number of challenges arise

Table 1
Some of the interdisciplinary challenges facing tissue engineers

Biological challenges	Engineering challenges	Clinical challenges
Cell source	Choice of scaffold material	Volume/shape retention
Quick expansion of cell number	Optimization of bioreactors	Integration of neotissue
Induction or maintenance of differentiated state	Production of functional tissue	Vascularization of neotissue

when using a patient's own cells. First, if the cells are taken from a mature tissue, the patient will suffer some degree of donor-site morbidity. This effect grows in importance when the donor site is of limited size or accessibility, such as the trachea. One option being explored by tissue engineers is the use of similar cells from a more accessible and less structurally important source. For example, Kojima et al [2] have shown that chondrocytes harvested from the nasal septum or tracheal tissue of sheep have similar abilities to generate new tracheal tissue. Another problem with the use of mature autologous cells has to do with the cell number. It is likely that the cells must be able to proliferate to an adequate number for transplantation without losing their differentiated phenotype. Chondrocytes have been shown to lose their phenotype and become more fibroblastlike upon expansion in monolayer with normal growth media [3]. Martin et al [4] have found that the addition of fibroblast growth factor-2 during monolayer expansion of chondrocytes makes them less likely to express fibroblastic markers and also enhances their responsiveness to chondrogenic factors, allowing them to produce normal cartilage extracellular matrix. In spite of these advances, mesenchymal stem cells (MSCs) may provide an attractive alternative to cells from a mature tissue.

The use of MSCs as a cell source for bone and cartilage tissue engineering brings a number of advantages. First, autologous MSCs can be obtained from a marrow sample, using a procedure that is less invasive than a cartilage or bone biopsy and does not result in donor-site morbidity. They also ultimately have the ability to differentiate down multiple lineages, including bone, cartilage, fat, muscle, and stromal cells [5–8]. Their ability to differentiate into both chondrocytes and osteoblasts enables them to be used to engineer cartilage, bone, or possibly a combination of the two. The particular factors that send MSCs down the differentiation paths to become chondrocytes or osteoblasts are the subject of intensive research because of the possibilities afforded by these cells.

Engineering aspects

In addition to the obstacle posed by cell source, a number of engineering challenges exist. Most important of these are selection of an appropriate cell scaffold and production of tissue that is a functional replacement. A scaffold must minimally allow for seeding or encapsulation of cells, as well as diffusion of nutrients and waste. In an ideal situation, the scaffold would be degraded or resorbed by the surrounding tissue as the neotissue forms. A number of natural and synthetic materials have been used as scaffolds for cartilage and bone tissue engineering. Characteristics and advantages of particular scaffolds are discussed in following sections.

It is important, especially in bone and cartilage applications, that engineered tissue replace mechanical function. Engineered bone must have similar mechanical properties to the tissue it is meant to replace, and the same is true for cartilage. Typically, the compressive modulus of cartilage tissues produced in vitro falls within a large range that extends both higher and lower than that of native cartilage [9–11]. This wide range has a great deal to do with cell source and culture conditions, but it is also very dependent on the initial scaffold stiffness and the degradability of the scaffold material. Depending on the application, other mechanical properties are also important. For example, auricular cartilage has a great deal of flexibility. Auricular cartilage is high in elastin content, and it is also surrounded by a perichondrium that gives it the ability to flex significantly without breaking. Researchers have recently begun designing specifically engineered systems with this characteristic in mind and have established methods for mechanical evaluation of these neotissues [12]. It may be necessary for engineered auricular cartilage to be seeded or encapsulated in multilayered scaffolds, so that a final tissue can include a perichondrium that complements the mechanical properties of the underlying neocartilage.

In response to the complexity associated with the growth of new tissues in vitro, many tissue engineers have explored the use of bioreactors to control cell seeding and culture conditions. Bioreactors as simple as spinner flasks have been used to increase the seeding efficiency of cells onto polymer meshes [13]. These flasks have needles to hold a number of scaffolds away from the bottom and sides of the flask and a mechanical stirrer to increase transport of cells during seeding and nutrients or waste during construct culture. Stirring or shaking has also been shown to improve the quality of tissue-engineered cartilage produced in vitro [14,15]. In addition to improving cell seeding and diffusion, more complex bioreactors have been fabricated that allow researchers to culture constructs under mechanical stresses meant to mimic the natural environment of the tissue being studied [16–18]. In general, the effects of culture with this type of bioreactor seem to vary greatly depending on scaffold choice, probably because the actual force transferred to the cells is a function of the bulk properties of the scaffold material [19].

Clinical aspects

Tissue engineering remains an emergent technology in clinical otolaryngologic practice. The myriad structural defects created and repaired in neurotology, facial plastics, laryngology, head and neck oncology, and other subsubspecialties dictate a vast array of bioengineered materials that will someday be available for the surgeon. Until that time, the best available tissue for reconstruction is autograft; however, this tissue (whether bone, cartilage, skin, or composite tissue) is fraught with problems of supply, harvest morbidity, and unfavorable biomechanical properties. Bioengineered tissue offers a potentially limitless supply of bioactive, biointegrating, and biofunctional materials that could be ready for implantation with minimal front-end cost, preparation, and patient morbidity. To date, orthopedics is the only surgical specialty for which bioengineered implants are commercially available and approved for use in humans by the Food and Drug Administration (FDA) [20]. Compared with orthopedic procedures, which involve highly sterile surgical environments, otolaryngologic procedures frequently involve surgical fields covered with normal bacterial and fungal flora and, as such, are considered clean or clean-contaminated wounds. Additionally, implant sites may have poor microvascular circulation because of the inherent perturbation that comes with soft-tissue surgery or from more damaging local therapies such as external beam radiation. It is understandable that the initial application of bioengineered materials in otolaryngology will probably involve implantation into surgical beds with robust vascularity and low bacterial load. Although encapsulation of growth factors, proangiogenesis factors, and other chemicals to promote graft incorporation would be beneficial in most tissue applications, these factors are contraindicated in reconstruction after oncologic resection. In addition, postradiated surgical fields may not be appropriate for bioengineered tissue until composite implants can be designed that incorporate complex aggregations of different tissue types including robust blood vessels.

Polymeric scaffolds for tissue engineering

Scaffold function and properties

The four primary functions of tissue engineering scaffolds are

1. To provide a three-dimensional shape onto which cells can attach
2. To direct and guide the production of extracellular matrix by the cells
3. To provide the mechanical strength necessary before the tissue has developed enough to support itself
4. In some cases, to deliver bioactive molecules

In addition to these fundamental functions of the scaffolds, properties such as biocompatibility, degradability, porosity, water content, transport, and cell adhesion, must be considered in the design of scaffolds (Table 2).

Table 2
Important scaffold properties and a comparison of scaffold types

	Scaffold material	
Property	PLA, PGA, PLGA	Hydrogels
Pore/mesh size	10–100s μm	10–100s Å
Water content	Low	High
Mechanics	Typically stronger	Typically weaker
Cell adhesiveness	High	Low
Biocompatibility	Yes	Yes
Degradability	Hydrolytic	Enzymatic, Hydrolytic

Abbreviations: PGA, polyglycolic acid; PLA, polylactic acid; PLGA, polylactic-co-glycolic acid.

Degradability allows newly synthesized tissue to replace the scaffold both physically and functionally as the scaffold resorbs. Degradation products are either metabolized or diffuse away from the scaffold and are cleared by the body. After complete degradation, only newly formed tissue remains, leaving no permanent foreign object. Care must be taken to match the rate of scaffold degradation to the rate of formation of new tissue. If the degradation occurs too fast, defects may develop in the scaffold where tissue is unable to form [21]; if the rate is too slow, it may prevent diffusion of newly synthesized matrix molecules through the scaffold [22].

Biocompatibility is of critical importance in a scaffold to ensure that the implant or its degradation products do not elicit an acute or chronic inflammatory immune response, thereby preventing any chance of successful repair. Porosity of scaffolds must be sufficiently large to allow diffusion of nutrients and waste products into and out of the scaffold to maintain cell viability. If the scaffold is initially unseeded or is seeded at a cell density low enough to require proliferation for tissue formation, the scaffold must be porous enough to allow cell migration or proliferation. Water content and cellular adhesion are important in providing a familiar setting for the cells. Chondrocytes, for instance, are exposed to a high water content in their native environment and produce better tissue when they remain in a rounded morphology. In contrast, osteoblasts prefer a lower water content and produce tissue best when they attach and spread out on the scaffold surface.

Bioactive molecules such as growth factors are known to enhance tissue production by inducing cell migration, proliferation, or matrix synthesis; therefore scaffolds are often designed to deliver these molecules locally during a prescribed time period. This sustained and local release can happen in a variety of ways, most commonly by physically entrapping the molecule in the polymer scaffold. With these considerations in mind, researchers have designed polymeric scaffolds out of materials that can be broadly grouped into two categories: prefabricated, porous scaffolds and in situ–forming scaffolds.

Prefabricated scaffolds

Materials commonly used for prefabricated, porous scaffolds include polyglycolic acid (PGA) [23], polylactic acid (PLA) [23–25], and their copolymers, polylactic-co-glycolic acid (PLGA) [25,26] (Table 3). These synthetic materials are attractive for scaffold fabrication largely because of their long history of application in human medicine (eg, as degradable sutures) and the ability to control material properties. Careful selection of the polymer composition and processing method allows control of degradation, pore size, hydrophilicity, and cell attachment [24]. In addition, manufacture of these scaffolds is highly reproducible [24]. These materials are biocompatible and are most commonly spun into fibers and either

Table 3
Commonly used polymers for scaffold fabrication

Scaffold type	Common materials	Selected references
Prefabricated	Polylactic acid (PLA)	[23]
	Polyglycolic acid (PGA)	[23–25]
	Polylactic-co-glycolic acid (PLGA)	[25,26]
In situ–forming hydrogels	Collagen	[50,51]
	Alginate	[38–41]
	Fibrin glue	[36,37]
	Polyethylene glycol	[71–73]
	Pluronics	[52]
	Hyaluronic acid	[74,75]

woven together or pressed into a nonwoven mesh [27]. These meshes do not always provide the desired properties of a scaffold, so researchers have learned to control scaffold shape as well as porosity through a variety of processing conditions. Commonly used processing conditions include porogen leaching [28,29], emulsion freeze-drying [30], gas foaming [31], and phase separation [32,33]. These techniques result in pores hundreds of microns in diameter with varying structures and interconnectivities (Fig. 2). Other techniques such as thermally induced phase separation result in pore tens of microns in diameter [27]. Both the pore size and overall porosity must be carefully selected for the intended application. Typically, scaffolds with 70% to 95% porosity and a pore size distribution between tens and hundreds of microns are used in tissue-engineering applications.

The polyα-hydroxy esters are hydrolytically degradable at physiologic pH, which means degradation relies on the local aqueous environment. PLA is more hydrophobic and sterically hindered than PGA and consequently degrades at a slower rate. In addition, these polymers are semicrystalline, and degradation is much slower in the crystalline regions than in the amorphous regions. The degree of crystallinity depends on both the polymer composition and processing method. Thus, both the chemistry and crystallinity allow control over the final degradation rate. When processed into highly porous structures, these scaffolds have high surface area to volume ratios and significant amounts of open space. These properties facilitate the seeding of the scaffolds with cells after they are formed, but care must be taken during processing to ensure that the pores are interconnected. Additionally, the water content in PLA, PGA, and PLGA is minimal, but transport of nutrients and waste products into and out of the macroscopic scaffold is facile because of the interconnected pore structure.

One common application of prefabricated scaffolds is in bone-tissue engineering, in which porous scaffolds are implanted into critical-sized bone defects [34,35]. The porous scaffolds facilitate clot formation and allow osteoprogenitor cells to migrate into the scaffold. Proteins adsorb to the hydrophobic scaffold and support the attachment and spreading of

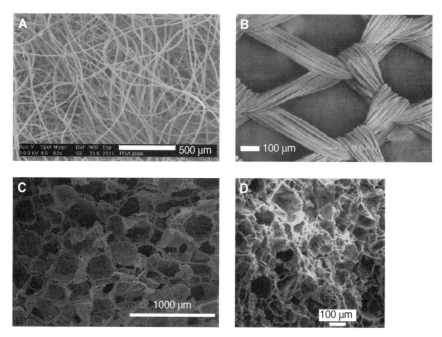

Fig. 2. Scanning electron microscopy images of (*A*) nonwoven PGA fiber mesh, (*B*) woven PLGA mesh [70], (*C*) PLGA scaffold fabricated through gas foaming, and (*D*) PLA scaffold prepared through porogen leaching. (*From* ref. [69]. (*A*) Fuchs JR, Nasseri BA, Vacanti JP. Tissue engineering: a 21st century solution to surgical reconstruction. Ann Thorac Surg 2001;72:577–91, with permission; *From* ref. [70]. (*B*) Chen G, Sato T, Ushida T, et al. The use of a novel PLGA fiber/collagen composite web as a scaffold for engineering of articular cartilage tissue with adjustable thickness. J Biomed Mater Res 2003;67A:1170–80, with permission.)

osteoprogenitor cells. The open pore structure encourages proliferation and matrix deposition. Finally, many scaffolds are stiff enough to provide some initial mechanical strength before the scaffold degrades away and is replaced by newly formed tissue.

In situ–forming scaffolds

There are numerous types of in situ–forming biomaterials. This discussion is restricted to hydrogel materials that are often used as cell-delivery vehicles for tissue regeneration. Hydrogel scaffolds can be further divided into three basic types depending on the cross linking mechanism: physical, ionic or covalent. Fibrin glue [36,37] is a commonly used biomaterial that gels through a series of ionic and hydrogen bond interactions. Alginate [38–41] and hyaluronic acid [42] are common materials that can gel through an ionic cross linking mechanism using multivalent cations. These naturally occurring materials avoid problems associated with biocompatibility and are inherently interactive with the cells. In addition, these gels degrade through the exchange of cross link–forming multivalent cations with monovalent cations that render the scaffold water soluble. Alginate [39,43] and hyaluronic acid [43,44] can also be modified to gel through covalent cross linking mechanisms that allow better control over the cross linking reaction. More recently, chondroitin sulfate [45] and chitosan [46] have been investigated for use as natural scaffold materials, and some researchers have investigated gels composed of multiple materials to enhance tissue formation [45,47].

Polyethylene glycol (PEG) is used in numerous medical and pharmacologic applications [48,49]. It is often considered a stealth biomaterial, because it resists protein adsorption and therefore delays the corresponding physiologic reaction. To create hydrogels with PEG, several groups have modified these molecules with polymerizable end groups, which lead to a covalently cross linked gel. The hydrophilic nature of these PEG-based gels makes them noninteractive with proteins and highly expandable in water. These gels can be made to degrade by incorporation of degradable units (eg, PLA) within the network cross links.

Physically cross-linked gels typically involve hydrogen bonding and interactions of hydrophobic groups, which become stronger with increasing temperature. These types of gels include collagen [50,51], which gels because of changes in temperature and pH, and Pluronics (BASF Group, Mount Olive, NJ) [52], which gels because of hydrophobic interactions between polypropylene oxide regions of the molecules. These scaffolds can be delivered either by injecting a liquid scaffold solution directly into the surgical site and subsequently inducing gelation under physiologic conditions [36,53] or, if a specific shape is needed, by gelling the scaffold in a mold before implantation [54].

Many of the properties of in situ–forming hydrogels are directly related to the density of cross links in the network. A high cross linking density results in a small mesh size, which limits the amount of water that the hydrogel imbibes, as well as the diffusion of large macromolecules. Hydrogels characteristically have high water content (50%–99% water) and a molecular-scale porosity that is sufficient for nutrient and waste diffusion but is too small for cell migration. As a result, these scaffolds are often mixed with a cell suspension before gelation, giving the advantage of homogenous cell distribution.

Mechanical properties of hydrogels can be controlled through both the cross linking density and cross linking mechanism. A higher cross linking density results in a stiffer, high modulus material; however, most physically and ionically cross-linked gels are relatively weak because the cross-links are easily broken under load. In contrast, covalently cross linked gels are stiffer, with moduli in the range of 1 to 1000 kPa. An important consideration in using gels for tissue engineering is the interdependence of diffusion, water content, and mechanical properties on the network cross-linking density. For example, high-strength gels may have desired mechanical properties but undesirably low diffusion coefficients.

When the hydrophilic nature of hydrogels is coupled with other hydrogel properties such as high stiffness and transport, their advantages in cartilage-tissue engineering become evident. Chondrocytes, the dominant cell type used in cartilage-tissue engineering, are not naturally proliferative or migratory and prefer a rounded morphology. Hydrogels are suitable because their hydrophilic nature prevents protein adsorption and cell attachment, and the chondrocytes remain embedded in their rounded morphology, encouraging extracellular matrix production. Additionally, the small mesh size prevents the chondrocytes from migrating, and the hydrogel degrades as the cells produce new cartilage.

Applications and future directions of bioengineered tissue in otolaryngology

Auricular reconstruction

Reconstruction of auricular defects arising from either congenital or traumatic causes requires that the implanted tissue maintain shape over time (structural fidelity) and closely mimic the biomechanical properties of elastic cartilage. Currently, costal (rib) cartilage provides a readily available source of hyaline cartilage that can be carved, shaped, and implanted for creation of a neoauricle. Generally, the process of microtia repair is segmented into two to five staged procedures that take place over many months to years and require considerable time and effort from both the patient and surgeon [55,56]. This technique remains the standard against which other techniques are evaluated and has been shown to have excellent structural fidelity and cosmetic results [55].

Although bioengineered implants for auricular reconstruction have not been developed for humans, the groundwork is being laid with in vitro cell culture and in vivo animal experiments. Bioengineered constructs have been developed using chondrocytes suspended in PGA/PLA scaffolds implanted into immune-incompetent mice. The implants maintained qualitative structural fidelity at 10 months [20,57]. When the same implants were inserted into immune-competent rabbits, construct rejection was seen, possibly because of cell-mediated attack against residual PGA/PLA in the scaffold. Recently, Pluronic F-127, a biocompatible copolymer hydrogel of polyethylene oxide and polypropylene oxide, was seeded with autograft chondrocytes and implanted into immune-competent pigs and sheep using an auricle-shaped pure gold mold containing thousands of microperforations to allow nutrient perfusion [58]. Explants showed robust cartilage formation without apparent cell-mediated immune rejection of the Pluronic F-127 scaffold. Some of the hydrogel-chondrocyte solution extruded through the microperforations, however, causing implant shrinkage and imperfect aesthetic results. In preparation for human implantation, future animal research must elucidate the issues of implant rejection and structural fidelity.

Human implementation of existing bioengineering technology could involve a minimally invasive harvest (needle-core or punch biopsy) of an autograft chondrocyte graft (septal or auricular cartilage) that could then be expanded in vitro before the expanded chondrocytes are incorporated into a nonimmunogenic hydrogel implant. Ideally, bioengineered implants would be composed of elastic cartilage so that the biomechanical properties of the neoauricle would be identical to the contralateral ear. Recent reports have shown it is possible to produce elastic cartilage in vitro [57,59]. Because most cartilage engineering has been with articular cartilage, elastic cartilage bioengineering will be necessary if this substrate is to be applied to facial plastic surgery [60]. Skin tension overlying the bioengineered implant presents a problem that could be overcome with the use of tissue expanders before implant insertion.

Nose and nasal septum reconstruction

Nasal reconstruction requires the use of local flaps and grafts such as the forehead (median or paramedian) flap, melolabial flap, full-thickness skin graft, and auricular composite (skin and cartilage) grafts. Contracture prevention is accomplished by creating an internal nasal lining. This lining is typically accomplished with local flaps such as the septal mucosa flap, bipedicled bucket-handle intranasal flap, hinged composite septal flap, inferior turbinate flap, epithelial turn-in flap, and, in more extreme cases, a pericranial flap or radial forearm free flap [61]. When there is loss of the bony and cartilaginous nasal structure, autologous auricular or costal cartilage and split calvarial bone graft provide a good scaffold on which to place soft tissue flaps. Bioimplants (eg, porous polyethylene) and alloplast (eg, purified acellular human dermis [Alloderm, LifeCell Corp., Branchburg, NJ] and purified acellular costal cartilage and pericardium [Tutoplast, Tutogen Medical Inc., Alachua, FL]) may serve as alternatives to autograft. Medical prosthetic implants are available for patients with unfavorable (postradiated) surgical fields. Future bioengineered implants could be constructed from in vitro expansion of elastic or hyaline cartilage chondrocyte populations that would then be encapsulated into a biodegradable hydrogel. Complete bioengineered composite tissue (containing skin, cartilage, bone, and blood vessels) is probably many decades from production because of the inherent problems of manufacturing thick cultured tissue, vascular supply, and structural fidelity. Bioengineered septal cartilage may be closer at hand if robust in vitro chondrocyte expansion can be accomplished. Recently, alginate beads were used for in vitro monolayer expansion of septal chondrocyte populations; however, although the cells produced significant amounts of sulfated glycosaminoglycans, total cell number did not increase significantly over 14 days [62].

Larynx and trachea

The laryngotracheal complex presents unique problems for the application of bioengineered materials because of the specialized function (phonation and maintenance of airway patency) of these tissues. Currently, reconstruction of the larynx following partial surgical resection involves the rotation of local muscle flaps to add tissue bulk to the glottic and supraglottic area to improve phonation (by opposing the contralateral vocal fold) and lessen aspiration. Medialization thyroplasty involves the injection (through percutaneous or direct approaches) of autograft (fat) or allograft (Cymetra, LifeCell Corp., Branchburg, NJ; Gelfoam, Pharmacia Corp., Peapack, NJ) and open implantation of nondegradable bioimplants (polymeric silicone [Silastic], titanium, and Teflon, DuPont Corp., Wilmington, DE) to restore phonation following hemilaryngeal paralysis. Polydimethylsiloxane gel (currently not FDA approved) has been used in Europe for medialization thryroplasty. Hyaluronic acid (hylan b gel, Hylaform, Inamed Corp., Santa Barbara, CA) is currently FDA approved for injection of facial rhytids. Injection medialization thyroplasty studies using animal models have shown hyaluronic acid has highly favorable viscoelastic properties in the glottis [63] and may be approved for future use in humans. In cases of subglottic or tracheal stenosis, surgical options include tracheotomy, cricoid split procedures, laryngotracheal reconstruction, and tracheal resection. Laryngotracheal reconstruction uses an anterior and (sometimes) posterior autologous cartilage graft to expand the critical area of stenosis. The autograft is usually harvested from costal cartilage, but other sites, such as the auricle and thyroid ala, have been used [64]. Costal cartilage harvest yields a large amount of high-quality cartilage but carries an inherent risk of pneumothorax and wound infection and leaves a noticeable chest scar. Application of bioengineered cartilage implants in laryngeal and tracheal reconstruction could involve preoperative in vitro expansion and production of chondrocyte-seeded biodegradable implants, eliminating the added surgical cost and risk of donor-site morbidity. Kojima et al [65] bioengineered a trachea in an animal model using sheep nasal septal chondrocytes and epithelium. In this study, a PGA mesh sheet seeded with chondrocytes was wrapped around a silicone cylinder and implanted into the back of an immune-incompetent nude mouse. After 6 weeks of incubation, the silicone cylinder was removed, and epithelial cells were injected into the lumen of the construct. Histologic analysis of explants at 4 weeks showed mature cartilage lined with pseudostratified columnar epithelium; grossly, the construct resembled native sheep trachea. The results from this study are encouraging: a tracheal segment 7 mm wide by 30 mm long was created with chondrocytes harvested (and expanded in vitro for 3 weeks) from only 25 mm^2 of septum.

Facial skeleton

Repair of bony defects in the facial skeleton usually requires considerable time, effort, and morbidity for bone graft harvest or free-tissue transfer. Tissue-engineered bone graft has been used to augment the posterior maxilla in humans using bone matrix from mandibular periosteum; 10 of 18 patients showed lamellar bone formation 3 months after implantation [66]. VivescOs (IsoTis, Bilthoven, Netherlands), a new tissue-engineered bone graft, should be available in 2004 or 2005 for use in revision surgery, spinal surgery, and dental implants. The process involves harvest of the patient's bone marrow from the mandible or pelvis, in vitro expansion of cell isolates, and cell seeding of a bone scaffold of appropriate shape. Final constructs are ready for patient implantation in 4 weeks [67]. Recently, a neomandible was constructed from bone mineral blocks, autologous bone marrow aspirate, and bone morphogenic protein packed into a titanium mesh tray that was surgically implanted into the patient's own latissimus dorsi muscle. Seven weeks after implantation, the neomandible was harvested and implanted as a free-tissue transfer into the surgical defect created from an earlier manidibulectomy for advanced oral cancer [68]. Although these results are quite promising, future advances in skeletal repair would benefit from the design of resorbable scaffolds that could restore partial or complete mechanical function immediately and then accelerate mineralized tissue formation along with vascular ingrowth.

References

[1] Langer R, Vacanti JP. Tissue engineering. Science 1993;260:920–6.
[2] Kojima K, Bonassar LJ, Ignotz RA, et al. Comparison of tracheal and nasal chondrocytes for tissue engineering of the trachea. Ann Thorac Surg 2003;76:1884–8.
[3] Mayne R, Vail MS, Mayne PM, et al. Changes in type of collagen synthesized as clones of chick chondrocytes grow and eventually lose division capacity. Proc Natl Acad Sci U S A 1976;73:1674–8.
[4] Martin I, Suetterlin R, Baschong W, et al. Enhanced cartilage tissue engineering by sequential exposure of chrondrocytes to FGF-2 during 2D expansion and BMP-2 during 3D cultivation. J Cell Biochem 2001;83:121–8.
[5] Pittenger MF, Mackay AM, Beck SC, et al. Multilineage potential of adult human mesenchymal stem cells. Science 1999;284:143–7.
[6] Wakitani S, Saito T, Caplan AI. Myogenic cells derived from rat bone marrow mesenchymal stem cells exposed to 5-azacytidine. Muscle Nerve 1995;18:1417–26.
[7] Dennis JE, Caplan AI. Differentiation potential of conditionally immortalized mesenchymal progenitor cells from adult marrow of a H-2Kb-tsA58 transgenic mouse. J Cell Physiol 1996; 167:523–38.
[8] Majumdar MP, Haynesworth SE, Thiede MA, et al. Culture-expanded human mesenchymal stem cells (MSCs) express cytokines and support hematopoiesis in vitro. Blood 1995;86: 494a.
[9] Miyata S, Furukawa KS, Ushida T, et al. Static and dynamic mechanical properties of extracellular matrix synthesized by cultured chondrocytes. Materials Science & Engineering C-Biomimetic and Supramolecular Systems 2004;24:425–9.
[10] Rotter N, Bonassar LJ, Tobias G, et al. Age dependence of biochemical and biomechanical properties of tissue-engineered human septal cartilage. Biomaterials 2002;23:3087–94.
[11] Ma PX, Schloo B, Mooney D, et al. Development of biomechanical properties and morphogenesis of in vitro tissue engineered cartilage. J Biomed Mater Res 1995;29:1587–95.
[12] Roy R, Kohles SS, Zaporojan V, et al. Analysis of bending behavior of native and engineered auricular and costal cartilage. J Biomed Mater Res 2004;68A:597–602.

[13] Vunjak-Novakovic G, Obradovic B, Martin I, et al. Dynamic cell seeding of polymer scaffolds for cartilage tissue engineering. Biotechnol Prog 1998;14:193–202.

[14] Freed LE, Hollander AP, Martin I, et al. Chondrogenesis in a cell-polymer-bioreactor system. Exp Cell Res 1998;240:58–65.

[15] Vunjak-Novakovic G, Martin I, Obradovic B, et al. Bioreactor cultivation conditions modulate the composition and mechanical properties of tissue-engineered cartilage. J Orthop Res 1999;17:130–8.

[16] Davisson T, Kunig S, Chen A, et al. Static and dynamic compression modulate matrix metabolism in tissue engineered cartilage. J Orthop Res 2002;20:842–8.

[17] Hunter CJ, Mouw JK, Levenston ME. Dynamic compression of chondrocyte-seeded fibrin gels: effects on matrix accumulation and mechanical stiffness. Osteoarthritis Cartilage 2004; 12:117–30.

[18] Lee CR, Grodzinsky AJ, Spector M. Biosynthetic response of passaged chondrocytes in a type II collagen scaffold to mechanical compression. J Biomed Mater Res 2003;64A: 560–9.

[19] Bryant SJ, Chowdhury TT, Lee DA, et al. Crosslinking density influences chondrocyte metabolism in dynamically loaded photocrosslinked poly(ethylene glycol) hydrogels. Ann Biomed Eng 2004;32:407–17.

[20] Nussenbaum B, Teknos Theodoros N, et al. Tissue engineering: the current status of this futuristic modality in head neck reconstruction. Curr Opin Otolaryngol Head Neck Surg 2004;12:311–5.

[21] Rice MA, Anseth KS. Encapsulating chondrocytes in copolymer gels: bimodal degradation kinetics influence cell phenotype and extracellular matrix development. J Biomed Mater Res 2004;70A:560–8.

[22] Bryant SJ, Anseth KS. Controlling the spatial distribution of ECM components in degradable PEG hydrogels for tissue engineering cartilage. J Biomed Mater Res 2003;64A: 70–9.

[23] Freed LE, Marquis JC, Nohria A, et al. Neocartilage formation in vitro and in vivo using cells cultured on synthetic biodegradable polymers. J Biomed Mater Res 1993;27: 11–23.

[24] Grad S, Zhou L, Gogolewski S, et al. Chondrocytes seeded onto poly (L/DL-lactide) 80%/ 20% porous scaffolds: a biochemical evaluation. J Biomed Mater Res 2003;66A:571–9.

[25] Rotter N, Aigner J, Naumann A, et al. Cartilage reconstruction in head and neck surgery: comparison of resorbable polymer scaffolds for tissue engineering of human septal cartilage. J Biomed Mater Res 1998;42:347–56.

[26] Moran JM, Pazzano D, Bonassar LJ. Characterization of polylactic acid polyglycolic acid composites for cartilage tissue engineering. Tissue Eng 2003;9:63–70.

[27] Nam YS, Park TG. Porous biodegradable polymeric scaffolds prepared by thermally induced phase separation. J Biomed Mater Res 1999;47:8–17.

[28] Mikos AG, Sarakinos G, Leite SM, et al. Laminated 3-dimensional biodegradable foams for use in tissue engineering. Biomaterials 1993;14:323–30.

[29] Mikos AG, Thorsen AJ, Czerwonka LA, et al. Preparation and characterization of poly(l-lactic acid) foams. Polymer 1994;35:1068–77.

[30] Whang K, Thomas CH, Healy KE, et al. A novel method to fabricate bioabsorbable scaffolds. Polymer 1995;36:837–42.

[31] Mooney DJ, Baldwin DF, Suh NP, et al. Novel approach to fabricate porous sponges of poly(D, L-lactic-co-glycolic acid) without the use of organic solvents. Biomaterials 1996;17: 1417–22.

[32] Schugens C, Maquet V, Grandfils C, et al. Polylactide macroporous biodegradable implants for cell transplantation. 2. Preparation of polylactide foams by liquid-liquid phase separation. J Biomed Mater Res 1996;30:449–61.

[33] Lo H, Kadiyala S, Guggino SE, et al. Poly(L-lactic acid) foams with cell seeding and controlled-release capacity. J Biomed Mater Res 1996;30:475–84.

[34] Burdick JA, Frankel D, Dernell WS, et al. An initial investigation of photocurable three-dimensional lactic acid based scaffolds in a critical-sized cranial defect. Biomaterials 2003;24: 1613–20.

[35] Hedberg EL, Kroese-Deutman HC, Shih CK, et al. Bone regenerative effect of varied release kinetics of the osteogenic thrombin peptide TP508 from biodegradable, polymeric scaffolds. J Biomed Mater Res, in press.

[36] Silverman RP, Passaretti D, Huang W, et al. Injectable tissue-engineered cartilage using a fibrin glue polymer. Plast Reconstr Surg 1999;103:1809–18.

[37] Sims CD, Butler PE, Cao YL, et al. Tissue engineered neocartilage using plasma derived polymer substrates and chondrocytes. Plast Reconstr Surg 1998;101:1580–5.

[38] Paige KT, Cima LG, Yaremchuk MJ, et al. De novo cartilage generation using calcium alginate-chondrocyte constructs. Plast Reconstr Surg 1996;97:168–78.

[39] Lee KY, Rowley JA, Eiselt P, et al. Controlling mechanical and swelling properties of alginate hydrogels independently by cross-linker type and cross-linking density. Macro-molecules 2000;33:4291–4.

[40] LeRoux MA, Guilak F, Setton LA. Compressive and shear properties of alginate gel: effects of sodium ions and alginate concentration. J Biomed Mater Res 1999;47:46–53.

[41] Fragonas E, Valente M, Pozzi-Mucelli M, et al. Articular cartilage repair in rabbits by using suspensions of allogenic chondrocytes in alginate. Biomaterials 2000;21:795–801.

[42] Taguchi T, Ikoma T, Tanaka J. An improved method to prepare hyaluronic acid and type II collagen composite matrices. J Biomed Mater Res 2002;61:330–6.

[43] Smeds KA, Pfister-Serres A, Miki D, et al. Photocrosslinkable polysaccharides for in situ hydrogel formation. J Biomed Mater Res 2001;54:115–21.

[44] Bulpitt P, Aeschlimann D. New strategy for chemical modification of hyaluronic acid: preparation of functionalized derivatives and their use in the formation of novel biocompatible hydrogels. J Biomed Mater Res 1999;47:152–69.

[45] van Susante JLC, Pieper J, Buma P, et al. Linkage of chondroitin-sulfate to type I collagen scaffolds stimulates the bioactivity of seeded chondrocytes in vitro. Biomaterials 2001;22: 2359–69.

[46] Kim SE, Park JH, Cho YW, et al. Porous chitosan scaffold containing microspheres loaded with transforming growth factor-beta 1: implications for cartilage tissue engineering. J Controlled Release 2003;91:365–74.

[47] Allemann F, Mizuno S, Eid K, et al. Effects of hyaluronan on engineered articular cartilage extracellular matrix gene expression in 3-dimensional collagen scaffolds. J Biomed Mater Res 2001;55:13–9.

[48] Bhadra D, Bhadra S, Jain P, et al. Pegnology: a review of PEG-ylated systems. Pharmazie 2002;57:5–29.

[49] Peppas NA, editor. Hydrogels in medicine and pharmacy, vol 2. Boca Raton (FL): CRC Press, Inc.; 1986.

[50] Nehrer S, Breinan HA, Ramappa A, et al. Canine chondrocytes seeded in type I and type II collagen implants investigated in vitro. J Biomed Mater Res 1997;38:95–104.

[51] Wakitani S, Goto T, Young RG, et al. Repair of large full-thickness articular cartilage defects with allograft articular chondrocytes embedded in a collagen gel. Tissue Eng 1998;4: 429–44.

[52] Cao YL, Rodriguez A, Vacanti M, et al. Comparative study of the use of poly(glycolic acid), calcium alginate and pluronics in the engineering of autologous porcine cartilage. J Biomater Sci Polym Ed 1998;9:475–87.

[53] Paige KT, Cima LG, Yaremchuk MJ, et al. Injectable cartilage. Plast Reconstr Surg 1995;96: 1390–8.

[54] Chang SCN, Rowley JA, Tobias G, et al. Injection molding of chondrocyte/alginate constructs in the shape of facial implants. J Biomed Mater Res 2001;55:503–11.

[55] Brent B. Auricular repair with autogenous rib cartilage grafts—2 decades of experience with 600 cases. Plast Reconstr Surg 1992;90:355–74.

[56] Walton RL, Beahm EK. Auricular reconstruction for microtia: part II. Surgical techniques. Plast Reconstr Surg 2002;110:234–49.
[57] Cao YL, Vacanti JP, Paige KT, et al. Transplantation of chondrocytes utilizing a polymer-cell construct to produce tissue-engineered cartilage in the shape of a human ear. Plast Reconstr Surg 1997;100:297–302.
[58] Kamil SH, Vacanti MP, Aminuddin BS, et al. Tissue engineering of a human sized and shaped auricle using a mold. Laryngoscope 2004;114:867–70.
[59] Rodriguez A, Cao YL, Ibarra C, et al. Characteristics of cartilage engineered from human pediatric auricular cartilage. Plast Reconstr Surg 1999;103:1111–9.
[60] Kaufman MR, Tobias GW. Engineering cartilage growth and development. Clin Plast Surg 2003;30:539.
[61] Chang JS, Becker SS, Park SS. Nasal reconstruction: the state of the art. Curr Opin Otolaryngol Head Neck Surg 2004;12:336–43.
[62] Homicz MR, Chia SH, Schumacher BL, et al. Human septal chondrocyte redifferentiation in alginate, polyglycolic acid scaffold, and monolayer culture. Laryngoscope 2003;113:25–32.
[63] Hertegard S, Dahlqvist A, Laurent C, et al. Viscoelastic properties of rabbit vocal folds after augmentation. Otolaryngol Head Neck Surg 2003;128:401–6.
[64] de Jong AL, Park AH, Raveh E, et al. Comparison of thyroid, auricular, and costal cartilage donor sites for laryngotracheal reconstruction in an animal model. Arch Otolaryngol Head Neck Surg 2000;126:49–53.
[65] Kojima K, Bonassar LJ, Roy AK, et al. A composite tissue-engineered trachea using sheep nasal chondrocyte and epithelial cells. FASEB J 2003;17:823–8.
[66] Schimming R, Schmelzeisen R. Tissue-engineered bone for maxillary sinus augmentation. J Oral Maxillofac Surg 2004;62:724–9.
[67] Parikh SN. Bone graft substitutes: past, present, future. J Postgrad Med 2002;48:142–8.
[68] Warnke PH, Springer ING, Wiltfang J, et al. Growth and transplantation of a custom vascularized bone graft in a man. Lancet 2004;364:766–70.
[69] Fuchs JR, Nasseri BA, Vacanti JP. Tissue engineering: a 21st century solution to surgical reconstruction. Ann Thorac Surg 2001;72:577–91.
[70] Chen G, Sato T, Ushida T, et al. The use of a novel PLGA fiber/collagen composite web as a scaffold for engineering of articular cartilage tissue with adjustable thickness. J Biomed Mater Res 2003;67A:1170–80.
[71] Elisseeff J, Anseth K, Sims D, et al. Transdermal photopolymerization for minimally invasive implantation. Proc Natl Acad Sci U S A 1999;96:3104–7.
[72] Anseth KS, Metters AT, Bryant SJ, et al. In situ forming degradable networks and their application in tissue engineering and drug delivery. J Control Release 2002;78:199–209.
[73] Bryant SJ, Anseth KS. Hydrogel properties influence ECM production by chondrocytes photoencapsulated in poly(ethylene glycol) hydrogels. J Biomed Mater Res 2002;59:63–72.
[74] Prestwich GD, Marecak DM, Marecek JF, et al. Controlled chemical modification of hyaluronic acid: synthesis, applications, and biodegradation of hydrazide derivatives. J Control Release 1998;53:93–103.
[75] Zheng Shu X, Liu Y, Palumbo FS, et al. In situ crosslinkable hyaluronan hydrogels for tissue engineering. Biomaterials 2004;25:1339–48.

ELSEVIER
SAUNDERS

Otolaryngol Clin N Am
38 (2005) 215–240

OTOLARYNGOLOGIC
CLINICS
OF NORTH AMERICA

Biophotonic and Other Physical Methods for Characterizing Oral Mucosa

Randall Tagg, PhD*, Masoud Asadi-Zeydabadi, PhD, Arlen D. Meyers, MD, MBA

University of Colorado, Denver, CO 80217, USA

Oral cancer is the sixth most common form of cancer in the United States. Five-year survival rates after therapy have held to approximately 50% for decades [1]. Improved prognosis is well known to result from earlier detection. The critical need for early detection of oral cancer and the accessibility of tissue in the mouth drive the development of noninvasive or minimally invasive methods of characterizing oral mucosa. A further inducement comes from the need for improved, rapid, and reliable identification of disease-free margins during surgical removal of cancerous tissue. For diagnosis, margin detection, and prognosis, a conventional biopsy or surgical excision followed by analysis of stained sections by experienced pathologists is the standard against which alternative measures are compared. The hope is that simpler, less expensive, and more quantitative procedures will be the basis for earlier and more widespread testing of suspected lesions before invasive approaches are required. Such methods should enable more systematic coverage of suspected tissue than is practical with random biopsies. Physical methods should also provide surgeons with real-time indications of disease margins and reduce the recurrence rate after resection.

By far the most developed approach to physical characterization of oral mucosa is the use of light and its interaction with tissue. Many biophotonic methods, either singly or in combination, have shown great promise for clinical use. These methods are the main topic of this article, with emphasis on detection and diagnosis rather than on therapy. Biophotonics is a rapidly expanding field, with several books published recently to guide further inquiry [2–5]. Therapeutic applications, including photodynamic activation

---

* Corresponding author. Box 114, University of Colorado-Denver, Denver, CO 80217.
E-mail address: randall.tagg@cudenver.edu (R. Tagg).

0030-6665/05/$ - see front matter © 2005 Elsevier Inc. All rights reserved.
doi:10.1016/j.otc.2004.10.004

of oxidants, laser hyperthermia, and laser ablation, are mentioned only briefly in their relation to photonic methods of tissue characterization. Such light-based therapies are amply reviewed elsewhere [6].

There is also a brief discussion of other physical methods that are under investigation, recognizing that the physical character of tissues is determined by a combination of optical, electrical, mechanical, and thermal properties. Imaging methods, such as radiography, CT, MRI, positron emission tomography (PET), and ultrasound imaging are important, well-established diagnostic tools [7,8]. It is important to find ways to correlate features seen in imaging systems with the physical characterizations described in this article. The article concludes by discussing an evolving picture of oral tissue as a dynamic system that largely succeeds in maintaining itself against a wide variety of internal and external stresses. The goal is to be able to evaluate, in a clinical setting, the interaction between underlying molecular composition—including genetic aberrations—and the complex spatial and dynamic behavior of tissue as it occasionally changes from a healthy to a malignant state.

Tissue variability

A challenge in characterizing the optical properties of oral mucosa is the variety of tissue that falls into this category, depending on the location in the mouth. As described by Müller et al [9], tissues of the buccal region, the soft palate, the floor of the mouth, and the inner lip are nonkeratinized and have a loose lamina propria. The hard palate, the gingiva, and the dorsal side of the tongue have a keratin layer, with a dense network of collagen fibers and bone under the hard palate and gingiva and papillary structures and taste buds on the dorsal surface of the tongue. All oral mucosa are characterized as stratified squamous cell epithelia, but the morphology and connection to underlying stroma are variable in a way that can affect optical properties.

Müller et al [9] made a systematic assay of diffuse reflectance and fluorescence spectra from seven types of tissue sites for 15 patients with varying states of malignancy (normal, dysplastic, and cancerous) along with tissue from eight healthy volunteers. To classify and detect diseased tissue, these investigators found it sufficient to distinguish only between keratinized and nonkeratinized tissues.

DeVeld et al [10] found that fluorescence spectra from 13 locations sampled from 96 lesion-free patients revealed that 11 of the 13 locations did not warrant separate reference spectra. Only the dorsal tongue and the vermillion border of the lip seemed to have sufficiently different spectra to require separate databases for comparison with diseased tissue. Two types of comparisons were proposed for diagnosis of suspected lesions: one with spectra from tissue at the contralateral location of the same region of the mouth in the same patient, and the other with the reference databases compiled from healthy volunteers. In a separate study, DeVeld et al [11] measured the influence of individual characteristics such as skin color, gender, use of dentures, alcohol consumption, and tobacco use. Although variations were found, the only variation pronounced enough to warrant separate classification of fluorescence spectra was skin color.

Visual inspection

One could argue that photonics has always been an element of oral oncology, because visual inspection is used to classify lesions according to color and texture. Indeed, primary categories of lesion are based on their color [7]:

1. Leukoplakia, with whitish surface reflection usually associated with hyperkeratosis, are often benign but call for further scrutiny.
2. Erythroleukoplakia, with reddish (erythematous) regions embedded in the leukoplakia, are clinically much more likely to undergo malignant transformations than other types of leukoplakia.
3. Erythroplasia, reddish regions by themselves, are also associated with greatly increased cancer risk.

Persistence of lesions of the latter two types is generally sufficient to warrant biopsies. All three types of lesion may be further characterized by different surface textures.

Mashberg [12] emphasizes the importance of visual discrimination of lesions: "The earliest and most significant visual sign of carcinoma in situ, microinvasive or early invasive squamous carcinoma is a persistent, asymptomatic, small, innocuous, red in appearance, inflammatory atrophic mucosal alteration of unknown etiology, with or without a keratinized component, in high-risk sites. Some of these early cancers may be 2–5 mm in size when first observed."

The challenge of identifying lesions is underscored by Betz et al [13]:

> [E]arly lesions are often hard to detect and are sometimes overlooked, even by experienced clinicians. These early invasive carcinomas in situ might simply appear as flat, inconspicuous irregularities of the mucosal surface and may lack typical morphologic characteristics of malignant tumors. At the same time, especially when tongue-like, submucosal spreading of malignancy or diffuse infiltration into surrounding tissue layers is present, superficial demarcation of the tumor borders via simple inspection or other common diagnostic procedures often remains unsatisfactory.

To allow a more definitive interpretation of such small lesions, contrast agents have been sought that selectively stain dysplastic tissue when applied topically or administered as an oral rinse. Chief among these is toluidine blue, a metachromatic thiazine dye that binds to DNA and RNA

[14]. Possible reasons for selective identification of suspect tissue include accentuated dye concentration caused by increased chromatin fractions, easier penetration of intercellular spaces, or increased permeability of cell membranes [15–17]. The potential for toluidine blue to identify malignant lesions has been known for some time [18–21] and is the basis of a 1982 patent by Mashburg [22]. Recent tests confirm genetic changes in cells identified by toluidine blue stain [23,24] as well as its effectiveness in detecting cancerous margins [25]. A commercially designed kit (OraTest, Zila Inc, Phoenix, Arizona) is in phase III clinical trials in the United States; an earlier test in Asia of a related Zila product cited a "remarkable sensitivity in the detection of invasive carcinoma" [26]. Another stain that has been investigated is Lugol's Iodine [27,28]. There are also indications that acetic acid induced whitening, similar to that found in cervical tissues [29–31], occurs in oral dysplasia [32].

Diffuse reflectance spectroscopy

Another approach to accentuating subtle changes in oral lesions is to measure quantitatively the spectroscopic composition of light reflected from tissue. Here it is necessary to distinguish two types of reflection. The first type is specular (mirrorlike) reflection of light at the moist tissue boundary; this reflection obeys the rule that the angle of reflection equals the angle of incidence. The light does not probe the underlying tissue, but it can give information about surface morphology. The second type of reflection occurs when light enters the tissue and eventually is scattered out again. Such multiply scattered light is strongly affected by tissue properties and is the basis of an approach called "diffuse reflectance spectroscopy." This type of spectroscopy has been under intense development in the last decade [33–35].

As light enters tissue, it undergoes a combination of absorption and scattering, both of which are wavelength dependent. Some of the scattered light re-emerges and can be readily analyzed with commercial spectrometers. Fiber optics conveys light to and from the tissue. The interaction of light with tissue is generally described by three parameters that are used to characterize strong, randomized scattering in so-called "turbid media" [36]. All of the parameters depend on the wavelength of the light. The first parameter is the absorption coefficient, μ_a, whose reciprocal, $1/\mu_a$ measures the average length a photon of light will travel before being absorbed. The second is the scattering coefficient, μ_s, whose reciprocal, $1/\mu_s$ measures the average length a photon of light will travel before being scattered into a new direction. The third is called the anisotropy factor, g, which measures how uniformly light is scattered in different directions: completely uniform scattering has an anisotropy factor ($g = 0$), whereas light that is scattered mostly into the forward direction has an anisotropy factor approaching unity. Taking this feature into account, a reduced scattering coefficient, μ_s' is defined by

$$\mu_s' = (1 - g)\mu_s$$

Media with large values of μ_s' are the type normally associated with strong scattering, because incoming light is quickly diverted into many different directions.

The principal type of molecules (chromophores) responsible for visible light absorption in tissue are hemoglobin and melanin. The hemoglobin absorption depends on its oxidative state and falls rapidly for wavelengths above 600 nm. At longer wavelengths in the near-infrared part of the spectrum, water begins to absorb strongly above 1000 nm. The intervening region of the spectrum is called the "therapeutic window" because light in this red-to-near-infrared range can penetrate deeply (several millimeters to centimeters) into tissue. Generally the epithelial layers of tissue have only a mild influence on absorption (a small value of μ_a), so that the underlying stromal tissue dominates the absorption characteristics of diffusively reflected light. Increased hemoglobin caused by changes in vascularization associated with cancer can thus have an important influence on light absorption.

Both the epithelium and the underlying connective tissue strongly scatter light. The cause of scattering in tissue is optical inhomogeneity: there are small but significant variations in the index of refraction. The index of refraction of water, 1.33, sets a lower limit for biologic materials. In simulations of optical scattering, Drezek et al [37] used values of 1.36 to 1.375 for cytoplasm, 1.38 to 1.41 for nuclei, 1.38 to 1.41 for organelles, and 1.46 for collagen. Phospholipid membranes have much higher index of 1.48 [38]; although thin, they can be significant components of enfolded structures such as the endoplasmic reticulum.

The details of the scattering depend on the relative size of the inhomogeneities compared with the light's wavelength. Organelles and membrane structures within cells and fibers in the extracellular matrix are much smaller than the wavelength and give rise to Rayleigh scattering. The strength of this scattering varies as the inverse fourth power of the wavelength, so that blue light scatters much more than red light. Cell nuclei have sizes equal to or greater than the wavelength, resulting in a pattern of scattering called "Mie scattering." The strength of this scattering has a weak but oscillatory dependence on wavelength and is strongly concentrated in the forward direction. Structures of intermediate size (ie, mitochondria and internal variations within nuclei, including the nucleolus) produce significant forward scattering but divert some light to larger angles [39]. Overall, the anisotropy factor of tissue is high, with values of g near 0.9 [40].

Light that scatters only a few times before being detected carries unique information about the scatterers that would be washed out if the light continued to propagate and scatter through the tissue. One approach to finding this component is to construct a model of the diffuse component of scattered light and then to subtract this diffuse component from measured data; the residual is presumed to be minimally scattered light from the upper cell layers of the tissue. Perelman et al [41] used this approach to estimate nuclear sizes in the epithelial layer. Unfortunately, it is difficult to obtain good signal-to-noise ratios with this procedure [9].

Light that scatters only once or a small number of times retains its initial polarization. Polarization is the feature of light that describes the orientation of the light's electric field. Filters can be used to select the polarization of incoming light and analyze the polarization of light that returns. If the measured intensity of randomly polarized light is subtracted from the total intensity of reflected light, the portion that remains corresponds to such minimally scattered light. This portion comes from the top 100 to 200 μm of tissue and thus preferentially samples the epithelial layer. It carries information about the size of the scatterers and thus might be useful for monitoring changes in a variety of subcellular structures [42–48].

Useful insight into the diagnostic potential of scattered light comes from experimental models that mimic the physical properties of tissue. The simplest model is a suspension of polystyrene beads with sizes and distributions similar to cells and cell structures. Increasingly more sophisticated models use the emerging technologies of tissue engineering to create multilayer structures built from collagen matrices and epithelial cell cultures [49]. (For a review of methods for making tissue phantoms, see [50].) Complementary to these artificial constructs is a variety of approaches using numerical simulation. For example, photon scattering through tissue can be modeled as a sequence of probabilistic events calculated for a large number of trials using the Monte Carlo method [51,52]. An understanding of the process of scattering from single cells can be obtained by direct solution of the underlying electromagnetic field equations using, for example, finite-difference time-domain methods [53,54].

Although the combined measurements of absorption, scattering, and polarization can indeed distinguish normal from dysplastic tissue, more definitive results have been achieved by combining such measurements with another method called "fluorescence spectroscopy" [9,55–57]. This topic is discussed next.

Fluorescence

When light is absorbed by molecules, the energy tends to be converted quickly into random molecular vibrations, that is, heat. The time scale for this process is usually picoseconds. For some molecules, however, the excitation that a photon of light causes within the molecule is retained for a longer time interval, perhaps a few nanoseconds [58–61]. This time interval, comparable to a computer clock tick, is short by everyday experience but is moderately long at the scale of molecular phenomena. During this interval a small portion of the energy is transferred to other modes, but then the molecule loses the remainder of the absorbed energy by emitting a new photon of light. This light is shifted to wavelengths longer than the wavelength of light that was initially absorbed. The absorption of light with subsequent re-emission at longer wavelength is called fluorescence. In some cases, internal dynamics involving changes in electron spin further delay the re-emission; the process is then called "phosphorescence." In these cases, the delay can range from milliseconds to seconds. Finally, in some situations, the initial excitation is efficiently transferred to another molecule (or to another part of the same molecule) before re-emission occurs; this transfer is called "fluorescent resonant energy transfer" (FRET). Such transfer occurs only when molecules are in close proximity or when a particular conformation of a protein allows transfer from one location to another. Thus FRET is useful for monitoring intermolecular processes such as cell signaling [62].

The combined measurement of fluorescence and light scattering has benefited greatly from recent advances in optoelectronics and photonics technology that have allowed the design of compact instruments at moderate cost. An example of such a system, similar to the design used by many research groups, is described by Gustafsson [63]. The components of such systems include optical fibers, filters, compact spectrometers, and low-cost light sources available over a spectrum ranging from near-infrared wavelengths down to near-ultraviolet wavelengths. For example, for autofluorescence studies Ueda and Kobayashi [64] recently used the Nichia NLH500A laser diode (Nichia Corporation, Tokyo, Japan) at a wavelength of 400 nm with a power of a few milliwatts. In addition, current microfabrication techniques allow the conversion of many bench-top optical systems into micro-optic formats that can be placed at the end of a fiber-optic cable or endoscope.

The origins of fluorescence used for diagnostic purposes fall into three categories:

1. Intrinsic fluorophores, that is, proteins and other molecules naturally present in the tissue that fluoresce at detectable levels (autofluorescence)
2. Fluorescence brought about by photosensitizers that are introduced externally to enhance the cellular production of fluorophores
3. Fluorescent markers attached to specific biomolecules that are introduced externally to bind to target molecules, for example through antibody attachment to membrane receptors or through selective binding to nucleotide sequences

Wilder-Smith [65] has recently reviewed the first two categories in the context of oral cancer. The third category is most commonly employed in microscopy and is discussed later in a separate section on molecular markers.

In biologic materials, a relatively small number of molecules intrinsically exhibit a high probability of absorption and fluorescent re-emission. These molecules include amino acids with aromatic rings (tryptophan, tyrosin, and phenylalanine), the metabolic co-enzymes NADH and FAD, extracellular materials (collagen and elastin), flavins, keratin, and porphyrins. For each type of molecule, a single wavelength of excitation light produces a spectrum of emitted light. Peaks in the spectrum are broad, with widths over 10 nanometers in optical wavelength. Compiling such spectra over a range of excitation wavelengths gives a complete profile of the fluorescence process, the excitation-emission matrix. This profile depends sensitively on the molecular environment (eg, whether a protein is in its normally folded state or if a molecule is attached to a substrate).

Autofluorescence has proven to be an effective discriminator of tissue health in the oral mucosa [9–11,16,64–94]. In particular, malignant transformation is thought to bring about alterations in the oxidative state and in the abundance of coenzymes NADH and FAD, degradation of collagen matrices, and changes in heme metabolism, thus changing the overall fluorescent characteristics of suspected tissue. The total fluorescence excitation-emission profile is complex because it consists of an overlap of effects from different fluorophores. Further complication in the spectral characteristics arises because both the excitation and emission light must diffuse through strongly scattering and absorbing tissue. Thus the successful deployment of methods to recognize precancerous and cancerous tissue with high sensitivity and specificity requires solving two classes of problem:

1. Separation of the various effects, often using models of the underlying optical characteristics of the tissue and the contributing fluorophores
2. Statistical categorization of spectra as arising from healthy, dysplastic, or malignant tissues

Müller et al [9] present one approach to solving these problems and creating a diagnostic approach for oral cancer, which they call "tri-modal spectroscopy." Measurements were made simultaneously of white light–scattering spectra and of fluorescence emission spectra at selected excitation wavelengths using a multifiber probe [95] and a fast excitation-emission matrix (fast-EEM) apparatus [96]. Five repeated measurements at a given tissue site only took seconds. Later, tissue samples were biopsied from the measurement sites in the patients with suspected lesions; these samples underwent standard histologic analysis and classification, and the results were used as training data for classifying the results of the physical measurements. Information from the white light diffuse reflectance spectroscopy was used to calculate parameters that described the tissue optical properties. These parameters were then used as a demarcation of suspected tissue by examining the clustering of data for pathologic tissue samples and normal samples. The parameters and the corresponding theoretic model of tissue scattering and absorption were also used to disentangle these effects from the fluorescence spectra [97]. This process converted the directly measured fluorescence spectra into rational estimates of the intrinsic spectra that would be obtained if scattering and absorption effects were absent. The instrinsic spectra were then decomposed into contributions from the specific fluorophores NADH and collagen using the statistical technique of multivariate curve resolution. Clustering of spectral components was used as a second demarcation of tissue condition. Finally, the wavelength dependence of the minimally scattered component of white light was used to infer changes in sizes of cell nuclei following the approach of Perelman [41]; this information provided a third basis for tissue evaluation. The combined techniques were applied to 91 tissue sites from 15 patients and eight healthy volunteers. Sensitivity of 96% and specificity of 96% were obtained in distinguishing cancerous or dysplastic tissue from normal tissue.

This work used fluorescence excited by 337-nm and 358-nm laser light and thought to result from NADH and collagen, with most of the intensity falling in the range of 375 to 525 nm. Recent work by Onizawa [98] measured the fluorescence caused by excitation at 404 nm in a cell line, an animal model, and in human swab samples. Emission spectra in the range of 450 of 750 nm were the focus of the study. Spectral peaks at 582 nm and 634 nm (among others) were attributed to Zn-protoporphyrin IX and protoporphyrin IX (PPIX), respectively. The ratio of the intensity of the 634-nm peak to the intensity of a peak at 582 nm was found to be a useful discriminator of tissue condition. Similar work by Inaguma and Hashimoto [99] also suggests that porphyrin-associated autofluorescence near 630 nm is diagnostic of cancer. Both groups attempted to confirm porphyrin presence using standard analytic techniques (capillary electrophoresis [99] and high performance liquid chromatography [100]) on eluted material from tissue samples. The results of the analysis were somewhat ambiguous, confirming the presence of protoporphyrin in only a fraction of the cases. There is controversy about the source of protoporphyrin-associated autofluorescence; it is often attributed to bacteria that might collect near cancerous lesions. The fluorophores seem to be concentrated near the surface and can sometimes be wiped off. Such fluorescence also occurs in normal tissue on the dorsal surface of the tongue. As discussed later, induced protoporphyrin fluorescence seems to avoid these ambiguities.

A variation on measuring autofluorescence at single points is to image the fluorescence across entire regions of tissue using modified video endoscopes. Detailed spectral information is traded for wider spatial coverage (see Andersson-Engels et al [101] and Wilder-Smith [65] for general reviews). The work by Onizawa [71], discussed previously, stemmed from earlier investigations into the use of fluorescence photography for delineating cancerous tissue in an animal model. An ultraviolet flash lamp provided a band of spectral light peaking at 360 nm; fluorescent light passed through a filter blocking wavelengths below 488 nm and was recorded on Polaroid type 339 instant film (Polaroid Corp., Waltham, MA). Lesions were identified when they appeared as orange fluorescence. This method gave 88% sensitivity and 94% specificity in distinguishing between healthy and neoplastic tissue.

Betz et al [16] performed electronic imaging of the mouth with a xenon lamp light source with a filtered output spanning a continuous range of wavelengths from 375 to 440 nm. Blocking filters restricted the light coming back to a charge-coupled device (CCD) camera to wavelengths greater than 515 nm so that none of the excitation light was detected. The images appeared green, and the cancerous lesions appeared darker, that is, they had lower fluorescence under these conditions of illumination and detection. The discrimination of lesions based on intensity values was relatively poor, however, because of the high variability among different locations in the mouth and even within given locations. Much better results were obtained when imaging was based on both autofluorescence and fluorescence induced by topical application of 5-aminolevulinic acid (5-ALA) [102]. The induction of fluorescence through exogenous agents is discussed in the next section. In these combined studies, red-to-green contrast separated lesions from healthy tissue.

Kulapadithorom and Boonkitticharoen [103,104] used a laser-induced fluorescence endoscopy (LIFE) system to measure ratios of red-to-green fluorescence under 442-nm excitation. This ratio gave sensitivity of 100% and specificity of 87.5% in identifying neoplasia. Svistun et al [105] explored the potential for wide clinical use of a particularly simple imaging system using the human eye with a viewing filter as a detector and a fiber-optic bundle carrying filtered xenon arc light as an illuminator. Optimal viewing occurred with excitation at 400 nm and observation at 530 nm. Several other autofluorescence imaging systems have been developed in the last 10 years [91,106–110].

Recently Wilder-Smith et al [111] used multiphoton fluorescence imaging to follow and grade cancer development in a hamster model. Such methods fall into the domain of nonlinear optics, in which more than one photon of light must be absorbed to elicit a fluorescent emission (multiphoton fluorescence) or two photons of light of identical frequency are converted to a single emitted photon at twice the frequency (second harmonic generation) [112]. The excitation light can be in the near-infrared range, thus penetrating the tissue more deeply. Also, certain biomolecules are particularly responsive as nonlinear media. The technique seems to be a particularly sensitive way to monitor the degradation and cellular infiltration of the collagen matrix in the tissue of the hamster cheek pouch.

Induced fluorescence

Certain exogenous agents stimulate fluorescence in tissue. Much of the recent work on induced fluorescence in oral cancer used the topical application of 5-ALA. This biochemical is a naturally occurring component in ordinary cell metabolism leading to heme production. Adding 5-ALA to tissue bypasses normal cell feedback mechanisms and results in an accumulation of PPIX, especially in malignant tissues. This fluorophore, discussed previously, has a distinctive red fluorescent emission. Van der Breggen et al [113] used excitation in a 60-nm band centered on 400 nm (near the 410 maximum in the PPIX excitation peak) to record spectra from cancer in the hamster cheek pouch. The ratio of the intensity of the fluorescent peak at 632 nm to the intensity at 595 nm was found to be a useful discriminator of tissue status. Leunig et al [114] used endoscopes to examine fluorescence from human oral tissue with similar illumination conditions and found that cancerous tissue is many times more intense than healthy tissue at the fluorescent peak near 630 nm. Moreover, the maximum contrast is achieved relatively quickly, 1 to 2 hours after application. The intensity of the fluorescence and the side effects of tissue photosensitivity faded within 24 hours. Leunig et al [102,115–118] and several other groups [119–122] have continued to evaluate and refine the use of 5-ALA induced fluorescence.

Another agent that has been used for many years to induce fluorescence in oral cancer tissues is a hematoporphyrin derivative [123–127]. It is also used for photodynamic therapy. Its fluorescence is weaker than ALA-induced PPIX fluorescence, and systemic application of hematoporphyrin derivative requires patients to remain in a darkened room for several weeks. Other agents used for induced fluorescence are tetracycline [128] and aluminum phthalocyanine disulphonate [129,130].

Infrared spectroscopy

Infrared light is typically absorbed and re-radiated as the result of changes in the vibrational energy of molecular bonds. Quantum theory shows that the energy exchanges and consequently the wavelengths of photons absorbed or emitted are restricted to discrete values (quanta) that depend on the particular molecular bond and its environment. Infrared spectroscopy can thus be a sensitive indicator of molecular species and is a common tool in the analytical chemistry laboratory.

Successful use of infrared spectroscopy in vivo to identify molecular changes in tissue is subject to considerations similar to those governing the use of fluorescence: Molecular species of interest must be present in sufficient abundance to be detected, and spectral signatures must be disentangled from overlapping effects. There are also instrumental challenges in finding optical materials and components that can transmit light across the range of wavelengths desired for infrared spectroscopy [131]. A particular problem is the increasing absorption by water in the tissue for wavelengths above 1 μm. One way to deal with high tissue absorption is to conduct the infrared light through a waveguide placed into or adjacent to the tissue so that a portion of the infrared energy exists just outside the waveguide, exponentially decaying with distance from the waveguide surface. Wavelength-dependent absorption of light in this so-called "evanescent portion" of the guided wave causes a measurable decrease in transmission through the waveguide. This decrease in transmission is the basis of attenuated total reflection (ATR) spectroscopy. When this principle is used with fiber optics, it is called "fiber-optic evanescent wave" spectroscopy.

It is customary to express infrared spectral components in wavenumber units, v, that are reciprocally related to the wavelength: $v = 1/\lambda$. The spectral range of interest for wavenumber v is typically from 3300 to 700 cm^{-1} and thus for this range of interest the wavelength λ is typically from 3 to 14 μm. Peak widths are relatively narrow, about a few cm^{-1}, and collectively provide "fingerprints" of various molecular bonds.

Ordinary glass does not transmit light in this spectral range, so special materials such as silver halides are required for optical fibers and other components [132]. A common method of extracting spectral information is to record interference intensities in a Michelson-interferometer, an approach that gives the Fourier-transform of the wavenumber spectrum. This method, Fourier-transform infrared spectroscopy (FTIR), has some advantages over conventional spectroscopy: Nondispersive optical components (mirrors) are used, and information about the entire spectrum can be recorded at any point in time.

The use of infrared spectroscopy for tissue characterization is still in an exploratory stage. Work so far has been largely been ex vivo with single cells, cell suspensions, or tissue samples. Schultz [133,134] used FTIR microspectroscopy to discriminate normal from malignant oral tissue, with emphasis on biochemical features associated with keratin production in cancerous cells. Mourant et al [135], working with fibroblast cell lines, demonstrated that changes in hydration, cell thickness, and cell mitotic stages can affect infrared spectra. They also measured spectra from major cell components (DNA/RNA, proteins, phospholipids, and glycogen) to show that whole cell cultures can be represented by linear combinations of spectra from the individual components. Working with oral mucosa tissue samples, Fukuyama et al [136] measured and assigned several subtle changes in infrared spectra from normal and malignant tissue. Wu et al [137] made measurements in vivo on oral mucosa using a fiber-optic probe. They found that a particularly useful discriminator in the spectra was a 1745-cm^{-1} band assigned to ester group $C = O$ vibrations in triglycerides. Yoshida and Yoshida [138] recently described the use of an ATR probe to measure changes in vivo of polyunsaturated fatty acids in oral mucosa; this measurement was based on special attention to an alkene C-H stretching band near 3010 cm^{-1}. Although intended for diagnostic purposes other than cancer detection, their work further demonstrated the feasibility of in vivo infrared diagnostics for oral mucosa. Experimental methods and data analysis techniques applicable to oral cancer detection are also described by Bindig et al [139] in studies of colon tissue and by Sukuta and Bruch [140] for skin cancer.

Raman spectroscopy

The same characteristic vibrational-mode information about biomolecules can be obtained using light in the ultraviolet/visible/near-infrared region of the spectrum. Light scatters off molecules in the tissue inelastically, depositing a small portion of energy into the vibrational modes of the molecules. The effect, discovered by C.V. Raman in 1928, is weak: typically, 1 photon in 10^9 is scattered with such energy loss. Lasers, efficient collection optics, and sensitive detectors allow precise spectral measurements to be made. Thorough reviews of the biomedical and instrumental aspects of Raman spectroscopy for cancer diagnosis have been written by Mahadevan-Jansen and Richards-Kortum [141] and by Hanlon et al [142].

One challenge in the use of Raman spectroscopy in vivo is that fluorescence from the tissue can overwhelm the received light. This problem is minimized by using light in the near-infrared range for Raman scattering. At such wavelengths, tissue fluorescence is minimized. Numerical fits to the background fluorescence can also be made and subtracted from the raw data to pull out the Raman component. Another problem is the Raman scattering from materials in the fiber optics used to convey light to and from the tissue. Filters are used to minimize this interference. Finally, a compromise must be made between the desire to maximize input laser power and limitations on tissue heating and data collection time. Technical advances in probe design [143] permit spectra to be obtained using 100 mW of laser power and 1- to 10-second collection times.

Limited but promising work has been done on the use of Raman spectroscopy for oral cancer. Yang et al [144] demonstrated that Raman spectra could distinguish normal head and neck tissue from squamous cell carcinoma. Venkatakrishna et al [145] collected more than 100 spectra from 51 oral tissue specimens, performed ex situ Raman spectroscopy with 785-nm light from a diode laser, and with statistical classification techniques achieved 85% sensitivity and 90% specificity in identifying lesions. The spectra were interpreted as indicating that normal tissues have a spectrum mostly indicative of lipid content, whereas malignant samples have proteinlike spectra. Similar studies with hamster cheek pouch tissue have been reported by de Oliveira et al [146]. Shim and Wilson [147] used human buccal mucosa to demonstrate the effectiveness of an in vivo Raman probe.

In vivo microscopy

Standard biopsy and histologic analysis reveal important structural and morphologic information that is not contained in spectroscopic data. Because the epithelium in oral mucosa is accessible and is relatively thin (200–500 μm), there is an inviting prospect to design microscopes that look at the tissue in the mouth without the need for biopsy. Sokolov [148,149] has reviewed technical developments by many research groups. It seems possible to see subcellular structure and to record dysplastic changes in cellular organization in vivo [150–156].

Two principal types of microscopes are currently being developed and tested. One is an endoscopic version of the confocal microscope [157]. It achieves spatial resolution and depth discrimination by using pinhole apertures (or the effective aperture of a small optical fiber) to select both the region of illumination and the region from which light is received by a detector. The successful use of such instruments on living tissue requires adequate contrast in the light returning from the specimen [158,29]. In ordinary reflectance microscopy, this contrast arises from variations in index of refraction and absorption of the cellular materials. These variations determine the amount of light that is scattered back into the microscope aperture. It is possible to enhance such contrast using stains, as has been discussed previously. It is also possible to use fluorescence to accentuate and identify cellular structures. Fluorescent molecular markers can be used to tag desired constituents of the cell. This approach is discussed in a separate, following section.

The other microscopic technique is optical coherence tomography (OCT) [159,160], which is intrinsically well suited to implementation using fiber optics. Laser light is divided by a beam splitter into two pathways. Light going down one of the fiber pathways impinges on the tissue, and some of it is reflected back through the same fiber. The other portion of light follows a reference pathway of precisely the same length and is reflected back by a mirror to mix with the light returning from the specimen. Only tissue that is at a depth where the two lengths precisely match will produce interference between the two light waves. The strength of this interference signal can be used to image features of the desired layer of tissue. Presently it is difficult to obtain depth discrimination better than 15 microns and lateral resolution better than 3 to 5 microns. Images from this kind of microscope mostly reveal the boundaries between the epithelium and the underlying stroma [161]. Thickening of the epithelial layer or loss of contrast with the underlying tissue can indicate pathology. McNichols et al [162] describe a fluorescent image–guided OCT probe for detection of oral cancer. A probe with similar function for application to colon cancer was designed by Tumlinson et al [163]. Other applications of OCT to oral cancer are described by Hsu et al [164], Bibas et al [165], and Fomina et al [166].

Molecular markers

Advances in molecular biology have revealed a large number of genetic and protein changes associated with cancer. Thus a goal of cancer diagnosis is to use this rapidly increasing store of information to identify, in vivo and in real time, molecular alterations associated with oncogenes, tumor suppressor genes, cell signaling molecules, membrane receptors, and enzymes that are implicated in cancer development. Many such molecular markers have been identified for oral cancer [167–173]. Some of the potential markers include epidermal growth factor receptor (EGFR, a transmembrane protein involved in cell proliferation) [174], *p53* (a tumor-suppressor/apoptosis-regulating protein), *p16* (a cyclin-dependent kinase inhibitor), cadherins and other cell adhesion molecules, and metalloproteinases that degrade the basement membrane and thus may be a factor in malignant invasion and metastasis.

One approach is to use rapid versions of conventional wet-bench techniques to amplify and detect molecular markers on a time scale that would be useful for detecting cancerous tissue margins during an operation [175]. The previously discussed advances in microscopy provide a promising possibility that such margins could be identified in vivo without tissue extraction [149]. Takes [176] has reviewed a variety of imaging techniques and a list of biomarkers for use in staging head and neck cancers. Cherry [177] provides an even broader review of molecular imaging, including distributed imaging throughout the body using molecule-specific contrast agents for various types of medical imaging systems.

One method of molecular imaging used for in situ microscopy [149] is fluorescent tagging of antibodies to selected molecules. The use of fluorescent tags is now well established in microscopy, and commercial sources of fluorophores are readily available [178]. Sokolov et al [149] used fluorescent markers conjugated to EGFR antibodies to observe expression of these receptor molecules in cells, fresh tissue slices, and organ cultures. Another approach used by this research group was to attach selected antibodies to luminous metallic nanoparticles or to semiconductor quantum dots. EGFR antibodies were again used, attached to colloidal gold particles or to semiconductor quantum dots. These tagged particles identified changes in EGFR expression on cell membranes. Metallic nanoparticles such as colloidal gold provide strong backscatter of light because of the resonant excitation of bound charge waves called "surface plasmons." Quantum dots enhance visibility in a different way: electrons in the confined geometry occupy states that can fluoresce with much higher efficiency than most molecular fluorophores. (See Prasad [179] for a discussion of these new technologies.) Such probes are nontoxic and can carry the same sort of molecular detectors used in microarray technology into cells for optical detection of desired target molecules [180].

Methods of measuring other physical properties

Many other physical properties of tissue could be measured in response to developing pathology [181]. In addition to optical properties, tissues—like any collection of matter—can be characterized by

1. Mechanical properties
2. Acoustic properties

3. Thermal properties
4. Electrical properties

Clinical usefulness depends on whether or not methods of measuring these properties can be made compact enough to work in vivo and definitive enough to detect changes associated with small lesions. Although work has been done to characterize cancerous tissue using these methods, the literature on applications to oral cancer is quite sparse in comparison with the photonic methods discussed in this article. Two such nonoptical methods are discussed here as examples of possible developments.

Tissue stiffness is a mechanical property that describes the resistance to deformation under an applied force. A measure of such stiffness is called "elasticity," and elasticity can be probed in a variety of ways. The simplest is palpitation, which in its most basic form is a common method for self-examination of the breast and testicles and is also a clinical approach for inspecting the liver, prostate, and thyroid. A method for measuring tissue stiffness that can probe deep into tissue uses ultrasound to measure local deformations in response to an externally imposed compression of the tissue. This imaging method is called "elastography" [182,183]. Ultrasound scans with and without the applied compression are cross-correlated to measure, as a function of distance from the probe, how the tissue distorts in response to the deforming force. Although this method is designed for probing tissue such as breast or leg muscle that is deeper than oral mucosa, a variation might be appropriate in cases where invasion deep into the stroma is suspected. Corresponding techniques have been developed using MRI [184]. It is also possible to measure the response of thin tissue layers to shearing rather than to compression. Such a probe recently has been developed to measure the stiffness of skin to dynamic shearing forces [185]. An ultrasound palpation system has been used by Zheng et al [186] to measure neck tissue fibrosis.

As cell shape, cell internal structure and intercellular space are modified by tissue transformation, the ease with which electric charge passes through tissue will vary. This is measured as "impedance", a factor indicating how much voltage is required to drive a given electric current through the tissue. This factor depends on frequency: direct current and low frequency currents are largely influenced by the ease with which charge flows through intercellular spaces. High frequency currents are also influenced by the charging and discharging of cellular membranes. When impedance is measured as a function of frequency of the applied voltage, an "impedance spectrum" is obtained that characterizes the tissue state. This has been applied to cervical tissue [187–189], where the low frequency impedance has been found to be especially responsive to changes in structure of precancerous tissue.

Summary: tissues as dynamic systems

Optical methods provide a wide range of diagnostic tools for discriminating cancerous tissue from healthy tissue. The most widely developed approaches use light scattering and fluorescence measurements together to detect changes in tissue structure and composition. Infrared or Raman spectroscopy can potentially provide specific information about proteins, lipids, sugars, and DNA molecules and their environments. A goal is to relate these observations to underlying molecular changes that are thought to be responsible for cancer progression. New in vivo microscopes and molecular tagging techniques promise to help make such molecular identifications possible in a routine clinical setting. Measurements of other physical properties can provide complementary information about tissue structure and function.

Cancer is, however, a complex disease that shows great variability from patient to patient. The isolation of one or a few indicators of suspected pathology will still require judgment on how to proceed with therapy. Future aids to such judgment will rely on greater integration of diagnostic tools. Such integration will need models of both healthy and malignant tissue that recognize the ways that tissue functions as a complex, dynamic system. Systems approaches are progressing at the cellular level as signaling networks and gene regulation processes become better understood [190–192]. Corresponding approaches at the tissue level will be needed to recognize combinations of events occurring in mild dysplasia that are likely to lead to malignancy and metastasis [193,194]. This need raises the possibility that a new class of diagnostic instruments might be developed to measure the collective response of populations of cells to stresses experienced by mucosal tissues. In this way, detection of local molecular and structural abnormalities might be placed in a context that allows earlier and more reliable prognosis and choice of therapy.

References

[1] Vokes EE, Weichselbaum RR, Lippman SM, et al. Head and neck cancer. N Engl J Med 1993;328(3):184–94.
[2] Vo-Dinh T, editor. Biomedical photonics handbook. Boca Raton (FL): SPIE Press; 2003.
[3] Tuchin VV, editor. Handbook of optical biomedical diagnostics. Bellingham (WA): SPIE Press; 2002.
[4] Prasad PN. Introduction to biophotonics. New York: Wiley; 2003.
[5] Mycek M-A, Pogue BW, editors. Handbook of biomedical fluorescence. New York: Marcel Dekker; 2003. p. 1–27.
[6] Niemz MH. Laser-tissue interactions: fundamentals and applications. Berlin: Springer; 2004.
[7] Silverman S Jr. Oral cancer. 5th edition. Hamilton (Ontario): B.C. Decker; 2003.
[8] Ahuja AT, Evans RM, King AD, et al. Imaging of head and neck cancer: a practical approach. London: Greenwich Medical Media; 2003.

[9] Müller MG, Valdez TA, Georgakoudi I, et al. Spectroscopic detection and evaluation of morphologic and biochemical changes in early human oral carcinoma. Cancer 2003;97(7): 1681–92.

[10] de Veld DCG, Skurichina M, Witjes MJ, et al. Autofluorescence characteristics of healthy oral mucosa at different anatomical sites. Lasers Surg Med 2003;32(5):367–76.

[11] de Veld DCG, Sterenborg HJCM, Roodenburg JLN, et al. Effects of individual characteristics on healthy oral mucosa autofluorescence spectra. Oral Oncol 2004;40:815–23.

[12] Mashberg A. Diagnosis of early oral and oropharyngeal squamous carcinoma: obstacles and their amelioration. Oral Oncol 2000;36(3):253–5.

[13] Betz C, Stepp H, Janda P, Arbogast S, et al. A comparative study of normal inspection, autofluorescence and 5-ALA-induced PPIX fluorescence for oral cancer diagnosis. Int J Cancer 2002;97:245–52.

[14] Kiernan JA. Histological and histochemical methods: theory and practice. London: Arnold; 1999.

[15] Epstein JB, Scully C, Spinelli J. Toluidine blue and Lugol's iodine application in the assessment of oral malignant disease and lesions at risk of malignancy. J Oral Pathol Med 1992;21(4):160–3.

[16] Betz CS, Mehlman M, Rick K, et al. Autofluorescence imaging and spectroscopy of normal and malignant mucosa in patients with head and neck cancer. Lasers Surg Med 1999;25(4): 323–4.

[17] Bornhop DJ, Contag CH, Licha K, et al. Advances in contrast agents, reporters, and detection. J Biomed Opt 2001;6(2):106–10.

[18] Niebel HN, Chomet B. In vivo staining test for delineation of oral intraepithelial of oral intraepithelial neoplastic change: preliminary report. J Am Dent Assoc 1964;63:801–6.

[19] Strong MS, Vaughan CW, Incze JS. Toluidine blue in the management of carcinoma of the oral cavity. Arch Otolaryngol 1968;87(5):527–31.

[20] Mashberg A. Reevaluation of toluidine blue application as a diagnostic adjunct in the detection of asymptomatic oral squamous carcinoma: a continuing prospective study of oral cancer III. Cancer 1980;46(4):758–63.

[21] Silverman S Jr, Migliorati C, Barbosa J. Toluidine blue staining in the detection of oral precancerous and malignant lesions. Oral Surg Oral Med Oral Pathol 1984;57(4):379–82.

[22] Mashberg A. Detection of malignant lesions of the oral cavity utilizing toluidine blue rinse. US Patent No. 4,321,251; 1982.

[23] Epstein JB, Zhang L, Poh C, Nakamura H, et al. Increased allelic loss in toluidine blue-positive oral premalignant lesions. Oral Surg Oral Med Oral Pathol Oral Radiol Endod 2003;95(1):45–50.

[24] Guo Z, Yamaguchi K, Sanchez-Cespedes M, et al. Allelic losses in OraTest-directed biopsies of patients with prior upper aerodigestive tract malignancy. Clin Cancer Res 2001; 7(7):1963–8.

[25] Portugal LG, Wilson KM, Biddinger PW, et al. The role of toluidine blue in assessing margin status after resection of squamous cell carcinomas of the upper aerodigestive tract. Arch Otolaryngol Head Neck Surg 1996;122(5):517–9.

[26] Warnakulasuriya KA, Johnson NW. Sensitivity and specificity of OraScan (R) toluidine blue mouthrinse in the detection of oral cancer and precancer. J Oral Pathol Med 1996; 25(3):97–103.

[27] Morgenroth K. Neue untersuchungen mit dem Kolposkop nach Hunselmann und der Vitalfarbung der Mundschleimhaut zur Fruhdiagnose von Tumoren im Kieferbereich. Dtsch Zahnaerztl Z 1957;12:192–201.

[28] Kurita H, Kurashina K. Vital staining with iodine solution in delineating the border of oral dysplastic lesions. Oral Surg Oral Med Oral Pathol Oral Radiol Endod 1996;81:275–80.

[29] Smithpeter C, Duan A, Drezek R, et al. Near real time confocal microscopy of cultured amelanotic cells: sources of signal, contrast agents and limits of contrast. J Biomed Opt 1998;3(4):429–36.

[30] Collier T, Shen P, De Pradier B, et al. Near real time confocal microscopy of amelanotic tissue: dynamics of aceto-whitening enable nuclear segmentation. Opt Express 2000;6(2): 40–8.

[31] Zuluaga AF, Drezek R, Collier T, et al. Contrast agents for confocal microscopy: how simple chemicals affect confocal images of normal and cancer cells in suspension. J Biomed Opt 2002;7(3):398–403.

[32] Huber MA, Bsoul SA, Terezhalmy GT. Acetic acid wash and chemiluminescent illumination as an adjunct to conventional oral soft tissue examination for the detection of dysplasia: a pilot study. Quintessence Int 2004;35(5):378–84.

[33] Mourant JR, Freyer JP, Hielscher AH, et al. Mechanisms of light scattering from biological cells relevant to noninvasive optical-tissue diagnostics. Appl Opt 1998;37(16):3586–93.

[34] Mourant JR, Bigio IJ. Elastic-scattering spectroscopy and diffuse reflectance. In: Vo-Dinh T, editor. Biomedical photonics handbook. Boca Raton (FL): SPIE Press; 2003. p. 29.1–22.

[35] Perelman LT, Backman V. Light scattering spectroscopy of epithelial tissues: principles and applications. In: Tuchin VV, editor. Handbook of optical biomedical diagnostics. Bellingham (WA): SPIE Press; 2002. p. 675–724.

[36] Ishimaru A. Diffusion of light in turbid media. Appl Opt 1989;28:2210–5.

[37] Drezek R, Dunn A, Richards-Kortum R. Light scattering from cells: finite-difference time-domain simulations and goniometric measurements. Appl Opt 1999;38(16): 3651–61.

[38] Beuthan J, Minet O, Helfmann J, et al. The spatial variation of the refractive index in biological cells. Phys Med Biol 1996;41:369–82.

[39] Drezek R, Guillaud M, Collier T, et al. Light scattering from cervical cells throughout neoplastic progression: influence of nuclear morphology, DNA content, and chromatin texture. J Biomed Opt 2003;8(1):7–16.

[40] Mobley J, Vo-Dinh T. Optical properties of tissues. In: Vo-Dinh T, editor. Biomedical photonics handbook. Boca Raton (FL): SPIE Press; 2003. p. 2.1–75.

[41] Perelman LT, Backman V, Wallace M, et al. Observation of periodic fine structure in reflectance from biological tissue: a new technique for measuring nuclear size distribution. Phys Rev Lett 1998;80:627–30.

[42] Backman V, Gurjar R, Badizadegan K, et al. Polarized light scattering spectroscopy for quantitative measurement of epithelial cellular structures in situ. IEEE J Sel Top Quantum Electron 1999;5(4):1019–26.

[43] Sokolov K, Drezek R, Gossage K, et al. Reflectance spectroscopy with polarized light: is it sensitive to cellular and nuclear morphology. Opt Express 1999;5:302–17.

[44] Gurjar RS, Backman V, Perelman LT, et al. Imaging human epithelial properties with polarized light scattering spectroscopy. Nat Med 2001;7:1245–8.

[45] Mourant JR, Johnson TM, Freyer JP. Characterizing mammalian cells and cell phantoms by polarized backscattering fiber-optic measurements. Appl Opt 2001;40(28): 5114–23.

[46] Mourant JR, Johnson TM, Carpenter S, et al. Polarized angular dependent spectroscopy of epithelial cells and epithelial cell nuclei to determine the size scale of scattering structures. J Biomed Opt 2002;7(3):378–87.

[47] Myakov A, Nieman L, Wicky L, et al. Fiber optic probe for polarized reflectance spectroscopy in vivo: design and performance. J Biomed Opt 2002;7(3):388–97.

[48] Bartlett M, Huang G, Larcom L, et al. Measurement of particle size distribution in mammalian cells in vitro by use of polarized light spectroscopy. Appl Opt 2004;43(6): 1296–307.

[49] Sokolov K, Galvan J, Myakov A, et al. Realistic three-dimensional epithelial tissue phantoms for biomedical optics. J Biomed Opt 2002;7(1):148–56.

[50] Pravdin AB, Chernova SP, Papazoglou TG, et al. Tissue phantoms. In: Tuchin VV, editor. Handbook of optical biomedical diagnostics. Bellingham (WA): SPIE Press; 2002. p. 311–52.

[51] Jaques SL, Wang L. Monte Carlo modeling of light transport in tissues. In: Welch AJ, van Gemert MJC, editors. Optical-thermal response of laser irradiated tissue. New York: Plenum; 1995. p. 73.

[52] Wang L, Jacques SL, Zheng L. MCML—Monte Carlo modeling of light transport in multi-layered tissues. Comput Methods Programs Biomed 1995;47:131.

[53] Dunn A, Richards-Kortum R. Three-dimensional computation of light scattering from cells. IEEE J Sel Top Quantum Electron 1996;2:898–905.

[54] Drezek R, Dunn A, Richards-Kortum R. Light scattering from cells: finite-difference time-domain simulations and goniometric measurements. Appl Opt 1999;38(16):3651–61.

[55] Richards-Kortum R, Sevick-Muraca E. Quantitative optical spectroscopy for tissue diagnosis. Annu Rev Phys Chem 1996;47:555–606.

[56] Bigio IJ, Mourant JR. Ultraviolet and visible spectroscopies for tissue diagnostics: fluorescence spectroscopy and elastic-scattering spectroscopy. Phys Med Biol 1997;42(5): 803–14.

[57] Sokolov K, Follen M, Richards-Kortum R. Optical spectroscopy for detection of neoplasia. Curr Opin Chem Biol 2002;6(5):651–8.

[58] Lakowicz JR. Principles of fluorescence spectroscopy. 2nd edition. New York: Kluwer Academic; 1999.

[59] Vo-Dinh T, Cullum BM. Fluorescence spectroscopy for biomedical diagnostics. In: Vo-Dinh T, editor. Biomedical photonics handbook. Boca Raton (FL): SPIE Press; 2003. p. 28.1–50.

[60] Schneckenburger H, Stock K, Steiner R, et al. Fluorescence technologies in biomedical diagnostics. In: Tuchin VV, editor. Handbook of optical biomedical diagnostics. Bellingham (WA): SPIE Press; 2002. p. 825–74.

[61] Redmond RW. Introduction to fluorescence and photophysics. In: Mycek M-A, Pogue BW, editors. Handbook of biomedical fluorescence. New York: Marcel Dekker; 2003. p. 1–27.

[62] Schmid JA, Sitte HH. Fluorescence resonance energy transfer in the study of cancer pathways. Curr Opin Oncol 2003;15(1):55–64.

[63] Gustafsson U, Palson S, Svanberg S. Compact fiber-optic fluorosensor using a continuous-wave violet diode laser and an integrated spectrometer. Rev Sci Instrum 2000;71(8):3004–8.

[64] Ueda Y, Kobayashi M. Spectroscopic studies of autofluorescence substances existing in human tissue: influences of lactic acid and porphyrins. Appl Opt 2004;43(20):3993–8.

[65] Wilder-Smith P. Fluorescence emission-based detection and diagnosis of malignancy. J Cell Biochem 2002;39(Suppl):54–9.

[66] Alfano RR, Tata DB, Cordero J, Tomashefsky P, et al. Laser induced fluorescence spectroscopy from native cancerous and normal tissue. IEEE J Quantum Electron 1984; QE-20(12):1507–11.

[67] Harries ML, Lam S, MacAulay C, et al. Diagnostic imaging of the larynx: auto-fluorescence of laryngeal tumours using the helium-cadmium laser. J Laryngol Otol 1995; 109(2):108–10.

[68] Kluftinger AM, Davis NL, Quenville NF, et al. Detection of squamous cell cancer and pre-cancerous lesions by imaging of tissue autofluorescence in the hamster cheek pouch model. Surg Oncol 1992;1(2):183–8.

[69] Silberberg MB, Savage HE, Tang GC, et al. Detecting retinoic acid-induced biochemical alterations in squamous cell carcinoma using intrinsic fluorescence spectroscopy. Laryngoscope 1994;104(3Pt1):278–82.

[70] Kolli VR, Savage HE, Yao TJ, et al. Native cellular fluorescence of neoplastic upper aerodigestive mucosa. Arch Otolaryngol Head Neck Surg 1995;121:1287–92.

[71] Onizawa K, Saginoya H, Furuya Y, et al. Fluorescence photography as a diagnostic method for oral cancer. Cancer Lett 1996;108(1):61–6.

[72] Sacks PG, Sacks PG, Savage HE, et al. Native cellular fluorescence identifies terminal squamous differentiation of normal oral epithelial cells in culture: a potential chemo-prevention biomarker. Cancer Lett 1996;104(2):171–81.

[73] Fryen A, Glanz H, Lohmann W, Dreyer T, et al. Significance of autofluorescence for the optical demarcation of field cancerisation in the upper aerodigestive tract. Acta Otolaryngol 1997;117(2):316–9.

[74] Ingrams DR, Dhingra JK, Roy K, et al. Autofluorescence characteristics of oral mucosa. Head Neck 1997;19(1):27–32.

[75] Schantz SP, Savage HE, Sacks P, et al. Native cellular fluorescence and its application to cancer prevention. Environ Health Perspect 1997;105(Suppl 4):941–4.

[76] Zargi M, Smid L, Fajdiga I, et al. Laser induced fluorescence in diagnostics of laryngeal cancer. Acta Otolaryngol Suppl 1997;527:125–7.

[77] Zargi M, Smid L, Fajdiga I, et al. Detection and localization of early laryngeal cancer with laser-induced fluorescence: preliminary report. Eur Arch Otorhinolaryngol 1997;254(Suppl 1):S113–6.

[78] Zhang JC, Savage HE, Sacks PG, et al. Innate cellular fluorescence reflects alterations in cellular proliferation. Lasers Surg Med 1997;20(3):319–31.

[79] Chen CT, Chiang HK, Chow SN, et al. Autofluorescence in normal and malignant human oral tissues and in DMBA-induced hamster buccal pouch carcinogenesis. J Oral Pathol Med 1998;27(10):470–4.

[80] Gillenwater A, Jacob R, Ganeshappa R, et al. Noninvasive diagnosis of oral neoplasia based on fluorescence spectroscopy and native tissue autofluorescence. Arch Otolaryngol Head Neck Surg 1998;124(11):1251–8.

[81] Gillenwater A, Jacob R, Richards-Kortum R. Fluorescence spectroscopy: a technique with potential to improve the early detection of aerodigestive tract neoplasia. Head Neck 1998; 20(6):556–62.

[82] Schantz SP, Kolli V, Savage HE, Yu G, et al. In vivo native cellular fluorescence and histological characteristics of head and neck cancer. Clin Cancer Res 1998;4(5):1177–82.

[83] Majumder SK, Gupta PK, Uppal A. Autofluorescence spectroscopy of tissues from human oral cavity for discriminating malignant from normal. Lasers in the Life Sciences 1999;8(4): 211–27.

[84] Onizawa K, Saginoya H, Furuya Y, et al. Usefulness of fluorescence photgraphy for diagnosis of oral cancer. Int J Oral Maxillofac Surg 1999;28:206–10.

[85] Wang CY, Chen CT, Chiang CP, et al. A probability-based multivariate statistical algorithm for autofluorescence spectroscopic identification of oral carcinogenesis. Photo-chem Photobiol 1999;69(4):471–7.

[86] Wang CY, Chiang HK, Chen CT, et al. Diagnosis of oral cancer by light-induced autofluorescence spectroscopy using double excitation wavelengths. Oral Oncol 1999;35(2): 144–50.

[87] Heintzelman DL, Utzinger U, Fuchs H, et al. Optimal excitation wavelengths for in vivo detection of oral neoplasia using fluorescence spectroscopy. Photochem Photobiol 2000; 72(1):103–13.

[88] Majumder SK, Mohanty SK, Ghosh N, et al. A pilot study on the use of autofluorescence spectroscopy for diagnosis of the cancer of human oral cavity. Curr Sci 2000;79(8):1089–94.

[89] Onizawa K, Yoshida H, Saginoya H. Chromatic analysis of autofluorescence emitted from squamous cell carcinomas arising in the oral cavity: a preliminary study. Int J Oral Maxillofac Surg 2000;29(1):42–6.

[90] van Staveren HJ, van Veen RL, Speelman OC, et al. Classification of clinical autofluorescence spectra of oral leukoplakia using an artificial neural network: a pilot study. Oral Oncol 2000;36(3):286–93.

[91] Katz A, Savage HE, Schantz SP, et al. Noninvasive native fluorescence imaging of head and neck tumors. Technol Cancer Res Treat 2002;1(1):9–15.

[92] Majumder SK, Ghosh N, Kataria S, et al. Nonlinear pattern recognition for laser-induced fluorescence diagnosis of cancer. Lasers Surg Med 2003;33(1):48–56.

[93] Tsai T, Chen HM, Wang CY, et al. In vivo autofluorescence spectroscopy of oral premalignant and malignant lesions: distortion of fluorescence intensity by submucous fibrosis. Lasers Surg Med 2003;33:40–7.

[94] Wang CY, Tsai T, Chen HM, et al. PLS-ANN based classification model for oral submucous fibrosis and oral carcinogenesis. Lasers Surg Med 2003;32:318–26.

[95] Cothren RM, Hayes GB, Kramer JR, et al. A multifiber catheter with an optical shield for laser angiosurgery. Lasers in the Life Sciences 1986;1:1–12.

[96] Zangaro RA, Silveira L, Manoharan R, et al. Rapid multiexcitation fluorescence spectroscopy system for in vivo tissue diagnosis. Appl Opt 1996;35:5211–9.

[97] Müller MG, Georgakoudi I, Zhang Q, et al. Instrinsic fluorescence spectroscopy in turbid media: disentangling effects of scattering and absorption. Appl Opt 2001;40(25):4633–46.

[98] Onizawa K, Okamura N, Saginoya H, et al. Analysis of fluorescence in oral squamous cell carcinoma. Oral Oncol 2002;38(4):343–8.

[99] Inaguma M, Hashimoto K. Porphyrin-like fluorescence in oral cancer: in vivo fluorescence spectral characterization of lesions by use of a near-ultraviolet excited autofluorescence diagnosis system and separation of fluorescent extracts by capillary electrophoresis. Cancer 1999;86(11):2201–11.

[100] Onizawa K, Okamura N, Saginoya H, et al. Characterization of autofluorescence in oral squamous cell carcinoma. Oral Oncol 2003;39(2):150–6.

[101] Andersson-Engels S, Klinteberg C, Svanberg K, et al. In vivo fluorescence imaging for tissue diagnostics. Phys Med Biol 1997;42(5):815–24.

[102] Betz C, Stepp H, Janda P, et al. A comparative study of normal inspection, autofluorescence and 5-ALA-induced PPIX fluorescence for oral cancer diagnosis. Int J Cancer 2002;97:245–52.

[103] Kulapaditharom B, Boonkitticharoen V. Performance characteristics of fluorescence endoscope in detection of head and neck cancers. Ann Otol Rhinol Laryngol 2001;110(1):45–52.

[104] Kulapaditharom B, Boonkitticharoen V. Laser-induced fluorescence imaging in localization of head and neck cancers. Ann Otol Rhinol Laryngol 1998;107(3):241–6.

[105] Svistun E, Alizadeh-Naderi R, El-Naggar A, et al. Vision enhancement system for detection of oral cavity neoplasia based on autofluorescence. Head Neck 2004;26:205–15.

[106] Lazerev VV, Roth RA, Kazakevich Y, et al. Detection of premalignant oral lesions in hamsters with an endoscopic fluorescence imaging system. Cancer 1999;85(7):1421–9.

[107] Paczona R, Temam S, Janot F, et al. Autofluorescence videoendoscopy for photodiagnosis of head and neck squamous cell carcinoma. Eur Arch Otorhinolaryngol 2003;260(10):544–8.

[108] Pathak I, Davis NL, Hsiang YN, et al. Detection of squamous neoplasia by fluorescence imaging comparing porfimer sodium fluorescence to tissue autofluorescence in the hamster cheek-pouch model. Am J Surg 1995;170(5):423–6.

[109] Tang J, Zeng F, Savage H, et al. Fluorescence spectroscopic imaging to detect changes in collagen and elastin following laser tissue welding. J Clin Laser Med Surg 2000;18:3–8.

[110] Zargi M, Fajdiga I, Smid L. Autofluorescence imaging in the diagnosis of laryngeal cancer. Eur Arch Otorhinolaryngol 2000;257(1):17–23.

[111] Wilder-Smith P, Osann K, Hanna N, et al. In vivo multiphoton fluorescence imaging: a novel approach to oral malignancy. Lasers Surg Med 2004;35(2):96–103.

[112] Denk W. Two-photon excitation in functional biological imaging. J Biomed Opt 1996;1(3):296–304.

[113] van der Breggen EWJ, Rem AI, Christian MM, et al. Spectroscopic detection of oral and skin tissue transformation in a model for squamous cell carcinoma: autofluorescence versus systemic aminolevulinic acid-induced fluorescence. IEEE J Sel Top Quantum Electron 1996;2(4):997–1007.

[114] Leunig A, Rick K, Stepp H, et al. Fluorescence imaging and spectroscopy of 5-aminolevulinic acid induced protoporphyrin IX for the detection of neoplastic lesions in the oral cavity. Am J Surg 1996;172(6):674–7.

[115] Betz CS, Lai JP, Xiang W, et al. In vitro photodynamic therapy of nasopharyngeal carcinoma using 5-aminolevulinic acid. Photochem Photobiol Sci 2002;1(5):315–9.

[116] Leunig A, Betz CS, Mehlmann M, et al. Detection of squamous cell carcinoma of the oral cavity by imaging 5-aminolevulinic acid-induced protoporphyrin IX fluorescence. Laryngoscope 2000;110(1):78–83.

[117] Leunig A, Mehlmann M, Betz C, et al. Fluorescence staining of oral cancer using a topical application of 5-aminolevulinic acid: fluorescence microscopic studies. J Photochem Photobiol B 2001;60(1):44–9.

[118] Mehlmann M, Betz CS, Stepp H, et al. Fluorescence staining of laryngeal neoplasms after topical application of 5-aminolevulinic acid: preliminary results. Lasers Surg Med 1999; 25(5):414–20.

[119] Charoenbanpachon S, Krasieva T, Ebihara A, et al. Acceleration of ALA-induced PpIX fluorescence development in the oral mucosa. Lasers Surg Med 2003;32:185–8.

[120] Ebihara A, Krasieva TB, Liaw LHL, et al. Detection and diagnosis of oral cancer by light-induced fluorescence. Lasers Surg Med 2003;32:17–24.

[121] Zheng W, Soo KC, Sivanandan R, et al. Detection of neoplasms in the oral cavity by digitized endoscopic imaging of 5-aminolevulinic acid-induced protoporphyrin IX fluorescence. Int J Oncol 2002;21(4):763–8.

[122] Zheng W, Soo KC, Sivanandan R, et al. Detection of squamous cell carcinomas and pre-cancerous lesions in the oral cavity by quantification of 5-aminolevulinic acid induced fluorescence endoscopic images. Lasers Surg Med 2002;31(3):151–7.

[123] Leonard JR, Beck W. Hematoporphyrin fluorescence: an aid in diagnosis of malignant neoplasms. Laryngoscope 1971;81:365–72.

[124] Profio AE. Laser excited fluorescence of hematoporphyrin derivative for diagnosis of cancer. IEEE J Quantum Elecron 1984;QE-20:1502–7.

[125] Burns RA, Klaunig JE, Shulo JR, et al. Tumour-localizing and photosensitizing properties of hematoporphyrin derivative in hamster buccal pouch carcinoma. Oral Surg 1986;61: 368–72.

[126] Wagnieres GA, Studzinski AP, Braichoote DR, et al. Clinical imaging fluorescence apparatus for the endoscopic photodetection of early cancers by the use of Photofrin II. Appl Opt 1997;36:5608–20.

[127] Wagnieres GM, Star WM, Wilson BC. In vivo fluorescence spectroscopy and imaging for oncological applications. Photochem Photobiol 1998;68:603–32.

[128] Dunn RJ, Devine KD. Tetracycline-induced fluorescence of laryngeal, pharyngeal and oral cancer. Layngoscope 1972;82:189–98.

[129] Witjes MJ, Speelman OC, Nikkels PG, et al. In vivo fluorescence kinetics and localisation of aluminum phthalocyanine disulphonate in an autologous tumour model. Br J Cancer 1996; 73(5):573–80.

[130] Witjes MJ, Mank AJ, Speelman OC, et al. Distribution of aluminum phthalocyanine disulfonate in an oral squamous cell carcinoma model. In vivo fluorescence imaging compared with ex vivo analytical methods. Photochem Photobiol 1997; 65(4):685–93.

[131] Gannot I. Current status of flexible waveguides for IR laser radiation transmission. IEEE J Sel Top Quantum Electron 1996;2(4):880–9.

[132] Moser F, Bunimovich D, DeRowe A, et al. Medical applications of infrared transmitting silver halide fibers. IEEE J Sel Top Quantum Electron 1996;2(4):872–9.

[133] Schultz CP, Mantsch HH. Biochemical imaging and 2D classification of keratin pearl structures in oral squamous cell carcinoma. Cell Mol Biol 1998;44(1):203–10.

[134] Schultz CP, Liu KZ, Kerr PD, et al. In situ infrared histopathology of keratinization in human oral/oropharyngeal squamous cell carcinoma. Oncol Res 1998;10(5):277–86.

[135] Mourant JR, Gibson RR, Johnson TM, et al. Methods for measuring the infrared spectra of biological cells. Phys Med Biol 2003;48(2):243–57.

[136] Fukuyama Y, Yoshida S, Yanagisawa S, et al. A study on the differences between oral squamous cell carcinomas and normal oral mucosas measured by Fourier transform infrared spectroscopy. Biospectroscopy 1999;5(2):117–26.

[137] Wu JG, Xu YZ, Sun CW, et al. Distinguishing malignant from normal oral tissues using FTIR fiber-optic techniques. Biopolymers 2001;62(4):185–92.

[138] Yoshida SY, Yoshida H. Noninvasive analyses of polyunsaturated fatty acids in human oral mucosa in vivo by Fourier-transform infrared spectroscopy. Biopolymers 2004;74: 403–12.

[139] Bindig U, Winter H, Wasche W, et al. Fiber-optical and microscopic detection of malignant tissue by use of infrared spectrometry. J Biomed Opt 2002;7(1):100–8.

[140] Sukuta S, Bruch R. Factor analysis of cancer Fourier transform infrared evanescent wave fiberoptical (FTIR-FEW) spectra. Lasers Surg Med 1999;24(5):382–8.

[141] Mahadevan-Jansen A, Richards-Kortum R. Raman spectroscopy for the detection of cancers and precancers. J Biomed Opt 1996;1(1):31–70.

[142] Hanlon EB, Manoharan R, Koo TW, et al. Prospects for in vivo Raman spectroscopy. Phys Med Biol 2000;45(2):R1–R59.

[143] Motz JT, Hunter M, Galindo LH, et al. Optical fiber probe for biomedical Raman spectroscopy. Appl Opt 2004;43(3):542–54.

[144] Yang Y, Liu CH, Savage HE, et al. Optical fluorescence and Raman biopsy of squamous cell carcinoma from the head and neck. Proc SPIE-Int Soc Opt Eng 1998;3250:68–71.

[145] Venkatakrishna K, Kurien J, Pai KM, et al. Optical pathology of oral tissue: a Raman spectroscopy diagnostic method. Curr Sci 2001;80(5):665–9.

[146] de Oliveira AP, Martin AA, Silveira L Jr, et al. Application of principal components analysis to diagnosis of hamster oral carcinogenesis: Raman study. Proc SPIE-Int Soc Opt Eng 2004;5321:111–6.

[147] Shim MG, Wilson BC. Development of an in vivo Raman spectroscopic system for diagnostic applications. Journal of Raman Spectroscopy 1997;28:131–42.

[148] Sokolov K, Sung KB, Collier T, et al. Endoscopic microscopy. Dis Markers 2002;18: 269–91.

[149] Sokolov K, Aaron J, Hsu B, et al. Optical systems for in vivo molecular imaging of cancer. Technol Cancer Res Treat 2003;2(6):491–504.

[150] White MW, Rajadhyaksha M, Gonzalez S, et al. Noninvasive imaging of human oral mucosa in vivo by confocal reflectance microscopy. Laryngoscope 1999;109(10):1709–17.

[151] White MW, Baldassano M, Rajadhyaksha M, et al. Confocal reflectance imaging of head and neck surgical specimens: a comparison with histologic analysis. Arch Otolaryngol Head Neck Surg 2004;130:923–8.

[152] Clark AL, Collier T, Lacy A, et al. Detection of dysplasia with near real time confocal microscopy. Biomed Sci Instrum 2002;38:393–8.

[153] Clark AL, Gillenwater AM, Collier TG, et al. Confocal microscopy for real-time detection of oral cavity neoplasia. Clin Cancer Res 2003;9(13):4714–21.

[154] Inoue H, Cho JY, Satodate H, et al. Development of virtual histology and virtual biopsy using laser-scanning confocal microscopy. Scand J Gastroenterol Suppl 2003;237:37–9.

[155] Sung KB, Liang C, Descour M, et al. Near real time in vivo fiber optic confocal microscopy: sub-cellular structure resolved. J Microsc 2002;207:137–45.

[156] Zheng W, Harris M, Kho KW, et al. Confocal endomicroscopic imaging of normal and neoplastic human tongue tissue using ALA-induced-PPIX fluorescence: a preliminary study. Oncol Rep 2004;12(2):397–401.

[157] Webb RH. Confocal optical microscopy. Reports on Progress in Physics 1996;59:427–71.

[158] Dunn AK, Smithpeter C, Welch AJ, et al. Sources of contrast in confocal reflectance imaging. Appl Opt 1996;35(19):3551–6.

[159] Fercher AF. Optical coherence tomography. J Biomed Opt 1996;1(2):157–73.

[160] Schmitt JM. Optical coherence tomography (OCT): a review. IEEE J Sel Top Quantum Electron 1999;5(4):1205–15.

[161] Yang Y, Whiteman S, Gey van Pittius D, et al. Use of optical coherence tomography in delineating airways microstructure: comparison of OCT images to histopathological sections. Phys Med Biol 2004;49:1247–55.

[162] McNichols RJ, Gowda A, Bell BA, et al. Development of an endoscopic fluorescence image guided OCT probe for oral cancer detection. Proc SPIE-Int Soc Opt Eng 2001; 4254:23–30.

[163] Tumlinson AR, Hariri LP, Utzinger U, et al. Miniature endoscope for simultaneous optical coherence tomography and laser-induced fluorescence measurement. Appl Opt 2004;43(1): 113–21.

[164] Hsu JJ, Lu CW, Yang CC, et al. High-resolution optical coherence tomography with fiber-induced broadband source and process algorithm for oral cancer study. Proc SPIE-Int Soc Opt Eng 2002;4619:95–7.

[165] Bibas AG, Podoleanu AG, Cucu RG, et al. OCT imaging of the larynx: a feasibility study. Proc SPIE-Int Soc Opt Eng 2003;4956:95–100.

[166] Fomina YV, Gladkova ND, Snopova LB, et al. In vivo OCT study of neoplastic alterations of the oral cavity mucosa. Proc SPIE-Int Soc Opt Eng 2004;5316.

[167] Batsakis JG. The molecular biology of oral cancer. In: Shah JP, Johnson NW, Batsakis JG, editors. Oral cancer. London: Martin Dunitz; 2003. p. 167–81.

[168] Lentsch EJ, Myers NJ. Pathogenesis and progression of squamous cell carcinoma of the head and neck. In: Myers EN, Suen JY, Myers JN, et al, editors. Cancer of the head and neck. 4th edition. Philadelphia: WB Saunders; 2004. p. 5–28.

[169] Nagpal JK, Das BR. Oral cancer: reviewing the present understanding of its molecular mechanism and exploring the future directions for its effective management. Oral Oncol 2003;39:213–21.

[170] Quon H, Liu FF, Cummings BJ. Potential molecular prognostic markers in head and neck squamous cell carcinomas. Head Neck 2001;23:147–59.

[171] Scully C, Field JK, Tanzawa H. Genetic aberrations in oral or head and neck squamous cell carcinoma (SCCHN): 1. Carcinogen metabolism, DNA repair and cell cycle control. Oral Oncol 2000;36:256–63.

[172] Scully C, Field JK, Tanzawa H. Genetic aberrations in oral or head and neck squamous cell carcinoma 2: chromosomal aberrations. Oral Oncol 2000;36:311–27.

[173] Scully C, Field JK, Tanzawa H. Genetic aberrations in oral or head and neck squamous cell carcinoma 3: clinico-pathological applications. Oral Oncol 2000;36:404–13.

[174] Ford AC, Gradnis JR. Targeting epidermal growth factor receptor in head and neck cancer. Head Neck 2003;25:67–73.

[175] Goldenberg D, Harden S, Masayesva BG, et al. Intraoperative molecular margin analysis in head and neck cancer. Arch Otolaryngol Head Neck Surg 2004;130:39–44.

[176] Takes RP. Staging of the neck in patients with head and neck squamous cell cancer: imaging techniques and biomarkers. Oral Oncol 2004;40:656–67.

[177] Cherry SR. In vivo molecular and genomic imaging: new challenges for imaging physics. Phys Med Biol 2004;49:R13–48.

[178] Haugland RP. Handbook of fluorescent probes and research products. 9th edition. Eugene (OR): Molecular Probes Inc.; 2002.

[179] Prasad P. Nanophotonics. New York: Wiley; 2004.

[180] Schena M. Microarray analysis. New York: Wiley-Liss; 2003.

[181] Duck FA. Physical properties of tissue: a comprehensive reference book. San Diego (CA): Academic; 1990.

[182] Ophir J, Céspedes I, Ponnekanti H, et al. Elastography: a quantitative method for imaging the elasticity of biological tissues. Ultrason Imaging 1991;13:111–34.

[183] Céspedes I, Ophir J, Ponnekanti H, et al. Elastography: elasticity imaging using ultrasound with application to muscle and breast in vivo. Ultrason Imaging 1993;15:73–88.

[184] Manduca A, Oliphant TE, Dresner MA, et al. Magnetic resonance elastography: non-invasive mapping of tissue elasticity. Med Image Anal 2001;5(4):237–54.

[185] Gennisson JL, Baldeweck T, Tanter M, et al. Assessment of elastic parameters of human skin using dynamic elastography. IEEE Trans Ultrason Ferroelectr Freq Control 2004; 51(8):980–9.

[186] Zheng YP, Leung SF, Mak AFT. Assessment of neck tissue fibrosis using an ultrasound palpation system: a feasibility study. Med Biol Eng Comp 2000;38(5):497–502.

[187] Brown BH, Tidy JA, Boston K, Blackett AD, Smallwood RH, Sharpe F. Relation between tissue structure and imposed electrical current flow in cervical neoplasia. Lancet 2000;355: 892–5.

[188] Walker DC, Brown BH, Hose DR, Smallwood RH. Modelling the electrical impedivity of normal and premalignant cervical tissue. Electronics Letters 2000;36:1603–4.

[189] Walker DC, Brown BH, Smallwood RH, Hose DR, Jones DM. Modelled current distribution in cervical squamous tissue. Physiol Meas 2002;23:159–68.

[190] Levchenko A. Dynamical and integrative cell signaling: challenges for the new biology. Biotechnol Bioeng 2003;84(7):773–82.

[191] Morel NM, Holland JM, van der Greef J, et al. Primer on medical genomics Part XIV: introduction to systems biology—a new approach to understanding disease and treatment. Mayo Clin Proc 2004;79:651–8.

[192] Weston AD, Hood L. Systems biology, proteomics, and the future of health care: toward predictive, preventative, and personalized medicine. J Proteome Res 2004;3:179–96.

[193] Michor F, Frank SA, May RM, et al. Somatic selection for and against cancer. J Theor Biol 2003;225:377–82.

[194] Ruiter DJ, van Krieken HJM, van Muijen GN. Tumour metastasis: is tissue an issue? Lancet Oncol 2001;2:109–12.

ELSEVIER
SAUNDERS

Otolaryngol Clin N Am
38 (2005) 241–254

OTOLARYNGOLOGIC
CLINICS
OF NORTH AMERICA

Selected Laser-based Therapies in Otolaryngology

Silvia Mioc, PhD, MBA[a,b,*], Mary-Ann Mycek, PhD[c,d]

[a]Colorado Photonics Industry Association, 105 South Sunset Street,
Suite G, Longmont, CO 80501, USA
[b]General Electric Healthcare Technologies, Louisville, CO, USA
[c]Applied Physics Program, Department of Biomedical Engineering, College of Engineering,
University of Michigan, 2200 Bonisteel Boulevard, Ann Arbor, MI 48109, USA
[d]Comprehensive Cancer Center, University of Michigan, Ann Arbor, MI, USA

Lasers have found a natural place in medicine for both therapeutic and diagnostic applications. Their use depends on the unique characteristics of the laser light and the on the interaction of the laser with tissue. In general, light incident on tissue can be absorbed, reflected, multiply scattered, or transmitted. Optical diagnostic modalities frequently use reflected and scattered light, whereas the energy from light needs to be absorbed to induce a clinical effect and achieve therapy. Reinisch [1] has written a comprehensive review of the fundamentals of laser properties and their interaction with biologic tissues.

This article provides an overview of selected laser-based therapies used in otolaryngology. The selection complements a recent review [2].

Because otolaryngologists are increasingly treating vascular lesions of the face, the first section of this article addresses the treatment of vascular lesions of the face with focus on the lesion most commonly treated using lasers, the port-wine stain (PWS). The discussion includes an introduction of laser–tissue interactions and recent clinical and modeling advances in the field.

The second section discusses the use of photodynamic therapy (PDT) in otolaryngology. The discussion of PDT includes an introduction to the basic theory of photodynamic action, including special considerations for in vivo tissue therapeutics; an illustration of the approach using representative clinical applications of PDT in otolaryngology, including recent advances in

---

* Corresponding author. Colorado Photonics Industry Association, 105 South Sunset Street, Suite G, Longmont, CO 80501, USA.
  E-mail address: Silvia.Mioc@comcast.net (S. Mioc).

the field; and a discussion of the cost-effectiveness of PDT relative to traditional therapies.

Recent advances in treatment of vascular lesions of the face with focus on port-wine stains

PWSs are benign vascular birthmarks consisting of superficial and deep dilated capillaries in the skin resulting in a reddish to purplish discoloration. They are present in 0.3% to 0.5% of newborns, initially are light in color, darken with age as capillaries continue to dilate, and can later progress to a raised and nodular surface. PWSs can cause significant psychologic trauma and often lead to a reduction in the quality of life. Treatment for PWS has included skin grafting, ionizing radiation, cryosurgery, tattooing, dermabrasion, and laser treatments [3]. Currently, lasers provide the treatment of choice for most PWS patients.

Interaction of laser light with skin tissue

The interaction of light with tissue is affected by two processes: absorption and scattering. Absorption is dominant in the epidermis, and scattering by collagen fibers is dominant in the dermis.

Anything that has color will preferentially absorb some region of visible light, and many objects that appear transparent absorb infrared light. For skin tissue, the main chromophores are proteins and DNA for short-wavelength UV light, melanin and hemoglobin for visible light, and water, the main component of tissue, for long-wavelength infrared light. The depth of light penetration is usually defined as the length over which the incident energy drops by $1/e$, or about 64%. Over the visible region of the spectrum, light penetration is inversely related to wavelength. On average, visible light penetrates tissue to a depth of 1 mm; light with a wavelength around 1 micron (Nd:YAG laser, 1.06 μm) penetrates most deeply, to a depth of about 4 mm; as the wavelength increases, the depth of penetration drops to 30 μm for the CO_2 laser (10.6 μm). (These numbers represent an average depth of penetration for several tissues, not for any particular tissue [1]).

When chromophores absorb light, their molecules become excited, and the absorbed energy can be dissipated as heat, a photothermal effect. A 5° to 10°C increase in temperature leads to cell injury, temperatures close to 100°C cause denaturation of DNA and proteins, temperatures above 100°C can ablate tissue through the vaporization of intracellular water, and further heating leads to desiccation and charring [4]. The heat deposited in the target chromophore will dissipate to adjacent areas, a process called "thermal relaxation." The rate of cooling depends on the thermal relaxation time, t, defined as the time required to cool the target to one half of its peak temperature immediately after laser irradiation. The extent of thermal damage depends on the temperature reached in the target tissue (which relates to the laser wavelength and fluence/energy density) and on the length of time that the tissue remains at that temperature (which relates to the duration of the laser pulse and t). The photothermal effect in its ablative manifestation is the main mechanism for the laser scalpel. In its nonablative manifestation, the photothermal effect is the mechanism used to treat vascular lesions, including PWSs, as discussed in more detail later in this article.

Localized heating caused by absorption can cause acoustic waves that mechanically destroy the absorbing tissue, a photomechanical effect. This effect may be the mechanism that leads to vascular rupture and purpura in PWS treatment with very short pulses (1 microsecond) and to pigment destruction in tattoo removal [4].

Last, absorbed laser energy can induce photochemical changes in tissues. This effect is the basis for photodynamic therapy (PDT), as discussed in the last part of this article.

Therapeutic mechanisms of lasers for port-wine stains

The goal in treating a PWS with a laser is to destroy the underlying blood vessels selectively (thus lightening the birth mark) without affecting the surrounding tissue and causing scarring. For this selective photothermolysis one must find a laser not absorbed by the skin and preferentially absorbed in the blood vessels at a rate faster than their cooling rate [5].

The main absorbers in the blood vessels are oxyhemoglobin and reduced hemoglobin. Oxyhemoglobin absorbs in the visible-light range, with peaks in the blue and yellow region (577 nm) of the spectrum. Reduced hemoglobin absorbs in the infrared range of the spectrum. Because venous saturation is approximately 70%, oxyhemoglobin is dominant, and visible lasers have generally been used for treatment. The yellow region happens to be a window of low absorption for melanin. Thus, in principle, for light-colored skin, a yellow laser will be absorbed preferentially by red blood cells, with minimal absorption in the skin. This preferential absorption is advantageous for two reasons. First, minimal direct thermal damage is caused to the epidermis, because only a small part of the energy is deposited there. Second, more light can reach the blood vessels to cause thrombosis and thus lightening of the PWS. To limit the thermal damage to the skin, the exposure of the skin to the laser should be shorter than t; therefore, pulsed lasers with pulse durations not longer than t are the treatment of choice. For dark skin, however, the melanin absorption is so high that thrombosis of the vessels is hard to obtain without damage to the skin. In this case, using infrared lasers, such as the Nd:YAG laser (1.06 µm), with light absorbed primarily by the reduced hemoglobin, is preferred.

The size of the vessels determines the amount of energy to be deposited for thrombosis to take place, and thus the combination of the energy density (fluence) and length of the pulse is important. Of course, every PWS has a distribution of vessel sizes, so an optimal compromise must be found: the fluence of the laser must be high enough to destroy the vessels within the exposure time. Thus, the wavelength, pulse duration, and fluence of a laser determine the critical balance between destruction of the target tissue and thermal damage of the surrounding area [6].

To minimize heating of the epidermis, various epidermal cooling techniques have been developed. The challenge is to cool the epidermis selectively while leaving the temperature of the underlying blood vessels unchanged. This epidermal cooling allows higher fluences to be delivered to the PWS and allows thus more photocoagulation of the vessels without thermal damage to the skin. The method that showed most improvement in blanching of PWSs, reduced incidence of adverse effects such as epidermal damage or pigmentary change, and increased patient comfort [7,8] is cryogen spray cooling (CSC) [9], in which spurts of cryogenic fluid are delivered to the skin for tens of milliseconds. In a recent study in Chinese patients, for whom the higher melanin content in the skin poses increased complications, CSC was shown to result in better therapeutic outcome than achieved with laser alone [10]. Cold-air cooling was also shown to be effective [11].

Therapy for port-wine stains

Various types of lasers have been used to treat PWS over the years: Argon (488 nm, 514 nm), Argon-pumped tunable dye laser (APTDL, 577 nm–585 nm), KTP (532 nm), Copper vapor/bromide (578 nm), Krypton (568 nm), and flashlamp-pumped pulsed dye laser (PDL, 585 nm). They ranged from continuous wave (CW) lasers (eg, the older Argon laser), to quasi-CW lasers (APTDL, KTP, Copper vapor/bromide, Krypton lasers), to pulsed PDLs [1,6,8,12].

The CW and quasi-CW lasers also have higher incidences of hypertrophic scarring, textural changes, and hyper- or hypo-pigmentation than occur with the PDL [6,8]. Complications of PDL treatment include purpura (bruising) caused by extravasation of red blood cells, postoperative swelling, and postinflammatory hyperpigmentation. These side effects usually resolve within a couple of weeks following treatment.

All laser treatments are performed under some type of anesthesia. Topical anesthesia is usually satisfactory for facial lesions, but sometimes local or regional anesthesia is required. Depending on the lesion size and site, children under 12 years of age may require general anesthesia. Postoperative pain, crusting, swelling, and erythema are alleviated by administering emollients and analgesics [12]. One laser treatment is not usually sufficient to destroy all the vessels that might respond to therapy, so several sessions are always used for best achievable blanching. These treatments are given some weeks apart, so that the epidermis has time to heal. Sixty percent to 80% improvement in the appearance of a PWS can be achieved after 4 to 12 treatments [12], but partial recurrence may occur because of the revitalization of incompletely damaged vessels. Few patients exhibit complete cure, because the threshold for epidermal damage is lower than for permanent blanching of PWS [7]. The site and size of the PWS have been shown to be good predictors of outcome, with small lesions and lesions on the central forehead responding most favorably. The color of the PWS and the age of patient showed conflicting results as predictors [3].

Today, the treatment of choice for PWSs is the PDL at wavelengths from 585 nm to 600 nm, pulsewidths of 0.4 to 1.5 milliseconds, at repetition rates up to 1 Hz, and fluences of 3 to 10 J/cm^2, with 3- to 10-mm exposure spots delivered through a fiber-optic handpiece with minimal overlap [1,3,8]. Newer laser systems incorporate cryogen cooling in the handpiece, making CSC easy to incorporate in therapy.

The 585-nm/0.45-ms PDL (short-pulse PDL) was developed as a direct result of the photothermolysis theory, based on a calculated t of less than 1 millisecond for vessel diameters of 10 to 50 μm [12]. Short-pulse PDL has become the standard mode for PWS treatment but is more effective in pediatric cases, where the vessels are relatively small, than in adult cases, where the vessels grow larger with age. The 560-nm/1.5-ms PDL (long-pulse PDL) was developed to treat deeper and thicker vessels. There are conflicting reports on the effectiveness of the 595-nm/1.5-ms system versus the 585-nm/0.45-ms system, most likely arising from the different morphology of the particular PWS treated. For deep vessels larger than 1 mm, near-infrared lasers may be effective as secondary therapy [3,8]. One of the most recent advances in PDL offers a tunable wavelength of 585 to 600 nm at 1.5 milliseconds or a tunable pulse length of 0.5 to 40 milliseconds at a fixed wavelength of 585 nm or 595 nm and higher fluences up to 28 J/cm^2.

The KTP laser, at the shorter wavelength of 532 nm and with pulse durations of 2 to 50 milliseconds, is still used for PWS treatment. Its main advantage is that it causes less purpura than PDL. It has less penetration in tissue, so it is not as effective in treating deeper vessels, and it is absorbed more by melanin and thus is of limited use for patients with darker skin types.

Recent findings on the effect of pulsed dye laser parameters on treatment of port-wine stains

One recent randomized, prospective study used the latest tunable PDL to compare PWS treatment with two wavelengths (585 nm and 595 nm) and two pulse durations (0.5 milliseconds and 20 milliseconds) in 15 patients with untreated PWS [13]. Three different laser settings were investigated at a spot size of 7 mm: 585nm/0.5ms/5.5J/cm^2, 595nm/0.5ms/5.5J/cm^2, and 595nm/20ms/13J/cm^2. Treatments were performed with cold-air cooling. The results showed that the traditional 585-nm/0.5-ms system yields a significantly greater clearance of PWSs but also the highest rate of adverse effects. Purple PWSs responded best to this treatment.

Another study evaluated by histologic observations the thermal damage to ex vivo epidermis samples after irradiation with a 595-nm PDL at various fluences and pulse durations, with and without CSC [14]. The samples were taken from 28 consenting women and had various degrees of pigmentation (Fitzpatrick types I–VI). The laser parameters investigated were incident fluences of 4, 6, 10, 15, and 20 J/cm^2 and pulse durations of 1.5, 10, and 40 milliseconds. CSC at 100 milliseconds was used. Results showed that under the same incident dosage, longer pulse durations led to decreased thermal injury to the epidermis. CSC allowed use of high incident dosages (15–20 J/cm^2) in skin types I through IV without damage to the epidermis. In skin type VI, however, thermal damage could not be prevented even with dosages as low as 4 J/cm^2 with CSC. The article lists the threshold values for irradiation parameters that resulted in thermal injury of each skin type with and without CSC.

Monte Carlo simulations of light–tissue interactions and analytical solutions to the diffusion approximation theory have been used to model PDL treatment of PWS by calculating the temperature distribution and the resulting coagulation pattern within specific blood vessels [15]. Wavelengths in the range of 577 nm to 587 nm were suggested as optimal, consistent with the success of PDL in treating PWS. Calculations also predicted that co-agulation across vessels was more uniform with 595 nm than with 585 nm and that at a depth of 1.2 mm vessels ranging from 50 to 100 μm in diameter would be coagulated from top to bottom, small vessels around 10 μm would not be coagulated, and vessels larger than 150 μm would be partially coagulated. Thus, this modeling showed that the optimal wavelength depends on the size of the vessel. Consequently, one expects different responses to same treatment from different patients: temperature profiles could be similar, but coagulation depends on the size of the vessels in each person. This variation could explain the widely varying reports in the literature regarding the effectiveness of 585-nm versus 595-nm treatment, which range from a strong preference for one or the other wavelength to seeing no difference between them.

Intense pulsed light source for treatment of port-wine stains

An alternative to lasers for treatment of PWS has been the intense pulsed light source (IPLS). The IPLS is not a laser, but it works on similar principles. The IPLS is a broadband flashlamp emitting light between 515 and 1200 nm that is used in conjunction with a series of wavelength-selecting filters. Software enables the operator to choose the treatment parameters, including wavelength and intensity delivered. The IPLS is versatile and can be tailored to various applications, but this versatility makes the establishing of ideal parameters for consistent and reproducible results difficult. Operator skill plays a great role in all laser treatments and an even greater role in IPLS treatment.

One recent study of 22 patients found that the IPLS can be useful in PWS treatment for Asian patients [16]. Fifteen of the patients had the PWS located over the head and neck region. Treatment consisted of three to eight sessions with 550-nm, 570-nm, and 590-nm cutoff filters in double-pulse or triple-pulse mode in conjunction with chilled gel to protect the epidermis. A longer cutoff filter was used for patients who tanned easily. More than 90% of patients showed better than 25% clearing; 40% of patients showed more than 50% blanching; and 9% achieved more than 75% clearing. No patient exhibited complete blanching. These results were better than the authors' experience with PDL without cooling and showed that IPLS can be effective therapy for PWS in Asian patients. The authors of that report had several years of experience with IPLS before starting this study.

Recent advances in understanding the causes for port-wine stains

The causes of PWS are not well understood, but in the late 1980s it was proposed that one cause could be the reduction of neural innervation around the vessels [17]. A recent article used a confocal microscope to determine nerve and blood vessel density and mean vessel size in PWSs [18]. A confocal microscope uses the coherent property of lasers (all photons being in phase in both time and space domain) to obtain high-resolution images with resolutions on the order of μm. Skin biopsies were taken from untreated PWS, PWS with good response to laser treatment, PWS with poor response to laser treatment, and uninvolved skin of three adult males. Additionally, biopsies of normal skin were obtained from three healthy volunteers of similar age as the patients. Results showed that nerve density was decreased in all evaluated PWS sites and thus could be a factor in lesion pathogenesis. PWS blood vessel size correlated well with response to PDL and might prove to be a useful prognostic indicator of therapeutic outcome.

Future of port-wine stain treatment: noninvasive in vivo imaging or a combination of photodynamic and photothermal treatment?

The average success rate for complete blanching of PWS is less than 25% [19]. A major limitation of current laser therapy is that there are no objective criteria to guide treatment plans. The color of the PWS and physician experience are two common subjective criteria. Knowledge of detailed skin parameters around the PWS and of the PWS itself could help optimize treatment. One recent article describes the development of a one-dimensional computational model for PWS depth profiling using pulsed photothermal radiometry (PPTR) [19]. PPTR measures the time-resolved changes in the blackbody emission of an object after irradiation with a laser pulse. PPTR has been applied by several groups for depth profiling of PWSs, but it also has some limitations [19]. As discussed earlier, light absorption dissipates as heat; thus, it increases the temperature and changes the blackbody emission spectrum. Light absorbed at the surface changes the emission immediately, whereas light absorbed deeper in the skin affects emission only after it diffuses toward the skin's surface. The model used a digitized histologic section of a PWS biopsy as the input skin geometry. Parameters extracted from the model were average epidermal thickness, maximum epidermal temperature rise, depth of PWS upper boundary, and depth of maximum PWS temperature increase. Comparison of actual and reconstructed profiles showed a good match for the four parameters. These results indicate that PPTR is promising for PWS depth profiling.

A drastically different approach to improving outcome is to use PDT in conjunction with standard PDL treatment [20]. (A general discussion of the principles of PDT is given later.) PDT shows potential because of unwanted side effects—red blood cell extravasation and local hemorrhage—that occur during treatment of tumors by this method. One of the main disadvantages of PDT is persistent skin photosensitivity, and second-generation drugs that overcome this photosensitivity by rapid metabolic clearance are under development. One such substance, Benzoporphyrin-derivative monoacid (BPD) is particularly useful for treatment of PWSs because of its strong absorbance at 576 nm and 690 nm. Sequential yellow and red light treatments can achieve progressively deeper PDT action and be useful for treatment of thick PWSs. PDT uses continuous low irradiance over exposures on the order of minutes, and thus the dose effect is cumulative as exposure time is increased. PDT destroys all vessels containing the drug, independent of their size, unlike PDL-induced coagulation, which spares vessels smaller than 20 um. Following subtherapeutic PDT exposure with yellow light, the red blood cells are more susceptible to photothermal damage because of transient changes that include thrombus formation at the vessel wall. PDL irradiation then preferentially heats the pretreated vessels already compromised by PDT. Thus, the combined use of PDT and PDL shows promise in the treatment of PWS. An in vivo study using the chick chorioallantoic membrane model resulted in significantly more severe vascular damage following PDT plus PDL than with either treatment alone [21]. Prospective, comparative, and controlled clinical studies against accepted treatment regimes are required to confirm these results.

Photodynamic therapy

Theory of photodynamic action and considerations for clinical tissue therapeutics

PDT is often described as a form of light-activated chemotherapy. In PDT, cell death and tissue necrosis result from the action of cytotoxic agents (eg, highly reactive singlet oxygen) that are created through the light-induced chemical reactions of an administered photosensitizer [22]. For example, in 2003 the United States Food and Drug Administration (FDA) approved the use of PDT with the injectable photosensitizer porfimer sodium (Photofrin, Wyeth-Ayerst Lederle, Inc., Pearl River, NY; dihematoporphyrin ether (DHE)) for the selective ablation of precancerous lesions in patients with Barrett's esophagus who do not undergo esophagectomy. Studies supporting the approval had demonstrated that patients receiving PDT had a 20% chance of developing cancer at 2 years after PDT, whereas the control group (those who did not undergo PDT) had a 50% chance of developing cancer within that time frame.

Several generations of photosensitizers under investigation, including first-generation mixtures such as porfimer sodium and second- and third-generation purified compounds such as 5-aminolevulinic acid (5-ALA) and meta-tetrahydroxyphenylchlorin (m-THPC). Advances in the development of chemically well-defined photosensitizers have enabled localized targeting of subcellular organelles, including mitochondria, for photodestruction [22]. Photosensitizers may be administered to a patient orally, intravenously, or topically. Given sufficient time for adequate biodistribution, photosensitizers tend to accumulate preferentially in target tissues, such as tumors and dysplastic lesions, relative to normal tissues, thereby enabling selective tissue destruction with light.

In addition to photosensitizer biodistribution, other considerations for successful therapeutic intervention using photodynamic action in tissues include light characteristics (wavelength, energy density, and power density) and the mode of light delivery to tissue. These factors can determine the depth to which light penetrates tissues and the overall efficiency of PDT; the ability to conduct quantitative dosimetry monitoring in vivo, which can enable patient-specific therapeutics; and the rate of photosensitizer clearance, which can help to minimize the risk of posttreatment side effects [23].

Selected applications of photodynamic therapy in otolaryngology

Several case reports and clinical studies regarding the effectiveness of PDT in otolaryngology employing a variety of photosensitizing agents have appeared in the literature. For example, a case report describing the treatment of infiltrating squamous cell carcinoma in the soft palate used PDT as an alternative to radiotherapy or surgery [24]. In this case, the photosensitizer m-THPC was administered intravenously at 0.15 mg/kg of body weight 96 hours before treatment. The laser used for PDT (a rhodamine dye laser pumped by a Copper-vapor laser) delivered a light dose of energy (density, 20 J/cm^2; power density, 100 mW/cm^2) at a wavelength of 652 nm and over a spot 3 cm in diameter. These treatment conditions were thought to be capable of achieving 1-cm tumor necrosis, a depth that was more than sufficient for treating the 2- to 3-mm tumor depth that was revealed on CT. After treatment and recovery, the patient experienced no loss of palatal function and had no recurrence of disease at 16 months after PDT. In this case, the only disadvantage of PDT, as opposed to conventional radiotherapy or surgery, was the need, typical of PDT interventions, to avoid direct sunlight for a period of time (in this case, 30 days) following administration of the photosensitizing agent to avoid a potentially serious photosensitive reaction.

Another study evaluated the efficacy of PDT for treatment of recurrent nasopharyngeal carcinoma (NPC) in a clinical trial of 12 patients [25], as an alternative to radiotherapy, surgery, or chemotherapy. The patients studied had recurrent NPC after completing a full course of radiotherapy and had no alternate curative therapy available. PDT treatment consisted of an intravenous injection of hematoporphyrin derivative (HPD) at 5 mg/kg of body weight followed by laser irradiation 48 to 72 hours later. The light source was a Gold vapor laser at a wavelength of 630 nm (power, 0.5–1.0 W) that delivered a total energy density of 150 to 200 J/cm^2 during treatment. Light delivery was achieved using an optical fiber with a rounded bulb-diffuser tip. Because the penetration of light into tissue was estimated to be approximately 1 cm, tumors with thicknesses greater than 1 cm were debulked 2 weeks before PDT. The authors noted four distinct phases of recovery after PDT: (1) an acute, local inflammatory reaction lasting 3 to 4 days; (2) an exudative phase lasting 2 weeks; (3) a crusting phase lasting 3 to 6 months; (4) re-epithelialization to normal-appearing mucosa. At 6 months after PDT all 12 patients showed tumor regression, as confirmed by CT or MRI, and 3 were disease-free at 9 to 12 months follow-up. The authors concluded that even a single treatment of PDT can result in useful palliation or cure for patients with recurrent NPC, with minimal complications (skin hypersensitivity; experienced by two patients).

Although side effects associated with PDT treatment are rare and are largely preventable by avoiding patient exposure to sunlight or bright room light, adverse reactions can occur, and the procedure is not without risk. For example, a case report describes a patient who received PDT for recurrent larynx papillomatosis using the photosensitizer Photosan 3 (DHE) that was administered intravenously at 2.5 mg/kg of body weight 24 hours before laser irradiation with light from an Argon-dye laser at wavelength 630 nm, administered with a cylindrical light applicator [26]. No complications arose during the procedure, but 3 hours after PDT the patient was inadvertently exposed to neon light and developed serious anaphylaxis, which was treated immediately and successfully in the ICU where the patient had been recovering. This case illustrates the potential seriousness of side effects associated with PDT and the importance of adequate post-PDT patient monitoring and care.

Indeed, large patient-to-patient variations in response to PDT were observed in a controlled study of tissue damage to both healthy mucosa and early squamous cell carcinoma (<2 mm infiltration depth) in the esophagus, bronchi, and mouth using the photosensitizer m-THPC [27]. The study examined 25 patients and found that the optimal conditions for PDT (ie, maximal tumor necrosis with minimal damage to normal tissue) in the bronchi and mouth included an intravenously injected dose of 0.15 mg/kg of body weight of m-THPC followed 4 days later by laser irradiation at wavelength 652 nm with an Argon-ion PDL with an energy density of 7 to 16 J/cm^2 (power density, 100–150 mW/cm^2). In the esophagus, light from an Argon-ion laser at wavelength 514 nm and at an energy density of 75 to 100 J/cm^2 (power density, 70–100 mW/cm^2) was found to be optimal. The second-generation photosensitizer m-THPC, a pure compound, was determined to have several advantages over first-generation porphyrin mixtures such as HPD and porfimer sodium (Photofrin II). These advantages included enhanced phototoxicity (100 times more phototoxic at 652 nm; 10 times more phototoxic at 514 nm) and a shorter duration of skin photosensitivity (one third the time). Of the 33 lesions treated, 28 exhibited no recurrence at 14 months after PDT, giving a recurrence rate similar to that of Photofrin II, approximately 15%. In determining the optimal conditions for PDT, the study found large interindividual variations in response (ranging from no reaction to tissue necrosis) for identical treatment conditions. This variation highlights the need for individualized patient dosimetry and monitoring in PDT. This study and others [23] have suggested the use of photosensitizer spectrofluorometry as a means of quantitatively and noninvasively monitoring photosensitizer concentration in living tissues to guide dosimetry and improve patient response to PDT interventions.

There is much interest in using PDT as an alternative to surgery or radiotherapy for the destruction of high-grade dysplasia and early carcinoma in the esophagus. Recent FDA approval for the first-generation photosensitizer, porfimer sodium, for PDT of precancerous lesions in the esophagus was described earlier. A prospective study of porfimer sodium PDT in 102 patients with advanced and early-stage esophageal cancer found that PDT offered significant improvement of symptoms in patients with advanced disease and was curative in some cases of early disease [28]. In the study, patients received an intravenous injection of porfimer sodium (Photofrin) at 2 mg/kg of body weight followed 24 to 72 hours later by laser irradiation at wavelength 630 nm. Complications following treatment included photosensitive reactions in the skin (in 5% of patients) and esophageal stricture (in 8% of patients). Patient response to PDT was compared with more than 1100 patients who were treated with other methods. For patients with advanced disease, PDT treatment was determined to be as beneficial as other palliative therapies, including esophageal resection, stents, and radiotherapy. For patients with early-stage disease, mean survival after PDT was long term (60.5 months). The study concluded that PDT can offer early-stage patients who are not candidates for esophageal resection the potential for cure.

Another study in the esophagus examined the second-generation photosensitizer 5-ALA for PDT in 27 patients with high-grade dysplasia and early carcinoma [29]. In the study, 5-ALA was administered orally at

60 mg/kg of body weight, and PDT was conducted 4 to 6 hours later using a dye laser operating at wavelength 635 nm. The laser was coupled to an optical fiber with a cylindrical light diffuser 2.0 cm in length and a light dose of energy (density, 150 J/cm^2; power density, 100 mW/cm^2) was employed for PDT. To avoid complications from skin photosensitivity, patients were protected from sunlight and bright room lights for 36 hours after photosensitizer administration. The pilot study found that high-grade dysplasia and superficial carcinoma (≤ 2 mm) could be completely eradicated by 5-ALA PDT without the serious complications (eg, esophageal strictures) observed in porfimer sodium PDT. This result was attributed to the highly specific accumulation of 5-ALA in dysplastic and malignant mucosa, in contrast to the less selective accumulation of porfimer sodium in esophageal tissues. It was suggested that under the experimental protocol employed in the study, 5-ALA PDT in the esophagus might be limited in effectiveness to mucosal penetration depths of 2 mm or less; patients with tumor thickness greater than 2 mm might be treated more successfully by using a different photosensitizer (ie, m-THPC).

Future directions for photodynamic therapy in otolaryngology

Several promising applications of PDT in otolaryngology have been described. First-generation photosensitizers have been approved by the FDA for use in selected PDT applications. With continued clinical research into the optimal conditions and protocols for using chemically defined second- and third-generation photosensitizers, and with the ability to employ photosensitizer spectrofluorometric methods in vivo to monitor dosimetry quantitatively and noninvasively, the efficiency, selectivity, and specificity of PDT interventions should continue to improve.

For PDT to develop from an experimental therapy to widespread clinical use, its cost effectiveness must also be considered. One prohibitive expense might be the relatively high costs of purchasing and maintaining the advanced laser systems employed to date in research studies. It is probable, however, that these technology costs will decline once laser specifications are well defined and mass production of solid-state laser systems becomes feasible.

In the United States, the costs of 5-ALA PDT and associated endoscopies for esophageal disease have been estimated to be approximately $6500 [29], much lower than costs associated with esophageal surgery. For patients with advanced head and neck cancer, a recent study in the United Kingdom compared the cost effectiveness of PDT with the photosensitizer Foscan (Biolitec Pharma, Ltd., Edinburgh, UK) (m-THPC) with palliative chemotherapy, extensive palliative surgery, and no treatment [30]. For each intervention the primary outcome for the study was defined as the incremental cost/life-year saved, relative to no treatment. In comparison with palliative chemotherapy and extensive palliative surgery, Foscan PDT was determined to be the most cost-effective intervention for patients with advanced head and neck cancer. The results of these types of analyses, coupled with promising clinical studies such as those described earlier, suggest that PDT might become a viable and cost-effective clinical intervention in otolaryngology.

Summary

This article has discussed selected applications of laser therapies in otolaryngology. Lasers are the treatment of choice for PWS lesions, but new advances are needed to achieve complete blanching in the majority of cases. Noninvasive in vivo imaging and laser therapy coupled with PDT are two areas showing promise to improve outcome. PDT has the potential to offer new, cost-effective treatment options, and possibly cure, to cancer patients who are not candidates for traditional surgery, chemotherapy, and radiotherapy.

References

[1] Reinisch L. Laser physics and tissue interactions. Otolaryngol Clin North Am 1996;29(6): 893–912.
[2] Reinisch L. Lasers in otolaryngology. In: Vo-Dinh T, editor. Biomedical photonics handbook. New York (NY): CRC Press; 2003. p. 44-1–44-10.
[3] Suthamjariya K, Anderson RR. Lasers in dermatology. In: Vo-Dinh T, editor. Biomedical photonics handbook. CRC Press; 2003. p. 40-1–40-28.
[4] Stratigos AJ, Dover JS. Overview of lasers and their properties. Dermatol Ther 2000;13: 2–16.
[5] Anderson RR, Parish JA. Selective photothermolysis: precise microsurgery by selective absorption of pulsed radiation. Science 1983;220:524–7.
[6] Alster TS, Lupton JR. Lasers in dermatology—an overview of types and indications. Am J Clin Dermatol 2000;2(5):291–303.
[7] Kelly KM, Nanda VS, Nelson JS. Treatment of port-wine stain birth marks using the 1.5 msec pulsed dye laser at high fluences in conjunction with cryogen spray cooling. Dermatol Surg 2002;28(4):309–13.
[8] Tanzi EL, Lupton JR, Alster TS. Lasers in dermatology: four decades of progress. J Am Acad Dermatol 2003;49:1–31.
[9] Nelson JS, Milner TE, Anvari B, et al. Dynamic cooling of the epidermis during laser port wine stain therapy. Lasers Surg Med 1994;6S:48.
[10] Chiu CH, Chan HHL, Ho WS, et al. Prospective study of pulsed dye laser in conjunction with cryogen spray cooling for treatment of port wine stains in Chinese patients. Dermatol Surg 2003;29:909–15.
[11] Greve B, Hammes S, Raulin C. The effect of cold air cooling on 585 nm pulsed dye laser treatment of port wine stain. Dermatol Surg 2001;27:633–6.
[12] Acland KM, Barlow RJ. Lasers for the dermatologist. Br J Dermatol 2000;143:244–55.
[13] Greve B, Raulin C. Prospective study of port wine stain treatment with dye laser: comparison of two wavelengths (585 nm vs. 595 nm) and two pulse durations (0.5 milliseconds vs. 20 milliseconds). Lasers Surg Med 2004;34:168–73.
[14] Dai T, Pikkul BM, Tunnell JW, et al. Thermal response of human skin epidermis in different skin types to 595-nm irradiation and cryogen spray cooling: an ex-vivo study. In: Bass LS, Kollias N, Malek RS, et al, editors. Lasers in surgery: advanced characterization, therapeutics, and systems XIII. Proceedings of the International Society of Optical Engineering 2003;4949:1–10.

[15] Shafirstein G, Baumler W, Lapidoth M, et al. A new mathematical approach to the diffusion approximation theory for selective photothermolysis modeling and its implication in laser treatment of port-wine stains. Lasers Surg Med 2004;34:335–47.

[16] Ho WS, Ying SY, Chan PC, et al. Treatment of port wine stains with intense pulsed light: a prospective study. Dermatol Surg 2004;30:887–91.

[17] Smoller BR, Rosen S. Port-wine stains: a disease of altered neural modulation of blood vessels? Arch Dermatol 1986;122:177–9.

[18] Selim MM, Kelly KM, Nelson JS, et al. Confocal microscopy study of nerves and blood vessels in untreated and treated port wine stains: preliminary observations. Dermatol Surg 2004;30:892–7.

[19] Choi B, Majaron B, Nelson JS. Computational model to evaluate port wine stain depth profiling using pulsed photothermal radiometry. J Biom Opt 2004;9(2):299–307.

[20] Kimel S, Svaasand LO, Kelly KM, et al. Synergistic photodynamic and photothermal treatment of port wine stain? Laser Surg Med 2004;34:80–2.

[21] Kelly KM, Kimel S, Smith T, et al. Combined photodynamic and photothermal induced injury enhances damage to in vivo model blood vessels. Laser Surg Med 2004;34:407–13.

[22] Henderson BW, Gollnick SO. Mechanistic principles of photodynamic therapy. In: Vo-Dinh T, editor. Biomedical photonics handbook. CRC Press; 2003. p. 36-1–36-27.

[23] Wilson BC, Weersink RA, Lilge L. Fluorescence in photodynamic therapy dosimetry. In: Mycek M-A, Pogue BW, editors. Handbook of biomedical fluorescence. New York: Marcel Dekker; 2003. p. 529–61.

[24] Poate TWJ, Dilkes MG, Kenyon GS. Use of photodynamic therapy for the treatment of squamous cell carcinoma of the soft palate. Br J Oral Maxillofac Surg 1996;34(1):66–8.

[25] Tong MCF, van Hasselt CA, Woo JKS. Preliminary results of photodynamic therapy for recurrent nasopharyngeal carcinoma. Eur Arch Otorhinolaryngol 1996;253:189–92.

[26] Öfner JG, Schlögl H, Kostron H. Unusual adverse reaction in a patient sensitized with Photosan 3. J Photochem Photobiol B Biol 1996;36:183–4.

[27] Savary J-F, Monnier P, Fontolliet C, et al. Photodynamic therapy for early squamous cell carcinomas of the esophagus, bronchi, and mouth with m-tetra(hydroxyphenyl) chlorine. Arch Otolaryngol Head Neck Surg 1997;123:162–8.

[28] Moghissi K, Dixon K. Photodynamic therapy (PDT) in esophageal cancer: a surgical view of its indication based on 14 years experience. Technol Cancer Res Treat 2003;2(4):319–26.

[29] Gossner L, May A, Sroka R, et al. Photodynamic destruction of high grade dysplasia and early carcinoma of the esophagus after the oral administration of 5-aminolevulinic acid. Cancer 1999;86(10):1921–8.

[30] Hopper C, Niziol C, Sidhu M. The cost effectiveness of Foscan mediated photodynamic therapy (Foscan-PDT) compared with extensive palliative surgery and palliative chemotherapy for patients with advanced head and neck cancer in the UK. Oral Oncol 2004;40: 372–82.

ELSEVIER
SAUNDERS

Otolaryngol Clin N Am
38 (2005) 255–272

OTOLARYNGOLOGIC
CLINICS
OF NORTH AMERICA

Bioengineering Solutions for Hearing Loss and Related Disorders

Dawn Burton Koch, PhD*, Steve Staller, PhD,
Kristen Jaax, MD, PhD, Elizabeth Martin, MA

Advanced Bionics Corp., 25129 Rye Canyon Loop, Valencia, CA 91355, USA

Technology development over the past 20 years has provided a number of unique treatments for the remediation of hearing loss and related disorders. Rapid advancements in microelectronics, battery technology, and mechanical packaging have allowed a number of effective and cosmetic solutions to be developed for individuals with hearing impairment. This article will review the various technologies that are currently available and provide insight into future developments.

Cochlear implants

History

A cochlear implant is a surgically implantable device that provides hearing sensation to individuals who have severe to profound hearing loss who cannot benefit from hearing aids. By electrically stimulating the auditory nerve directly, a cochlear implant bypasses damaged or undeveloped sensory structures in the cochlea, thereby providing usable information about sound to the central auditory nervous system.

Although it has been known since the late 1700s that electrical stimulation can produce hearing sensations [1], it was not until the 1950s that the potential for true speech understanding was demonstrated. In 1957, two French surgeons placed an electrode on the auditory nerve of a deaf man during an operation for facial nerve repair [2]. When current was passed through the electrode, the patient could discriminate some sounds and understand a few simple words. Based on that observation, several

---

* Corresponding author.
E-mail address: DawnK@advancedbionics.com (D.B. Koch).

research groups around the world began exploring the feasibility of an implantable electrical stimulator that could be used on a long-term basis by hearing-impaired individuals [3–5].

By the 1980s, cochlear implants had become an accepted treatment, providing safe and effective communication benefit to adults with profound hearing impairment. Since that time, cochlear implants have evolved from single-channel devices that primarily served as lipreading aids to sophisticated signal-processing systems that allow average implant users to communicate over the telephone. The population that can benefit from implants has expanded to include children and adults who have some residual hearing sensitivity. To date, there are over 60,000 cochlear-implant users worldwide, 20,000 of them children.

Technology

In a normal ear, sound energy is converted to mechanical energy by the middle ear, which then is converted to mechanical fluid motion in the cochlea. Within the cochlea, the sensory cells (the inner and outer hair cells) are sensitive transducers that convert the mechanical fluid motion into electrical impulses in the auditory nerve. Cochlear implants are designed to substitute for the function of the middle ear, cochlear mechanical motion, and sensory cells, transforming sound energy into electrical energy that will initiate impulses in the auditory nerve.

All cochlear implant systems consist of internal and external components (Fig. 1). The external components, which are worn on the head over or next to the ear, include a microphone that converts sound into an electrical signal, a speech/sound processor that manipulates and converts the signal into a special code (ie, sound-processing strategy), and a transmitter that sends the coded electrical signal to the internal components. The internal components are those parts of the system that are surgically implanted under the skin behind the ear. They include a receiver that decodes the signal from the speech processor, and an electrode array that stimulates the cochlea with electrical current. The entire system is powered by batteries located in the speech processor. Magnets located in the external transmitter

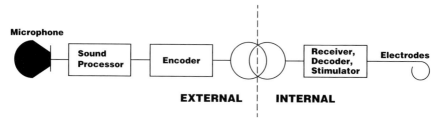

Fig. 1. External and internal components of a cochlear implant system.

and the implanted receiver facilitate transmission of data and power across the skin.

Currently, three cochlear-implant systems are available for children and adults in the United States and Canada: the HiResolution Bionic Ear (Advanced Bionics Corporation, Valencia, CA), the Nucleus 3 system (Cochlear Ltd., Lane Cove, NSW, Australia), and the COMBI 40/40+ device (Med-el, Innsbruck, Austria). All three manufacturers offer body-worn and behind-the-ear (BTE) speech processors. The BTE processors are similar to a BTE hearing aid. The processors vary in size, weight, style, colors available, and type of battery used. The electrodes, which are inserted into scala tympani, are either precoiled or flexible and thin. The precoiled types are spiral shaped and designed to hug the modiolus. The flexible arrays are designed to follow the curve of the cochlea. The number of intracochlear stimulus contacts on the electrode varies by manufacturer. The precoiled Advanced Bionics HiFocus Helix electrode (Advanced Bionics Corporation, Valencia, CA) has 16 stimulus contacts and the precoiled Nucleus Contour (Cochlear Ltd., Lane Cove, NSW, Australia) has 22 contacts. The flexible COMBI 40+ electrode (Med-el, Innsbruck, Austria) has 24 contacts arranged as 12 connected pairs.

Sound-processing strategies, which differ among devices, convert acoustic signals into electrical stimulation patterns that are delivered to the electrode contacts. In general, sound-processing algorithms filter the incoming acoustic signal into frequency bands. For each band, the envelope of the output of each filter is used to modulate trains of biphasic pulses that are sent to the electrodes. Information from the low-frequency bands are sent to more apical electrode contacts, whereas information from high-frequency bands are sent to more basal electrode contacts. In that way, the implant system preserves the tonotopic map of a normal cochlea. Contemporary cochlear-implant systems differ in a number of parameters, including the number of analysis filters, the bandwidth of the envelope extracted from the output of each filter, how many filter outputs are used to modulate the pulse trains (all or limited to those with highest energy), and the stimulation pulse rate. Ideally, patients should be able to be upgraded to new sound-processing strategies through software modifications without undergoing additional surgery. For example, patients who have the CII platform (Advanced Bionics Corporation, Valencia, CA) have already been converted from conventional to HiResolution sound processing, and will be able to use future algorithms that take advantage of the untapped capabilities of the implanted CII electronics without requiring a new implant.

Indications

Cochlear implants are approved for children aged 2 months through 17 years and for adults. Adult candidates must have severe to profound bilateral sensorineural hearing loss (average pure-tone audiometric [PTA] thresholds for 500, 1000, and 2000 Hz greater than 70 dB sound pressure level [SPL]). Appropriate candidates also must demonstrate through speech recognition tests with hearing aids that they are unable to benefit from conventional amplification. In addition, they must have no anatomical deformities that would preclude implantation of the device and must be able to undergo general anesthesia.

Pediatric cochlear-implant candidates also must demonstrate severe to profound sensorineural hearing loss. Children must have reached a plateau or show limited progress in acquisition of auditory skills with appropriate hearing aids and rehabilitation. Documentation of the level of hearing-aid benefit and auditory skills can be assessed using age-appropriate speech tests in older children and by using tools such as the Infant-Toddler Meaningful Auditory Integration Scale (a parent/guardian interview format) for young children [6,7]. Children should have no medical contraindications for surgery and their families should be counseled regarding appropriate expectations and follow-up treatment.

Surgery

Cochlear implant surgery is performed under general anesthesia and ordinarily takes between 1.5 and 3 hours. The procedure is performed typically in an outpatient setting. Cochlear implant surgical techniques are modifications of the widely used procedures for managing chronic infections of the middle ear and mastoid [8]. Skin incisions are designed to provide coverage of the external portion of the implant receiver while preserving the blood supply of the postauricular flap. Following the incision, a simple mastoidectomy is performed, and a bed for the receiver is drilled. The facial recess is opened and a cochleostomy is performed, followed by insertion of the electrode array into the scala tympani. Fascia is packed around the electrode at the cochleostomy, the receiver is securely affixed to the skull with sutures, and the incision is closed.

Medical and surgical complications, including device failures, are rare, with an occurrence of less than 1% [9], making cochlear implant reliability greater than that of cardiac pacemakers. Replacements of failed devices with new implants have not resulted in any significant decrement in benefit after the second surgery [10].

Outcomes

The benefits experienced by cochlear-implant recipients have continued to increase as the technology has developed and as the criteria for implantation have changed to include individuals with more residual hearing.

Adults

All adults are able to detect sound at lower intensities than with hearing aids and almost all are able to lipread better with the auditory information provided by the implant. Many postlinguistically deafened adults develop significant open-set word recognition ability and over half can converse to some degree on the telephone. Some adults are even able to score 100% on clinical tests of word recognition. The distributions of word and sentence recognition scores in a recent clinical trial of the Advanced Bionics device after 6 months of listening experience is shown in Fig. 2 [11]. All but one of the 51 users were able to understand some single words using only the auditory input from the device. A ceiling effect occurred with the sentence materials for most users. Adult recipients also reported a sense of greater independence and an increase in their social interactions.

Although a wide range of speech recognition scores exist, there are some factors that can predict the level of benefit that may be experienced. A

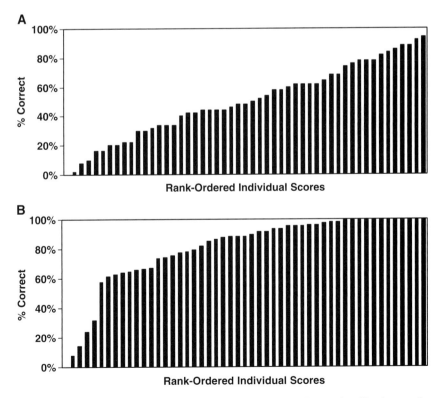

Fig. 2. Rank-ordered word and sentence recognition scores after six months of implant use for 51 adults who use the HiResolution Bionic Ear. (*A*) Monosyllabic words in quiet. (*B*) HINT sentences in quiet. (*Data from* refs [80,81].)

shorter duration of deafness, longer duration of implant use, and preimplant hearing ability are mild predictors of postimplant speech perception [12,13]. An individual's personality type and the need to use auditory communication can influence the degree of benefit, in addition to a host of other physiological, cognitive, and psychological factors. Age at implantation for adults, however, is not a major factor. The benefit experienced by older adults is not significantly different from younger adults, provided there are no other significant health issues [14–16].

Prelinguistically deafened adults also report significant benefit from a cochlear implant. Although speech scores for these users typically are poorer than postlinguistically deafened adults, they nonetheless report improvements in quality of life and communication abilities [17–20].

Children

Like adults, pediatric recipients are able to detect sound at lower levels with their implants than with hearing aids. Unlike adults, however, the age at implantation (or duration of auditory deprivation) has a significant influence on implant benefit. Children who are implanted at very young ages (ie, under 2 years of age) can experience normal or near-normal rates of auditory-skill and oral-language development [21,22]. Because of the early plasticity of the auditory system, the auditory input provided by a cochlear implant allows very young children to acquire age-appropriate language skills with much less effort than profoundly deaf children who use hearing aids. The brain's plasticity decreases dramatically after 3 years of age. Therefore, children who are implanted at older ages may not reach the same level of benefit as younger children because the parts of the brain that would normally receive auditory input have been taken over by input from other sensory modalities [23]. Even so, the oral language and speech benefit is substantial even in older children who have some residual hearing because they are able to hear more speech and sound information with the cochlear implant than with a hearing aid [24,25].

Other factors also can affect the success of implantation in children. The educational environment must support the use of oral language and be flexible as the auditory skills of an implanted child grow [26]. Young children who use oral communication exhibit better oral language and speech development than children who use total communication [27]. The expectations and involvement of parents or guardians also greatly affect how well a child uses a cochlear implant.

Quality of life and cost effectiveness

Studies of cost-to-usefulness ratios associated with cochlear implantation indicate that cost effectiveness (ie, acceptable value for money spent) is very high for adults [28–30] and children [31,32].

Electro-acoustic (hybrid) cochlear implants

History

The long intracochlear electrodes used in cochlear implants may cause loss of any residual hearing. Because the indications for cochlear implants now include people with PTAs as low as 70 dB SPL, significant usable low-frequency hearing may exist in those individuals. Nonetheless, patients who have residual low-frequency hearing in concert with precipitous high-frequency hearing loss often do not hear well with conventional hearing aids. These individuals are unable to distinguish the higher frequency sounds of speech (eg, consonants) and struggle particularly with speech perception in noisy and difficult listening conditions.

Technology and outcomes

In an attempt to meet the needs of those patients, Gantz and colleagues [33,34] proposed inserting a short atraumatic electrode into the scala tympani to provide electrical stimulation to the base of the cochlea, where high frequencies normally are processed. Concurrently, patients would use acoustic amplification in the same ear to aid residual low-frequency hearing. The goal was to provide high-frequency speech cues electrically in combination with low-frequency speech cues acoustically. Initial pilot work at the University of Iowa with a 6-mm electrode demonstrated that hearing thresholds were preserved consistently within 20 dB of preoperative levels in a handful of patients. However, patients reported that the sound quality was too high-pitched with the 6-mm electrode. When the electrode was lengthened to 10 mm, patients reported improved sound quality, and similar hearing preservation was observed. With hearing aids alone, word and sentence recognition was the same before and after implantation. However, all patients demonstrated better speech perception using the electrical stimulation from the short electrode than they did with hearing aids alone. Also, when the implant and hearing aids were used together, speech perception improved even more and continued to improve over time. Thus, these individuals were able to integrate acoustically and electrically processed speech successfully.

A different approach has been implemented in Europe where a 20-mm intracochlear electrode has been developed in which only the basal contacts are stimulated [35,36]. This approach has been shown to preserve some low-frequency acoustic hearing. However, the greater insertion depth poses an increased risk for hearing loss than does a shorter electrode. The electrode length, however, allows the clinician to activate additional apical electrodes should hearing continue to deteriorate over time.

Additional clinical data will determine the appropriate indications for each electrode type. For example, a short electrode may be more suitable for patients who have normal or near-normal low-frequency hearing whereas the longer electrode may be more suitable for patients who have moderate low-frequency losses. Clinical trials using both approaches are underway in the United States and Europe.

Auditory brainstem implants

History

Neurofibromatosis Type 2 (NF2) is a genetic disorder in which patients manifest bilateral benign tumors on the vestibular branch of the auditory nerve. Although the tumors can be removed surgically, the auditory nerve is often severed during the procedure, resulting in bilateral deafness. Because these patients do not have functioning auditory nerves, they are unable to benefit from a cochlear implant. Therefore, any electrical stimulation attempting to restore usable hearing must be directed to the next higher level of auditory processing.

In 1979, following his pioneering work with single-channel cochlear implants, Dr. William House proposed electrically stimulating the auditory system of NF2 patients with an electrode placed in the lateral recess of the fourth ventricle over the surface of the cochlear nucleus. In collaboration with Dr. William Hitselberger [37], Dr. House placed a ball electrode in the lateral recess of a patient who then was able to perceive sound from sinusoidal electrical stimulation similar to that provided by the single-channel cochlear implants of that era. Based on the initial success, a custom electrode was fabricated at the House Ear Institute, designed to facilitate fibrous integration and improve stability.

Technology and outcomes

In the early 1990s, Dr. Derald Brackmann and the House Ear Institute [37] initiated industrial collaborations with the Huntington Medical Research Institute and Cochlear Corporation to commercialize the then-named Auditory Brainstem Implant (ABI). Based on the Nucleus multichannel cochlear implant platform (Cochlear Ltd., Lane Cove, NSW, Australia), the electrode array is a Silastic pad with 21 disc electrodes organized in three rows (Fig. 3). The pad is backed with Dacron to facilitate fibrous tissue integration. The pad is placed surgically into the lateral recess of the fourth ventricle, which lies on the surface of the cochlear nucleus.

Patients using this 21-electrode device are able to detect sound and to lipread, although they have much poorer speech-perception abilities than multi-channel cochlear-implant users because they are not able to take advantage of the multiple channels of spectral information provided by the ABI. Typically, these patients perform similarly to users of single-channel cochlear implants [38,39]. Fewer than 10% of patients are able to understand limited words in sentences. Furthermore, 15% of patients

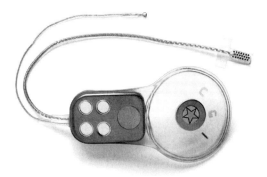

Fig. 3. Implanted components of the auditory brainstem implant (courtesy of Cochlear Ltd., Lane Cove, NSW, Australia).

cannot be stimulated adequately because the electrode array cannot be placed optimally or moves after surgery. In spite of these limitations, the ABI provides important hearing sensation to many NF2 patients who would otherwise be completely deaf.

The inability to use the pitch information may result from an inability to map pitch in a consistent fashion along the electrode array. The absence of a consistent pitch-place map may exist because the tonotopic arrangement of the cochlear nucleus is orthogonal to the surface, whereas the electrode array is parallel to the surface. To address the tonotopic mismatch, a new ABI is under development in which the electrodes penetrate the surface of the cochlear nucleus [40]. The electrodes are different lengths so they can be aimed at different frequency regions of the structure.

Middle ear implants

History

Conventional acoustic hearing aids have several disadvantages, including ear canal occlusion, acoustic feedback, sound distortion, and cosmesis. Over the past several decades, middle ear implants (MEIs) have been developed in an attempt to overcome some of these disadvantages. Although much of the research and development of MEIs followed on the successful application of cochlear implants, commercial success of these devices has been limited by reliability problems and the lack of third-party reimbursement.

Technology and indications

MEIs are designed for adults with moderate to severe hearing loss with normal middle ear function, good aided-speech perception (>50%), and prior experience with conventional amplification. The specific indications vary somewhat for different devices. All commercially available MEI systems are partially implantable and deliver sound by driving the middle ear ossicles mechanically, rather than acoustically, through either electromagnetic or piezoelectric transducers.

Two devices have been approved by the Food and Drug Administration (FDA) for marketing in the United States, the Vibrant Soundbridge (Med-el, Innsbruck, Austria) and the Soundtec system (Soundtec, Oklahama City, OK). Both devices use implanted electronics or transducers with external sound processors similar to cochlear implants. The Soundbridge sound processor is worn behind the ear. An external microphone transduces sound into an electrical signal that is transmitted across the skin by radio-frequency or piezoelectric transducers to the implanted receiver. The Soundbridge uses a floating magnet surrounded by a coil that is crimped to the incus. This electromagnet receives signals from the implanted receiver and then vibrates the ossicular chain.

The Soundtec external electronics are housed in a deep-canal earmold. At the tip of the earmold is a coil located 1.5 mm from the tympanic membrane, which provides appropriate distance and direction to communicate successfully with the implanted magnet transducer. The external coil sends an electromagnetic signal that initiates vibration of a magnet placed on the incus. Unique to this system, the middle ear magnet is placed by way of a tympano-meatal flap under local anesthesia. This procedure allows the surgery to be done in an outpatient setting. The ossicular chain is temporarily disarticulated to place a ring around the incudostapedial joint, which suspends the magnet. The joint is then reattached. Studies are presently underway to allow attachment of the magnet without requiring disarticulation of the incus.

Outcomes

Individuals implanted with middle ear implants typically show an average threshold improvement of approximately 10 dB from 500 Hz to 4000 Hz. At 6000 Hz, the functional gain is improved by approximately 20 dB compared with optimally fitted hearing aids. No difference has been observed between word recognition in quiet and in noise compared with conventional acoustic hearing aids. However, patients have reported reduction of acoustic feedback, reduction of the occlusion effect and distortion, and increased satisfaction [41].

Bone-anchored hearing aids

History

In the 1950s, European researchers discovered that when titanium is exposed to air, it develops an oxide layer that forms an active biological field that promotes living tissue to grow and bond permanently with the titanium

[42]. This process, called osseointegration, was first used in dental implants. The same process has been adapted and used to develop a bone-anchored hearing aid (BAHA), a system for delivering acoustic information to the inner ear through direct bone conduction.

Technology

The commercial BAHA system (Entific Medical Systems, Gothenburg, Sweden) is an implantable osseointegrated temporal bone prosthetic device specifically designed for patients who have mixed or conductive hearing loss, or unilateral sensorineural hearing loss, also known as Single Sided Deafness (SSD). The BAHA system is comprised of three parts: a titanium fixture, a connecting abutment, and a detachable sound processor. The fixture is implanted into the temporal bone during a 30- to 60-minute outpatient surgical procedure. After 3 months (6 months for children), which allows for thorough osseointegration, the sound processor is fitted by way of a snap abutment. The processor receives sound through the abutment and sends it to the functioning cochlea using the skull as a pathway to bypass the outer and middle ears. Currently, there are two ear-level processors available, one a linear system and one with automatic gain control and a directional microphone. A body-worn processor also is available that provides an additional 13 dB of gain over the ear-level processors.

Indications

The BAHA system was first approved by the FDA in 1996 to treat mixed and conductive hearing loss in patients aged 18 and older. In 1999, FDA indications were expanded to include children aged 5 years and older. In 2001, the system was approved for bilateral implantation and in 2002, it was approved for treatment of unilateral profound sensorineural hearing loss.

Patients who have a mixed or conductive hearing loss who cannot benefit from conventional air-conduction amplification may benefit from the BAHA. Chronic otitis media, congenital aural atresia and microtia, cholesteatoma, middle ear dysfunction or disease, and external otitis are examples of conductive hearing losses where conventional amplification may not prove beneficial. Candidates must be 5 years of age or older, have a mixed or conductive hearing loss where the bone conduction pure-tone average in the indicated ear is better than or equal to 45 dB HL, and have a monosyllabic word discrimination score of 60% or better. For bilateral fittings, candidates must have symmetrical bone conduction pure-tone averages between ears, defined as less than a 10-dB difference in bone conduction pure-tone averages or less than 15-dB differences in bone-conduction thresholds at 500, 1000, 2000, and 4000 Hz.

For patients who have SSD, candidates for the BAHA must have normal hearing in one ear, defined as an air conduction pure-tone average of 20 dB HL or better, along with a profound hearing loss in the other ear. In these patients, the BAHA system uses transcranial routing to send sound received by the sound processor on the deaf side to the cochlea in the normal-hearing ear. Common causes of SSD include acoustic neuroma tumors or tumor removal surgery, sudden deafness, neurological degenerative disease, Meniere's disease, viral infection, and trauma.

Outcomes

For patients who have conductive or mixed hearing loss, bone-conduction thresholds with the BAHA are lower than with conventional bone-conduction aids [42–44]. The direct bone conduction provided by the BAHA reduces attenuation from soft tissue and hair and can improve audiometric thresholds by as much as 10 to 20 dB [45]. For patients who have SSD, a contralateral routing of signal (CROS) hearing-aid system, where a hearing aid is placed in the deaf ear and the signal is routed to a hearing aid in the good ear, was once the only treatment option before the BAHA. Clinical studies comparing the BAHA to CROS amplification [46,47] show that patients experience a higher level of subjective benefit with the BAHA, as measured by the Abbreviated Profile of Hearing Aid Benefit [48], and that they have improved speech perception in noise.

Tinnitus suppression devices

Tinnitus is a disorder that has remained refractory to treatment in the majority of patients despite the advances of modern medicine. It is estimated that for 12 million Americans, tinnitus interferes with daily activities, and that 2 million Americans suffering from tinnitus are unable to function on a normal day-to-day basis [49].

The symptom of tinnitus results from a myriad of pathologies. Somatic sounds produced in the vicinity of the cochlea will elicit the perception of tinnitus. Sources of sound include vascular structures (eg, venous hum, vascular tumors, arteriovenous malformations), musculoskeletal structures (eg, myoclonus of the palatal muscles), and patulous eustachian tubes [50]. Sensorineural tinnitus, in which the symptom arises from the auditory system itself, represents the majority of tinnitus cases. Causes of sensorineural tinnitus include tumors that compress the auditory nerve and hearing loss that results from various sources including noise, ototoxic medications, and otosclerosis.

Therapeutic options for tinnitus sufferers are limited. In the minority of patients, treatment can be directed at the underlying pathology (eg, treatment of an arteriovenous malformation). For the majority of tinnitus patients, and in particular sensorineural tinnitus patients, treatment is aimed at modulating the patient's response to the tinnitus, rather than treating the tinnitus itself. Modalities include masking devices that generate a low-level sound to minimize the perception of tinnitus while the device is on, tinnitus retraining therapy that aims to induce habituation to the tinnitus [51], and biofeedback and stress reduction programs aimed at minimizing the body's reaction to the tinnitus.

For sensorineural tinnitus, electrical stimulation has the potential to go beyond the current state of the art to provide relief from the symptom of tinnitus. One theory of the pathogenesis of tinnitus is loss of suppression of activity in the auditory system secondary to either loss of normal input from the periphery or distortion of the behavior of pathways in the central auditory system, analogous to phantom limb pain [52–54]. It is proposed that electrical stimulation may suppress tinnitus by either modulating abnormal spontaneous firing patterns in the cochlear nerve [55], or changing the functional state of auditory nuclei and disrupting a potential source of tinnitus in the brainstem [56]. Early studies with direct current (DC) stimulation showed promising results, but tissue toxicity with DC exposure limits the clinical application of electrical stimulation to charge-balanced alternating current (AC) stimulation.

Many routes for applying electrical stimulation have been attempted for treatment of tinnitus, with varying degrees of success. Attempted sites include transcutaneous electrical stimulation (TENS), tympanic membrane stimulation, round window and promontory stimulation, and intracochlear stimulation.

It remains unclear whether TENS applied to a site distant from the cochlea could elicit suppression of tinnitus. Investigators have applied both AC and DC current to sites, including the auricle [57–59], behind the ear [60], and the mastoid process [61]. Although some techniques have yielded encouraging results on initial investigation, no technique has consistently been proven effective over repeated studies at multiple centers.

Preliminary studies suggest stimulation of the tympanic membrane may be effective in approximately 50% of patients. AC current applied to the tympanic membrane suppressed tinnitus in five of ten patients in one study [62] and in 34 of 65 patients in a second study [63]. The second study also demonstrated a positive correlation between treatment response and changes in the compound action potential and electrically evoked auditory brainstem response. The promontory and round window have also been popular targets for electrical stimulation, allowing proximity to the cochlear nerve and hair cells without requiring penetration of the inner ear. Recent acute studies have shown promising results in suppressing tinnitus in patients who have sensorineural hearing loss [64–68].

With 81% to 85% of cochlear implant patients reporting tinnitus before receiving their implant [69,70], cochlear implant patients have provided a rich source of knowledge regarding electrical stimulation for treatment of tinnitus. Multichannel implant studies consistently show that normal use of cochlear implants can reduce or eliminate symptoms in patients who have preexisting tinnitus [55,69–72]. Only 3% to 5% of patients typically experience worsening of tinnitus following cochlear implantation [56].

From these data, it seems likely that an implantable device that can provide chronic electrical stimulation in the middle ear in close proximity to the cochlea may offer the best solution for suppressing sensorineural tinnitus without jeopardizing residual hearing.

The recently developed bion microstimulator (Advanced Bionics Corporation, Valencia, California) may be an attractive method for implementing this solution [73]. The bion is a miniature, self-contained, rechargeable neurostimulator 27 mm long and 3 mm in diameter. It was designed as a platform device for the treatment of numerous diseases through direct electrical stimulation of nerves and muscles. The bion system is composed of four main components: (1) an implantable pulse generator, (2) a recharging system, (3) a remote control, and (4) a clinician's programmer. The implantable pulse generator contains a rechargeable battery, a radio and antenna for bidirectional telemetry, a programmable microchip, and stimulating electrodes. Its output can be connected to an electrode lead specifically designed to address the anatomical and electrophysiological requirements of the target nerve.

The remote control is a hand-held device that allows patients to control the basic functions of their bion. Features of the remote control include the ability to control stimulation amplitude, turn stimulation on and off, and check the battery level. The recharging system is comprised of recharging circuitry connected to a metal coil, which generates the electromagnetic field that charges the bion. The coil form-factor can be customized to the anatomical demands of the target nerve. For example, a chair cushion design is used to recharge bions implanted deep in the pelvis for treatment of incontinence. Recharging is anticipated to take 15 minutes per day or 60 minutes one to two times per week, on average. The clinician's programmer is a laptop interface that gives the clinician control of the bion's stimulation parameters, including frequency (range, 10–1000 pps), pulse width (range, 50–1550 µsec), current amplitude minimum and maximum settings (range, 0–10 mA), and bursting pattern.

To achieve the goal of chronically suppressing tinnitus, the bion could be implanted behind the ear with an electrode running subcutaneously to the middle ear to stimulate the round window or promontory with charge-balanced AC stimulation. A BTE-based recharging system could be designed to recharge the battery once a week. Using the remote control, patients would be able to customize the therapy to their needs, either stimulating continuously or turning it on for short intervals throughout the day.

Future technology directions

There are several new applications and research studies underway to improve and expand the benefit of implantable hearing technology, particularly cochlear implants. Studies in patients who use bilateral cochlear implants have shown improved understanding of speech in noise, better localization ability with two implants than with one alone, and improved sound quality [74–76]. Development of new sound-processing algorithms that mimic the nonlinear processes and compression of the normal cochlea may improve the signal delivered to the auditory nerve [77]. Frequency resolution may be enhanced by steering current to discrete sites along the cochlea, thereby increasing the number of spectral channels that can be perceived [78]. It may be possible for drugs that can preserve neural tissue or induce neural growth toward the electrode to be delivered through the cochlear implant electrode [79]. And finally, as technology develops, fully implantable cochlear devices should become available in the next few years.

Summary

Advances in digital signal processing, microelectronics, and power technology have produced devices that have contributed significantly to the quality of life and communication abilities of individuals with hearing impairment and tinnitus. Future technological developments will expand the benefits of current devices and offer new treatments for otologic disorders.

References

[1] Simmons FB. Electrical stimulation of the auditory nerve in man. Arch Otolaryngol 1966;84: 2–54.
[2] Djourno A, Eyries C. Prosthese auditive par excitation electrique a distance du nerf sensoriel a l'aide d'un bobinage inclus a demeure [Auditory prosthesis by means of a distant electrical stimulation of the sensory nerve with the use of an indwelt coiling]. Presse Med 1957;65:1417 [in French].
[3] Beiter AL, Shallop JK. Cochlear implants: past, present, and future. In: Estabrooks W, editor. Cochlear implants in kids. Washington, DC: Alexander Graham Bell Association; 1998. p. 3–29.
[4] Loizou PC. Mimicking the human ear. IEEE Sig Proc Mag. September 1998;101–30.
[5] Zeng FG. Auditory prostheses: past, present, and future. In: Zeng F, Popper A, Fay RR, editors. Cochlear implants: auditory prostheses and electric hearing. New York: Springer; 2004. p. 1–13.
[6] Robbins AM, Renshaw JJ, Berry SW. Evaluating meaningful auditory integration in profoundly hearing-impaired children. Am J Otol 1991;12(Suppl):151–64.
[7] Zimmerman-Phillips S, Robbins AM, Osberger MJ. Infant-toddler meaningful auditory integration scale. Valencia, CA: Advanced Bionics Corporation; 2001.
[8] Niparko J. Cochlear implants: clinical applications. In: Zeng F, Popper A, Fay RR, editors. Cochlear implants: auditory prostheses and electric hearing. New York: Springer; 2004. p. 53–100.
[9] Cohen NL, Hoffman RA. Complications of cochlear implant surgery in adults and children. Ann Otol Rhinol Laryngol 1991;100:131–6.
[10] Rubinstein JT, Parkinson WS, Lowder MW, et al. Single-channel to multichannel conversions in adult cochlear implant subjects. Am J Otolaryngol 1997;19:461–6.
[11] Koch DB, Osberger MJ, Segel P, et al. HiResolution and conventional sound processing in the HiResolution bionic ear: using appropriate outcome measures to assess speech recognition ability. Audiol Neurootol 2004;9:214–23.
[12] Rubinstein JT, Parkinson WS, Tyler RS, et al. Residual speech recognition and cochlear implant performance: effects of implantation criteria. Am J Otol 1999;20:445–52.

[13] Waltzman S, Fisher S, Niparko J, et al. Predictors of postoperative performance with cochlear implants. Ann Otol Rhinol Laryngol 1995;104(Suppl 165):S15–8.

[14] Buchman CA, Fucci MJ, Luxford WM. Cochlear implants in the geriatric population: benefits outweigh risks. Ear Nose Throat J 1999;78(7):489–94.

[15] Chatelin V, Kim EJ, Driscoll C, et al. Cochlear implant outcomes in the elderly. Otol Neurotol 2004;25(3):298–301.

[16] Herzog M, Mueller J, Milewski C, et al. Cochlear implantation in the elderly. Adv Otorhinolaryngol 2000;57:393–6.

[17] Koch DB, King CD, Vujanovic I, et al. Everyday cochlear-implant benefit in prelingually deafened adults [abstract]. Paper presented at: American Auditory Society; March 9, 2004; Scottsdale, AZ.

[18] Schramm D, Fitzpatrick E, Seguin C. Cochlear implantation for adolescents and adults with prelinguistic deafness. Otol Neurotol 2002;23:698–703.

[19] Waltzman SB, Cohen NL. Implantation of patients with prelingual long-term deafness. Ann Otol Rhinol Laryngol 1999;108(Suppl 177):S84–8.

[20] Zwolan TA, Kileny PR, Telian SA. Self-report of cochlear implant use and satisfaction by prelingually deafened adults. Ear Hear 1996;17:198–210.

[21] Miyamoto RT, Houston DM, Kirk KI, et al. Language development in deaf infants following cochlear implantation. Acta Otolaryngol 2003;123:241–4.

[22] McConkey Robbins A, Koch DB, Osberger MJ, et al. Effect of age at implantation on auditory skill development in infants and toddlers. Arch Otolaryngol Head Neck Surg 2004; 130:570–4.

[23] Lee DS, Lee JS, Oh SH, et al. Cross-modal plasticity and cochlear implants. Nature 2001; 409:149–50.

[24] Gantz B, Rubinstein J, Tyler R, et al. Long-term results of cochlear implants in children with residual hearing. Ann Otol Rhinol Laryngol 2000;185:33–6.

[25] Osberger MJ, Miyamoto RT, Zimmerman-Phillips S, et al. Independent evaluation of the speech perception abilities of children with the Nucleus 22-channel cochlear implant system. Ear Hear 1991;12(Suppl 4):S66–80.

[26] Koch M, Wyatt JR, Francis H, et al. A model of educational resource use by children with cochlear implants. Otolaryngol Head Neck Surg 1997;117:174–9.

[27] Osberger MJ, Zimmerman-Phillips S, Koch DB. Cochlear implant candidacy and performance trends in children. Ann Otol Rhinol Laryngol 2002;111(Suppl 189):S62–5.

[28] Cheng A, Niparko J. Cost-utility of the cochlear implant in adults: a meta-analysis. Arch Otolaryngol Head Neck Surg 1999;125:1214–8.

[29] Summerfield A, Marshall D. Cochlear implantation in the UK 1990–1994. Nottingham, England: Medical Research Council Institute of Hearing Research; 1995. p. 199–236.

[30] Wyatt JR, Niparko Jk, Rothman ML, et al. Cost utility of multichannel cochlear implants in 258 profoundly deaf individuals. Laryngoscope 1996;106:816–21.

[31] Cheng A, Rubin H, Powe N, et al. Cost-utility analysis of the cochlear implant in children. JAMA 2000;284:850–6.

[32] O'Neill C, O'Donoghue GM, Archbold SM, et al. A cost-utility analysis of pediatric cochlear implantation. Laryngoscope 2000;110:156–60.

[33] Gantz BJ, Turner CW. Combining acoustic and electrical speech processing: Iowa/Nucleus hybrid implant. Acta Otolaryngol 2004;124(4):344–7.

[34] Gantz BJ, Turner CW. Combining acoustic and electrical hearing. Laryngoscope 2003; 113(10):1726–30.

[35] Kiefer J, Tillein J, von Ilberg C, et al. Fundamental aspects and first results of the clinical application of combined electric and acoustic stimulation of the auditory system. In: Kubo T, Takahashi Y, Iwaki T, editors. Cochlear implants-an update. The Hague, The Netherlands: Kugler Publications; 2002. p. 569–76.

[36] von Ilberg C, Kiefer J, Tillein J, et al. Electric-acoustic stimulation of the auditory system. New technology for severe hearing loss. ORL J Otorhinolaryngol Relat Spec 1999;61(6): 334–40.

[37] Brackmann DE, Hitselberger WE, Nelson RA, et al. Auditory brainstem implant: I. Issues in surgical implantation. Otolaryngol Head Neck Surg 1993;108(6):624–33.
[38] Otto SR, Shannon RV, Brackmann DE, et al. The multichannel auditory brainstem implant: performance in twenty patients. Otolaryngol Head Neck Surg 1998;118:291–303.
[39] Otto SR, Brackmann DE, Hitselberger WE, et al. The multichannel auditory brainstem implant: update on performance in 61 patients. J Neurosurg 2002;96:1063–71.
[40] McCreery DG, Shannon RV, Moore JK, et al. Accessing the tonotopic organization of the ventral cochlear nucleus by intranuclear microstimulation. IEEE Trans Rehabil Eng 1998;6: 391–9.
[41] Roland PS, Shoup AG, Shea MC, et al. Verification of improved patient outcomes with a partially implantable hearing aid, the SOUNDTEC direct hearing system. Laryngoscope 2001;111(10):1682–6.
[42] Tjellstrom A, Hakansson B. The bone-anchored hearing aid. Design principles, indications, and long-term clinical results. Otolaryngol Clin North Am 1995;28(1):593–8.
[43] Tietze L, Papsin B. Utilization of bone-anchored hearing aids in children. Int J Pediatr Otorhinolaryngol 2001;58:75–80.
[44] Cremers CW, Snik FM, Beynon AJ. Hearing with the bone-anchored hearing aid (BAHA, HC 200) compared to a conventional bone-conduction hearing aid. Clin Otolaryngol 1992; 17:225–79.
[45] Hakansson B, Tjellstrom A, Rosenhall U. Hearing thresholds with direct bone conduction versus conventional bone conduction. Scand Audiol 1984;13:3–13.
[46] Niparko JK, Cox K, Lustig L. Comparison of the bone anchored hearing aid implantable hearing device with contralateral routing of offside signal amplification in the rehabilitation of unilateral deafness. Otol Neurotol 2003;24:73–8.
[47] Wazem J, Spitzer J, Ghossaini SN, et al. Transcranial contralateral cochlear stimulation in unilateral deafness. Otolaryngol Head Neck Surg 2003;129:248–54.
[48] Cox RM, Alexander GC. The abbreviated profile of hearing aid benefit. Ear Hear 1995;16: 176–86.
[49] American Tinnitus Association. Available at: http://www.ata.org/about_tinnitus/consumer/ faq.html. Accessed September 28, 2004.
[50] Fortune DS, Haynes DS, Hall JW 3rd. Tinnitus. Current evaluation and management. Med Clin North Am 1999;83:153.
[51] Jastreboff PJ, Gray WC, Gold SL. Neurophysiological approach to tinnitus patients. Am J Otol 1996;17:236.
[52] Lockwood A, Salvi R, Burkard R, et al. Neuroanatomy of tinnitus. Scand Audiol Suppl 1999;51:47.
[53] Moller A. Similarities between chronic pain and tinnitus. Am J Otol 1997;18:577.
[54] Muhlnickel W, Elbert T, Taub E, et al. Reorganization of auditory cortex in tinnitus. Proc Natl Acad Sci USA 1998;95:10340–3.
[55] Ito J, Sakakihara J. Suppression of tinnitus by cochlear implantation. Am J Otolaryngol 1994;15:145–8.
[56] Dauman R. Electrical stimulation for tinnitus suppression. In: Tyler R, editor. Tinnitus handbook. San Diego, CA: Singular Thomson Learning; 2000. p. 377–98.
[57] Chouard C, Meyer B, Maridat D. Transcutaneous electrotherapy for severe tinnitus. Acta Otolaryngol 1981;91:415–22.
[58] Engelberg M, Bauer W. Transcutaneous electrical stimulation for tinnitus. Laryngoscope 1985;95:1167–73.
[59] Vernon J, Fenwick J. Attempts to suppress tinnitus with transcutaneous electrical stimulation. Otolaryngol Head Neck Surg 1985;93:385–9.
[60] Maini S, Deogaonkar S. Transdermal electrical stimulation in sensorineural tinnitus. Indian J Otolaryngol 1999;51(2):37–9.
[61] Shulman A. External electrical stimulation in tinnitus control. Am J Otol 1985;6:110–5.

[62] Kuk F, Tyler R, Rustad N, et al. Alternating current at the eardrum for tinnitus reduction. J Speech Hear Res 1989;32:393–400.

[63] Mahmoudian S, Moosavi A, Daneshi A, et al. Comparative study of ECochG and ABR in tinnitus patients before and after auditory electrical stimulation (AES) [abstract]. Presented at the XVIII Biennial Symposium of the International Evoked Response Audiometry Study Group (IERASG). Las Palmas, Spain, June 8–12, 2003.

[64] Hazell J, Jastreboff P, Meerton L, et al. Electrical tinnitus suppression: frequency dependence of effects. Audiology 1993;32:68–77.

[65] Matsushima J, Fujimura H, Sakai N, et al. A study of electrical promontory stimulation in tinnitus patients. Auris Nasus Larynx 1994;21(1):17–24.

[66] Matsushima J, Sakai N, Uemi N, et al. Evaluation of implanted tinnitus suppressor based on tinnitus stress test. Int Tinnitus J 1997;3(2):123–31.

[67] Rubinstein J, Tyler R, Johnson A, et al. Electrical suppression of tinnitus with high-rate pulse trains. Otol Neurotol 2003;24(3):478–85.

[68] Ruiz-Rico R, Sainz M, de la Torre A, et al. Reduction of the incidence of tinnitus in patients treated with cochlear implants [abstract]. Presented at the 6th European Symposium on Paediatric Cochlear Implantation. Las Palmas, Spain, February 24–26, 2002.

[69] Gibson W. The effect of electrical stimulation and cochlear implantation on tinnitus. In: Aran J, Dauman R, editors. Proceedings of the Fourth International Tinnitus Seminar. New York: Kugler; 1992.

[70] Tyler R, Kelsay D. Advantages and disadvantages reported by some of the better cochlear-implant patients. Am J Otol 1990;11:282–9.

[71] Tyler R. Tinnitus in the profoundly hearing-impaired and the effects of cochlear implants. Ann Otol Rhinol Laryngol 1995;104:25–30.

[72] Zwolan T, Kileny P, Souliere C, et al. Tinnitus suppression following cochlear implantation. In: Aran J, Dauman R, editors. Proceedings of the Fourth International Tinnitus Seminar. New York: Kugler; 1992.

[73] Carbunaru R, Whitehurst T, Jaax K, et al. Battery-Powered bion microstimulators for neuromodulation [abstract]. Presented at the 6th Annual International Conference IEEE Engineering in Medicine and Biology Society (EMBS). San Francisco, September 1–5, 2004.

[74] Gantz BJ, Tyler RS, Rubinstein JT, et al. Binaural cochlear implants placed during the same operation. Otol Neurotol 2002;23:169–80.

[75] Litovsky R, Parkinson A, Arcaroli J, et al. Bilateral cochlear implants in adults and children. Arch Otolaryngol Head Neck Surg 2004;130:648–55.

[76] Muller J, Schon F, Helms J. Speech understanding in quiet and noise in bilateral users of the MED-EL COMBI 40/40+ cochlear implant system. Ear Hear 2002;23:198–206.

[77] Wilson B, Lawson D, Muller J, et al. Cochlear implants: some likely next steps. Annu Rev Biomed Eng 2003;5:207–49.

[78] Litvak L, Overstreet E, Mishra L. Steering current through simultaneous activation of intracochlear electrodes in the Clarion CII cochlear implant: frequency resolution [abstract]. Presented at the Conference on Implantable Auditory Prostheses. Pacific Grove, CA, August 20, 2003.

[79] Qun LX, Pirvola U, Saarma M, et al. Neurotrophic factors in the auditory periphery. Ann N Y Acad Sci 1999;884:292–304.

[80] Peterson GE, Lehiste I. Revised CNC lists for auditory tests. J Speech Hear Disord 1962; 27:62–70.

[81] Nilsson MJ, Soli S, Sullivan J. Development of the Hearing in Noise Test for the measurement of speech reception thresholds in quiet and in noise. J Acoust Soc Am 1994; 95:1085–99.

ELSEVIER
SAUNDERS

Otolaryngol Clin N Am
38 (2005) 273–293

OTOLARYNGOLOGIC
CLINICS
OF NORTH AMERICA

Nanotechnology in Otolaryngology

G. Louis Hornyak, PhD*

Department of Physics and Astronomy, University of Denver, Denver, CO 80208, USA
Colorado Nanotechnology Initiative, Inc., 12600 West Colfax Avenue,
Lakewood, CO 80215, USA

I would like to describe a field, in which little has been done, but in which an enormous amount can be done in principle. This field is not quite the same as the others in that it will not tell us much of fundamental physics (in the sense of, "What are the strange particles"?) but it is more like solid-state physics in the sense that it might tell us much of great interest about the strange phenomena that occur in complex situations. Furthermore, a point that is most important is that it would have an enormous number of technical applications. What I want to talk about is the problem of manipulating and controlling things on a small scale.

—Richard Feynman, "There's Plenty of Room at the Bottom," given December 29, 1959, at the annual meeting of the American Physical Society at the California Institute of Technology, Pasadena, California

What do the terms "nanoscience," "nanotechnology," "nanobiology," "nanobiotechnology," and "nanomedicine" have in common, and why are they relevant today? Hardly a day goes by without some mention of nano-technology in television commercials, and television specials on the topic are becoming more common. The number of scientific papers, conferences, workshops, and conventions centered on the commercial exploitation is gaining momentum as more and more remarkable discoveries wend their way into the mainstream. A major movie about nanotechnology, Michael Crichton's "Prey," is expected to debut in the near future, and the concomitant publicity is expected to reach stratospheric proportions. Investors are warned to be on the alert for "nanopretenders." This article, however, is concerned with the promise of nanotechnology, nanomedicine in particular. The author hopes to introduce the reader to an amazing world

---

* Colorado Nanotechnology Initiative, Inc., Suite C-440, 12600 West Colfax Avenue, Lakewood, CO 80215.
E-mail address: lhornyak@du.edu

defined by nanoscale proportions. In the process, he hopes to instill a deep appreciation and intrinsic understanding of the importance of the research and development currently being accomplished that will dramatically affect patients' future health and well-being.

Definition

The etymology of the prefix *nano* is based on the Greek *nanos*, which means "dwarf" or "little old man" [1]. *Nanos* is the root of words such as "nanna" and "nun" and of the prefix in *nanotechnology*. The meaning, however, has essentially evolved into an indication of extreme smallness [2] and, more particularly, in certain measurements, to mean one billionth [3]. Nanotechnology is based on the nanometer, that is, a measurement equivalent to one billionth of a meter (10^{-9} m), and the National Science Foundation defines the nanoscale as the domain between 1 and 100 nanometers [4]. For example, 10 hydrogen atoms in a line make 1 nm. An often-used comparison that lends perspective to the nanoscale is based on the thickness of the human hair, which ranges from 40 to 100 microns (one micron, 1 μm, is equivalent to one millionth of a meter, 10^{-6} m, or 1000 nm). A nanometer, therefore, is 1/40,000 to 1/100,000 as thick as a human hair. Good working definitions of the nanoscale, nanoscience, and nanotechnology are the following [5]:

- The nanoscale exists between 1 and 100 nm. In the more general sense, materials with at least one dimension below 1000 nm but greater than 1 nm are considered to be nanoscale materials.
- Nanoscience is the study of nanoscale materials with novel properties and functions.
- Nanotechnology, based on the manipulation, control, and integration of atoms and molecules to form materials, structures, devices, and systems at the nanoscale, is the application of nanoscience, especially to industrial and commercial objectives.

Nanotechnology is enabling, interdisciplinary, convergent, horizontal, and disruptive and will comprise the next industrial revolution with a pervasive impact on all future manufactured products. In many ways, nanotechnology is a platform similar to materials science, another broad-based interdisciplinary platform. Nanotechnology, however, differs from purist materials science in its whole-scale embrace of biology. Nanotechnology is horizontal in that it enables all current forms of technology. Examples include biotechnology, energy, photonics, electronics, and, of central interest in this article, medicine.

According the National Science Foundation, nanotechnology is expected to contribute 1 trillion dollars to the global economy within the next decade [6]. For this expectation to be realized, nanotechnology developers must overcome a high entry barrier. In the hey-day of the dot.com era, it was possible to create companies out of thin air, but nanotechnology developers must establish a manufacturing base in the economy. Therefore developments in nanotechnology require the deliberate formation of innovative partnerships among academia, business, and government [7]. Several well-established examples of such partnerships exist [8]. Fierce global competition is underway to commercialize nanotechnology, and other governments (eg, those of the European Union, China, and Japan) are subsidizing research and development at levels similar to or higher than the commitment of the United States.

To the unaware, or for that matter even to those who understand what it is, nanotechnology is not an easy sell. Many ask, "If nanotechnology embraces everything, what then is it"? [9]. In spite of this nebulous characterization, the potential and promise of nanoscience and technology have been embraced fully by leaders and decision-makers in academia, business, and government the world over. Nanotechnology is here and in a big way. Those quicker to realize its potential will position themselves strategically to reap its rewards. The rewards, however, always come with a concomitant penalty, and the social implications of nanotechnology cannot be understated. These social implications include ethical, legal, social, political, military, economic, and environmental considerations. An example is the worldwide controversy about genetically modified organisms. Serious efforts are underway to stay well ahead of the technology [10]. The United States government, in particular, through the National Nanotechnology Initiative (NNI), is striving to educate leaders from all sectors about the need to understand nanotechnology and its expected impact on society.

Historical perspective

Applications of nanotechnology have been in evidence since ancient times. For example, the spectacular Lycurgus cup, housed in the British Museum, was fabricated by the Romans in the fourth century A.D. Not until 1990, by means of transmission electron microscopic analysis, was the secret behind the dichroic character of the glass uncovered. Specifically, it was found that the ruby-crimson color upon transmission and the green color on reflection resulted from the presence of 70-nm gold/silver particles embedded in the soda-lime glass matrix [11]. The Greek philosophers Democritus and Leucippus in the fifth century B.C. proposed that matter was made of atoms, matter on a scale somewhat below the realm of nanotechnology. In 1661, Robert Boyle proposed the concept of corpuscles, referring to them as "minute masses or clusters that were not easily dissipable [sic] into such particles that composed them" [12]. In 1857, Michael Faraday [13] presented the following explanation for the causes of colored glass: "[G]old is reduced in exceedingly fine particles, which becoming diffused, produces a ruby fluid. The various preparations of gold, whether ruby, green, violet or blue, consist of that substance in a metallic divided state." Chemists, of course, and smugly so, claim that they have been nanoscientists for centuries.

In more recent times, examples of synthetic nanomaterials are plentiful. For example, anodically formed porous aluminum oxide films containing hexagonal arrays of nanometer-sized cells were first used more than 100 years ago to protect aluminum surfaces from corrosion [14]. These surfaces are now considered useful and adaptable templates in the fabrication of nanostructured materials [14]. Fig. 1 shows an atomic force microscope image of a porous alumina film. Titanium dioxide, responsible for the white pigment in paints, was discovered in 1821 and contains 200- to 400-nm diameter particles. Nanometer-sized carbon black particles have improved the performance of tires for several decades. In 1980, astronomers noticed a broad, red-fluorescent dust component of the Red Rectangle Nebula. In 1998, it was suggested that the red color is caused by the presence of quantum dots [15,16]. The optical behavior of quantum dots (QDs) depends on particle size. Although some QDs contain hundreds to thousands of atoms, electronic properties can resemble those of single atoms. Incidentally, gold nanoparticles are widely used in immunohistochemistry to identify protein–protein interactions [17]. Optically active gold nanoshells, much smaller than Faraday's gold particles (approximately 3 nm in diameter), have been used in targeted photothermal therapy to help kill tumor cells [18–20].

The onset of modern nanotechnology is widely credited to the late Richard Feynman of the California Institute of Technology. In his 1959 lecture "There's Plenty of Room at the Bottom: An Invitation to Enter

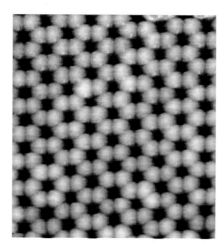

Fig. 1. Anodic alumina membrane with 50-nm pores. The membrane was imaged with an atomic force microscope (Courtesy of the National Renewable Energy Laboratory, Golden, CO).

a New Phase of Physics," Feynman asked, "Why cannot we write the entire 24 volumes of the *Encyclopedia Britannica* on the head of a pin?" [21].

Feynman's foresight is soon to become reality with memory devices ready to breach the terabyte-cm^{-2} threshold. For example, the head of a pin, 1 to 2 mm in diameter, has enough space to publish all 30,000 pages of the *Encyclopedia, Britannica* if characters were 10 nm in height [22]. In 1981, Nobel Prize winners Gerd Binnig and Heinrich Rohrer invented the scanning tunneling microscope (STM); and on April 5, 1990, two scientists at the IBM Almaden Research Center in San Jose, California, used an STM to position 35 individual xenon atoms on a surface to spell out "IBM" (Fig. 2). Later, they used that technique to build structures one atom at a time [23]. With the development of the atomic force microscope, STM, and other remarkable tools, the nano-age has arrived in full force. In the late 1980s and early 1990s, Carl Drexler [24] did much to promote awareness about the need for development of nanotechnology, especially with regard to military applications.

In 1996, a United States government interagency council was formed to determine what should be done at the federal level to promote the development of nanotechnology, and in 1998, the Interagency Working Group on Nanotechnology was established. The Clinton administration's budget submission for 2001 raised nanotechnology to the level of a federal initiative, and as a result the NNI was formed. On December 3, 2003, the Twenty-first Century Nanotechnology Research and Development Act was signed into law. In 2002, the National Institute of Health (NIH), under the direction of Elias A. Zerhouni, decided to develop a "roadmap" for medical research for the twenty-first century. The NIH is in the process of establishing nanomedicine development centers across the country to serve as "the intellectual and technological centerpiece of the Nanomedicine Roadmap Initiative." As mentioned earlier in this article, nanotechnology is developing on an exponential curve, similar to that seen in the information age.

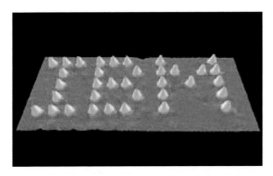

Fig. 2. "IBM" spelled out with Xenon atoms using a scanning tunneling microscope.

The nanoscale

Nanomaterials possess novel phenomena and properties. What is it about the 1-to-100-nanometer size that warrants such special distinction? The world of bulk materials is well understood, as is the quantum world of atoms and molecules; as a result, scientists have no difficulties in making bulk materials from atoms and molecules. It is only recently that scientists have begun to gain a perspective on the nanoscale world, and only recently has it been possible manufacture stable nanoscale materials on a routine basis (personal communication, Colby Foss, 2004). Micron-sized materials still exhibit properties characteristic of bulk materials [14,25], but at the threshold of the nanoscale those properties transform in fantastic ways. The onset of advanced procedures such as nanometer-scale lithography, focused ion beam fabrication, and purification methods have contributed significantly to overcoming the intrinsic barriers to nanoscale fabrication. The refinement of analytical tools such as scanning tunneling microscopy and atomic force microscopy has also made characterization and analysis with atomic resolution a routine process.

In part, nanomaterials possess physical properties that can be very different from their bulk-material counterparts because of characteristics resulting from confinement, predominance of interfacial phenomena, and quantum mechanics [25]. Size matters in the nanoworld. For example, as a result of confinement during the course of miniaturization, conducting materials transform into semiconductors, semiconducting materials transform into insulators, crystals melt at significantly lower temperatures, ferromagnetic materials lose ferromagnetic properties, and solubility properties can dramatically be altered. A straightforward consequence of miniaturization is a dramatic increase in chip storage density.

Nanomaterials possess a large fraction of surface atoms per unit volume. An example can illustrate the impact of such an increase in the number of surface atoms: with successive divisions into smaller and smaller cubes, the surface area of 1 g of sodium chloride increases from 3.6 cm^2 to 2.8×10^7 cm^2, with a concomitant increase in surface energy from 7.2×10^{-5} J/g to 560 J/g, a increase of seven orders of magnitude [26]! Because of the significant increase in surface energy, nanomaterials become inherently metastable and tend toward agglomeration. The reaction of Gold-55 quantum dot structures with phosphine ligands, for example, is one means of stabilizing the tiny clusters [27]. Gold, although generally not thought of as a catalytic material, is able to show catalytic behavior at the nanoscale. If significant amounts of material exchange or transformation need to be accomplished in nanoseconds, the properties of increased surface area must be included in design considerations.

There are numerous examples of the novel and phenomenal properties that nanomaterials exhibit. Carbon nanotubes, for example, have been reported to be 100 times stronger than steel. Storage of one bit of information with one electron is another. The formation of materials harder and more scratch resistant than silicon carbide is yet another example. Although any further detailed discussion of the remarkable physical characteristics of nanoscale materials is beyond the scope of this article, examples of naturally occurring nanoscale phenomena are discussed in some detail in the following section.

Nanobiology

Nanobiology is the application of nanoscience to biology. Nature is the best nanotechnologist. Within the realm of nanobiology exist the most basic and functional structures and mechanisms that make life what it is. Nature's fundamental mechanisms and chemical processes occur at the nanoscale. Why was this size domain selected for to conduct the business of life in all of its complexity? Was it because of the need for fast manufacture and distribution of nutrients and energy? Was it that phenomena at the nanoscale actually opened doors for the first living things? Below or near the nanoscale exist atoms and molecules, which by themselves react stochastically and, as it were, without direction. Above the nanoscale, moving into the realm of the micron, the time scale of reaction slows, and total surface area becomes drastically reduced. The nanoscale is the first domain in which there is manipulation, control, and integration of atoms and molecules to form materials, structures, devices, and systems.

Were the structures required to manipulate, control, and integrate atoms and molecules involved in the Krebs cycle, the Calvin cycle, the electron transport system, photosystems I and II, protein synthesis, and the phosphorylation of ADP to ATP by necessity bionanomaterials? For example, all metabolic pathways are regulated by enzymes that exist at the nanoscale. Genetic materials comprise a unique class of nanomaterials. An example of a system or hierarchy on the macroscopic level is given by structural tendon fascicles comprised of microfibrils (3.5 nm) that wrap into subfibrils (10–20 nm) that finally form fibrils (50–500 nm). The macroscopic expression of these nanocomponents results in a tendon that can range from 10 to 50 cm in length [28]. Apatite (calcium phosphate) crystals with a 5-nm diameter and ranging from 20 to 200 nm in length are bound by collagen fibers that comprise bone tissue [28].

Some commonly known molecular nanoscale structures that occur in living things are amino acids (0.42–0.67 nm), nucleotides (0.81–0.87 nm), monosaccharides (1 nm), heme (1 nm), and phosphatidylcholine (2–3 nm) [28]. Examples of proteins include insulin (2.2 nm), hemoglobin (7.0 nm), ATP synthase (10 nm) [29], RNA polymerase (15 nm) [30], ribosomes (20–25 nm) [31], γ-globulin (26 nm), fibrinogen (50 nm), and glycogen (150 nm) [28]. Examples of mesoscopic structures, some with dimensions measured in nanometers, that house the bionanomaterials listed previously include mitochondria (500 nm–3 μm) [9], chloroplasts (4 μm), viruses (10–200 nm), lysosomes (700 nm), and red blood cells (8 μm) [28]. Micelles and vesicles, major components of plasma membranes that control diffusion functions, exist at the nanoscale and also are nanoscale materials.

The functional complexes of thylakoid membranes in chloroplasts range from 8 to 13 nm in size [32]. Chlorophyll, a member of an important class of molecules known as porphyrins, is the central component of photosynthesis and is approximately 1.1 nm in size [28]. Porphyrins in the form of light-harvesting mechanisms [33] and as capacitors for storage systems in computers [34] are already playing a major role in the development of nanotechnologies. Porphyrins also have been placed in arrays called "nonamers" that self-organize into nanoscale optical and magnetic materials [35]. In essence, nine free-base porphyrins were placed in a 3 × 3 columnar array by self-assembly with the intent of creating a precursor to device formation [35]. The photophysical properties of the array are controlled by selection of the coordinating metal and the choice of surface. Fig. 3 illustrates such a self-assembled porphyrin nonamers structure.

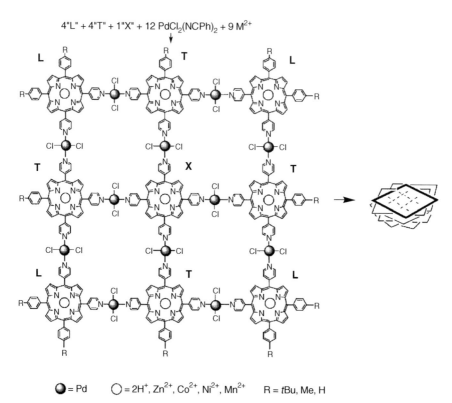

Fig. 3. Self-assembled porphyrin structure, a nonamer layer and stacks. (*From* Drain CM, Batteas JD, Flynn GW, et al. Designing supramolecular porphyrin arrays that self-organize into nanoscale optical and magnetic materials. Proc Natl Acad Sci U S A 2002;99:6498; with permission.)

Biomimetics is the study of synthetic structures that mimic or imitate structures found in biologic systems [28]. DNA, a useful and adaptable nanomaterial, is approximately 2.2 nm in thickness (the breadth of the complete helix), and each turn of the helix is approximately 3.3 nm in length [28]. Applications of DNA in nanotechnology include its use as templates [36], as nanosprings, and as components in biosensors [37]. Seemans [38] of New York University developed the concept of using DNA as a structural element. The two members of the helix are unraveled at the ends and then are spliced with another DNA molecule. In this way, arrays of DNA molecules can be assembled in a specific manner in two or three dimensions. According to researchers at Duke University, the development of structures based on DNA as a "general assembly method for nanopatterned materials" is expected to impact electronics, sensors, medicine, and other technologies [38]. Nanoparticles are also used to package DNA [39]. Shell cross-linked polymers, nanoscale biomimetic materials similar to globular proteins, have been shown to compact DNA effectively. The purpose of the packaging is to develop materials for gene-therapy applications [39]. In another study, the DNA of *Drosophila melanogaster* has been labeled by ultrabright silver plasmon resonant-particle optical reporters 60 to 100 nm in diameter [40]. Fig. 4 depicts the 3C band of the *Drosophila* chromosome without additional enhancement of the signal [40]. Incidentally, single-metal nanoparticle imaging can be accomplished by using an all-optical method [41].

Synthesis of multilayer films can be applied in biomineralization processes that involve incorporating calcium into soft living tissue to make bone, thereby reversing the degenerative effects of osteoporosis [25]. The animal and plant worlds have manufactured biocomposites from the nanometer to the macroscopic scale [42]. According to M. Sarikaya [42],

> It may ultimately be possible to construct a molecular erector set in which different types of proteins, each designed to perform a desired function, eg, nucleation or growth modification, could assemble into intricate, hybrid structures composed of minerals and proteins. This type of construction

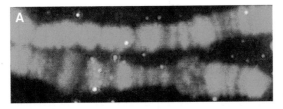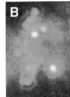

Fig. 4. Photographs of the region of the *Drosophila* X chromosome (band 3C) specifically labeled with colloidally prepared blue plasmon resonant particles (PRPs) using the in situ hybridization protocol. (*A*) The 3C band of the X-chromosome with PRP labels. (*B*) A close-up of the 3C band showing a high density of PRP labels. (*From* Schultz S, Smith DR, Mock JJ, et al. Single-target molecule detection with non-bleaching multicolor optical immunolabels. Proc Natl Acad Sci U S A 2000;97:996; with permission.)

would be a giant leap toward realizing genetically engineered technological materials.

Liu et al [43] present a nanoengineering approach to supramolecular chemistry by demonstrating protein positioning on surfaces. The authors state that so-called "bottom-up" approaches that mimic nature have resulted in creative syntheses of small molecular units and large molecular motifs [43,44]. The reactivity of immobilized proteins was demonstrated by testing a nanopattern consisting of rabbit IgG (Fig. 5). Injections of mouse anti-rabbit IgG showed an increase in height, thereby indicating successful absorption of the anti-IgG [43].

Micro- and nanocontacts in biologic attachment devices are another area of biomimetic study [45]. Geckos, for example, have the ability to cling to almost any surface. Geckos exploit capillary forces (sticking to wet surfaces) and van der Waals forces (sticking to dry surfaces) between the clinging mechanism and the specific surface. The clinging mechanism is comprised of

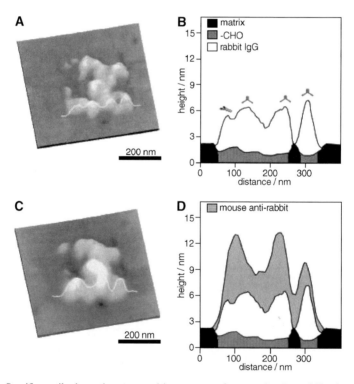

Fig. 5. Specific antibody–antigen recognition process for proteins immobilized on nano-patterns. (*A,B*) Rabbit IgG immobilized on a nanosquare and cursor profile. (*C,D*) The same area after the introduction of mouse anti-rabbit IgG and cursor profile. The increase in height indicates a positive reaction with the anti-rabbit IgG. (*From* Liu G-Y, Amro NA. Positioning protein molecules on surfaces: nanoengineering approach to supramolecular chemistry. Proc Natl Acad Sci U S A 2002:99:5165; with permission.)

200-nm keratin hairs densely packed on the feet of the gecko [46]. Researchers from the Center for Mesoscience and Nanotechnology at the University of Manchester (Manchester, UK) created a similar array comprised of fibers manufactured by electron beam lithography, and it generated an adhesion nearly 30% as good as that of the gecko [46]. Fig. 6 shows a comparison of natural gecko and biomimetic systems.

Nature has capitalized on the physical properties of nanoscale biologic materials. Materials and systems at the nanoscale operate to perform the vital functions required by living things, so it is no wonder that scientists are attempting to mimic nature's accomplishments. The next step in the nanotechnology adventure is in the realm of nanomedicine, where nanotechnology is expected to contribute to significant developments improving the health of human beings.

Nanomedicine

According to the NIH "roadmap"

> Nanomedicine, an offshoot of nanotechnology, refers to highly specific medical intervention at the molecular scale for curing disease or repairing damaged tissues, such as bone, muscle, or nerve. A nanometer is one-billionth of a meter, too small to be seen with a conventional lab microscope. It is at this size scale—about 100 nanometers or less—that biological molecules and structures inside living cells operate.

Freitas [47] the definition to include nanodevices:

> Nanomedicine may be defined as the monitoring, repair, construction and control of human biological systems at the molecular level, using engineered nanodevices and nanostructures.

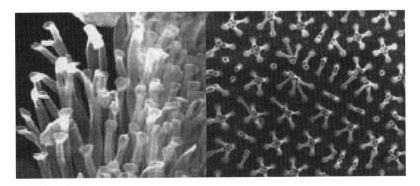

Fig. 6. (*Left*) Because of the 200-nm keratin hairs on their feet, Geckos can cling even to dry surfaces when upside down because of van der Waals forces and to wet surfaces because of capillary action. (*Right*) Thirty percent adhesion attained with plastic fibers made by electron beam lithography: a good example of biomimetic technology. (*From* The Center for Mesoscience and Nanotechnology, University of Manchester, Manchester, UK; with permission).

This statement, however, is somewhat restrictive. The definition should be expanded to include the "monitoring, repair, construction, and control of human biologic systems at the molecular and macroscopic levels." Replacement tissues and organs and biologic sensors made of nanomaterials will play a major role in medical therapeutic devices. For example, synthetic muscles comprised of carbon nanotubes [48] and synthetic larynx systems are currently under investigation (personal communication, Arlen Meyers, MD, School of Medicine, University of Colorado Health Sciences Center, 2004).

The realm of nanomedicine includes delivery systems for drug and gene therapies, body or organ imaging and labeling with nanostructured materials, surgical tools (eg, nanotweezers), nanoprobes aiding diagnostic procedures, molecular recognition, smart nanosensors with communication capability, and synthetic implantable therapeutic devices. Ancillary nano-tech developments in the computer field will enhance data gathering and modeling capabilities. Another category of technologies, nano- or molec-ular-scale machines ("nanobots"), is farther in the future and is not addressed in this article. According to the nanomedicine initiatives in the NIH "Roadmap," the benefits of nanomedicine are expected to be realized within 10 years [49]. The objectives of therapeutic nanodevices are to provide minimally invasive therapies with high functionality [9], site-specific targeting of disease, and, ultimately, reporting capability for efficient monitoring. The National Aeronautics and Space Administration (working in minimal-mass therapeutics) and the National Cancer Institute (working on early-detection programs) recently agreed to a collaborative relationship to investigate the creation of nanoscale therapeutic platforms [50].

According to Mario I. Romero of the University of Texas Southwest Medical Center and the Texas Scottish Rite Hospital (personal communi-cation, Dr. Mario I. Romero, Director, Scottish Rite Hospital for Children, Dallas, TX, July 2004), the development of strategies to foster axonal regrowth and target reinnervation could markedly improve functional recovery in persons who suffer from traumatic nerve injuries and various nerve diseases. At these institutions, studies have been conducted to understand and manipulate neuron regrowth and reconnection mechanisms. To that end, neurotrophin gene therapy, mouse genetics, and, more recently, bioengineering tissue repair have been under investigation. The understand-ing of the cellular and molecular mechanisms that mediate the neuronal response to injury and influence axonal grow is incomplete. The recent developments of nano-sized materials and systems (eg, QDs) may lead to the development of better imaging and analytic tools for the study of nerve injury and to the development of novel repair strategies. QDs can be used as unique fluorescent tags of specific cellular and molecular events and can be used to analyze temporal dynamics in living cells. In addition, nanoparticles and nanocapsules could be effective delivery systems for drug and gene therapies, possibly providing a viable alternative to current methods.

Wu et al [51], also a researcher at the University of Texas Southwest Medical Center, and his collaborators describe a strategy using poly (butylcyanoacryolate) nanospheres of approximately 30-nm diameter for use in "controlled and targeted drug delivery." A potential application of the proposed mechanism in the battle against Alzheimer's disease is to deliver therapeutics across the blood–brain barrier and to determine the location of the abnormal protein plaques or tangles that lead to impaired transmission of nerve signals in the brain. According to Lockman et al [52] of the Department of Pharmaceutical Science at the Texas Tech Health Sciences Center, the advantages of nanoparticle carrier technology are its ability (1) to penetrate the blood–brain barrier, and (2) to deliver the drugs at a slower rate. Slower and controlled delivery of the therapeutic drug has the potential to eliminate whole-scale peripheral toxicity. The authors also review nanoparticle strategies, synthesis, and transport mechanisms [52].

Perhaps one of the most significant proposed applications of nanomedicine is in the domain of cancer diagnosis and treatment. The National Cancer Institute's (NCI) Alliance for Nanotechnology in Cancer (http://nano. cancer.gov/) is testimony to the seriousness with which nanotechnology's promise is taken. The following excerpt is taken from the NCI's Web site:

> The NCI Alliance for Nanotechnology in Cancer is a comprehensive, systematized initiative encompassing the public and private sectors, designed to accelerate the application of the best capabilities of nanotechnology to cancer. Toward the end of eliminating suffering and death from cancer, the National Cancer Institute is engaged in efforts to harness the power of nanotechnology to radically change the way we diagnose, image and treat cancer. Nanotechnology can provide the technical power and tools that will enable those developing new diagnostics, therapeutics, and preventives to keep pace with today's explosion in knowledge.

In July 2004 the NCI has developed a comprehensive plan called the "Cancer Nanotechnology Plan" [53]. Molecular imaging and early detection, in vivo imaging, multifunctional therapeutics, and nanotechnology as a research enabler are some of the areas discussed in the plan.

A recent article by Gao et al [54] summarizes research focused on in vivo cancer targeting and imaging. The use of QDs is intended to facilitate the imaging of molecular, cellular, structural, and functional entities [55,56]. Semiconductor particles with nanometer dimensions have been tethered successfully to biomolecules that have biorecognition capability, such as nucleic acids, polypeptides, and immune-active moieties for use as fluorescent probes [54,57–59]. Gao et al [54] were the first to demonstrate combined QD targeting and imaging in live animals. They developed a multifunctional nanoparticle QD probe for targeting and imaging cancer in live animals. The researchers managed to encapsulate luminescent QDs with a polymer and link them to "tumor-targeting ligands and drug delivery functionalities" [54]. Research continues to investigate the metabolic effects and clearance of the QD probes injected into the live animals. The authors propose that the polymer-coated QDs could be cleared from the body by slow filtration and excretion by the kidneys [54].

Applications of nanomedicine will eventually be used in all fields of medical study, devices, and applications. Learning the lessons from nature through biomimetic studies and understanding the breadth and scope of the convergent character of nanomedicine can help investigators arrive at the destination quicker. Physics, chemistry, biology, and engineering all come together in the present and emerging field of nanomedicine. One of the uses of nanophotonics, for example, is the application of nanotechnology to the imaging of biologic and medical systems. Nanomedicine will change the way medical goals are accomplished. Is nanomedicine disruptive? Yes. Is it convergent? Absolutely yes.

Nanotechnology and otology, otolaryngology, and otorhinolaryngology

Nanotechnology is expected to have comprehensive effects on all fields of medicine, and otolaryngology is no exception. Nano-otology is the application of nanomedicine to diseases and disorders of the ear. The fields of otolaryngology (ear and throat) and otorhinolaryngology (ear, nose, and throat, or more commonly ENT) also involve study of ear disorders. Nearly every use of nanomaterials and nanotechnology from biology or medicine can be applied in otolaryngology. Some of the topics have been presented in this article. Salata [17] of the Sir William Dunn School of Pathology at Oxford University compiled a list of the applications of nanomaterials in biology and medicine, all of which are applicable in otolaryngology. The list includes fluorescent biologic labels, drug and gene delivery, biodetection of pathogens, detection of proteins, probing of DNA structures, tissue engineering, thermal ablation of tumors, separation and purification of molecules and cells, and MRI contrast enhancement.

With regard to otologic developments, technology for cochlear implants was developed by Dormer [60] in 1987 at the University of Oklahoma. Since then, Dormer [61] has been involved in testing the external magnetic field response of nanomaterials in the middle ear epithelium. NIH-funded programs in the Dormer laboratory currently focus on the use of nano-technology in otologic therapies [60]. Recent developments include the applications of silica-coated supramagnetic magnetite nanoparticles (MNPs) [62]. MRI enhancement, intravascular targeted delivery of therapeutics, and biosensor applications are some of the applications of supra-paramagnetic nanoparticles [60].

The study was done in collaboration with NanoBioMagnetics, Inc, (NBMI), of Oklahoma City, Oklahoma (www.nanobmi.com). NBMI is engaged in the development and commercialization of magnetically responsive nanoparticle technologies for human health applications, particularly in the emerging area of organ-assisting devices. In otologic applications, MNPs can be externally implanted and thereby cause tissue movement when an oscillating magnetic field is applied. The result is amplification of the auditory response [59]. In addition, MNPs can be used as a vectored drug-delivery system in the site-specific targeting of inner ear diseases and disorders. The middle ear epithelium consists of a tympanic membrane or ossicles. In one application, MNP particles were internalized by of magnetic force–enhanced endocytosis in which a rare-earth magnet was used to fix the MNP nanoparticles into the tissue [61]. Dormer et al [61] showed that a "physiologically relevant biomechanical function" mitigated by the MNP is produced in response to an external magnetic field. Fig. 7 illustrates an MNP application.

The presence of the silica-coated magnetic nanoparticles caused no indication of pathologic response although long-term toxicity is a concern should the silica shielding fail [61]. In concluding, Dormer et al [61] stated that silica-encapsulated magnetite nanoparticles can be used in conjunction with an external magnetic field to produce biomechanical forces in the middle ear, can be implanted in epithelia without producing toxic effects, and remain viable for at least 15 days. The amplitudes of displacements in ossicular chain displacements are comparable to those produced at the tympanic membrane in fresh-frozen human temporal bones [61]. An in vivo sound experiment using nanoparticles has been accomplished.

Oral cancer is a major area of research for otolaryngologists. One means of mitigating oral cancers within range of a radiation source is thermal ablation. This field has made significant strides as the result of advances in nanotechnology [63]. For example, gold-silica nanoshells have been recently exploited to destroy tumors with near-infrared (NIR) thermal therapy. Because therapeutic doses of heat are applied by an external NIR source, the procedure is suitable for treatment of oral cancer. The metal nanoshells are

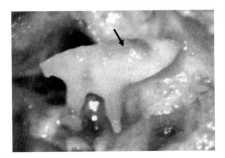

Fig. 7. The K. Dormer group's work on the incus of guinea pigs is illustrated in this figure. The arrow shows where MNPs were placed and internalized by the external magnetic field. No inflammatory response was noted after implantation. (*From* Dormer KJ, Seeney CE, Lewelling K, et al. Internalization of nanoparticles in middle ear epithelium and response to external magnetic field. Biomaterials, in press; with permission.)

nanoparticles with tunable optical resonance [63]. Experiments with human breast carcinoma cells irradiated with NIR radiation showed morbidity for cells incubated with metal nanoshells. Cells not containing nanoshells survived the NIR exposure intact. Fig. 8 shows gross pathology after in vivo treatment with nanoshells and NIR laser [63]. According to the authors, the combination of NIR radiation and nanoshells, both relatively benign in nature, has achieved localized irreversible photothermal ablation of tumor tissue both in vivo and in vitro [63].

The nose is also receiving attention. Research into olfactory systems is being conducted at the University of Colorado. The vision of the Cellular Engineering Microsystems (CEMS) Center at the University of Colorado is as follows [64]:

> To conduct path finding research at the intersection of Micro/Nano Technology and Molecular/Cellular Biology with the specific purpose of inventing and developing enabling technologies based on Micro and Nano engineering to enable research for enhancing the detection, monitoring, and treatment of disease.

One of the projects that involve CEMS researchers can be certainly classified as otorhinolarygologic in nature. Restrepo and his group [64] at the University of Colorado Health Sciences Center and Mahajan at the University of Colorado at Boulder Department of Mechanical Engineering have conducted research into the design and implementation of neuronal

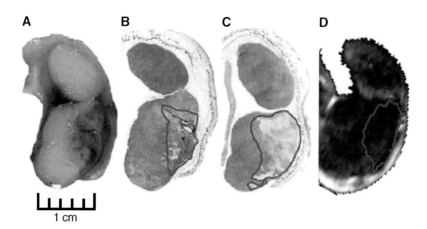

1 cm

Fig. 8. Following nanoshell and near-infrared laser treatment, the tumor tissue shows signs of thermal damage such as coagulation, cell shrinkage, and loss of nuclear staining. (*A*) Gross pathology reveals hemorrhaging and loss of tissue birefringence. (*B*) Detection of nanoshells by silver staining (outlined in red). (*C*) Tissue damage within the area occupied by nanoshells shown by hematoxylin/eosin staining. (*D*) MRTI (temperature sensitive magnetic resonance imaging) calculations revealed an area of irreversible thermal damage. (*From* Hirsch LR, Stafford RJ, Bankson JA, et al. Nanoshell-mediated near infrared thermal therapy of tumors under magnetic resonance guidance. Proc Natl Acad Sci U S A 2003;100:13549; with permission.)

implants with intent to develop a hybrid-brain interface. The research team used the olfactory system of mice as the test-bed for CEMS-based implants. The use of CEMS-based implants in the olfactory bulb will allow testing of the mechanisms that allow ensembles of neurons to respond to odors in awake, normally behaving mice undergoing learning [64].

Nearly every development in nanomedicine is expected to impact otology, otolaryngology, and otorhinolaryngology. This article has discussed only a few possible applications. Plastic surgery will certainly be affected by nanotechnology. For example, research is currently being conducted on the generation of nanofacets for bone regeneration [65]. Advances in neural fusion using micro- and nanoelectrodes may have the ability to reconnect nerves and restore functionality. Alaryngeal speech mechanisms and devices are currently under consideration (personal communication, Arlen Meyers, MD, School of Medicine, University of Colorado Health Sciences Center, 2004). Many more applications will be developed.

Summary and future considerations

This article has attempted to provide a useful overview of the new and exciting world of nanotechnology. It has attempted to define nanotechnology, has traced the history of nanotechnology, and has discussed the most recent advances in nanomaterials. It has demonstrated how nature has been the premier nanotechnology system and how investigators should follow suit. Nanotechnologic advances in medicine will surely affect health and longevity. Will there be a cure for cancer from nanomedical research? The hope of delivering that cure certainly is a driving force in nanomedical research. Will nanomedicine aid physicians in diagnosis, prevention, and cure? Will advances in nanomedicine lower the cost of maintaining good health? All these questions should be answered within the reader's lifetime. Cancer, Alzheimer'sdisease, hearing loss, and numerous other ailments now await an aging individual. The nano-cavalry may cut them off at the pass.

The first wide-scale application of nanoparticles will probably be in drug delivery [51,52]. QD and particle targeting and imaging technology are well developed and are receiving considerable attention from the commercial sector. Nano-ceramic applications in tissue engineering and orthopedics have also made headway into the commercial realm [65]. The concomitant development of photonics technology, another enabling technology, has a natural synergy with nanotechnology. Great discoveries are expected because of this synergy.

The age of nanobots that can scour artery walls and remove plaque buildup and others that can perform local surgery or cellular repair may be further down the road. An enormous technologic sophistication is required to produce such nanobots, especially devices that can function viably in an aqueous system. Someday, perhaps, they will become players in the health care arena, but a huge leap in the technologic paradigm will be required. The current state of the art of the more mundane nanomaterials is quite exciting as it is. The reader is urged to continue reading, listening, discussing, and, indeed, researching. The literature is burgeoning with such rich research in targeting gene delivery systems [66]; the viral assembly of oriented QD nanowires [67]; applications of bacterial spores in nanobiotechnology [68]; ultrasensitive magnetic biosensors for homogeneous immunoassay [69]; building nanostructures from the bottom up to emulate biologic processes [70]; large, porous, Trojan-horse particle carriers of nanoparticles for drug delivery [71]; nanopatterned molecular arrays from fusion protein templates [72]; and the inhibition of chymotrypsin by surface-bound nanoparticle-based receptors [73].

It is important to consider the societal implications of nanoscience, nanotechnology, and nanomedicine. New issues will arise. What if everyone lives to an age of 110 years? Will there be a population of healthy and robust 110-year-olds, or will it be one made feeble by other diseases not yet conquered by nanomedicine—or new diseases brought on by these technologic advances? Will investigators find the fountain of youth or open a Pandora's box [74]? Will the population of the earth exceed its carrying capacity? Sohail Inayatullah [74] asks

> Q. What are the pulls of the future, the images that define where we are going? A. The images are obvious, a long healthy, high quality life. Q. What are the pushes, the quantifiable drivers? A. Economics, an aging society, funding for high-tech interventions, globalization. Q. What are the weights, the structures or patterns that make change difficult? A. Class, gender, the medical system and of course evolution.

Many questions must be advanced and discussed in a public forum. Nanomedicine is the logical and natural path in the development of science and technology—to make things better by making them smaller. Are investigators now on the threshold of unraveling nature's secrets? They should proceed with caution—but not wait too long. It is important to form the partnerships necessary to encourage research. The technology will advance in any case. Medical professionals should participate as well-informed partners in what will certainly comprise the next industrial revolution.

References

[1] The American heritage dictionary of the English language. New York: Houghton Mifflin; 1969.
[2] Webster's third new international dictionary. Springfield (MA): Merriam-Webster; 1986.
[3] Webster's encyclopedic unabridged dictionary of the English language. New York: Random House; 1994.
[4] National Nanotechnology Initiative. Available at: www.nano.gov. Accessed September 2004.

[5] Fisher E, Bennett-Woods D, Hornyak L, et al. for the Task Force on Nano-Ethics and Societal Impacts. Welcoming the nano age. Colorado Nanotechnology Initiative, September 2003.

[6] Roco MC. Senior Adviser for Nanotechnology, National Science Foundation (NSF), Chair US Nanoscale Science, Engineering and Technology (NSTC's NSET), Dec. 2003.

[7] Modzelewski M. President, National Nanobusiness Alliance, 2003.

[8] Murdock S, Crosby S, Stein B, editors. Regional, state, and local initiatives in nanotechnology. Report of the National Nanotechnology Initiative Workshop. Arlington, Virginia, September 30–October 1, 2003.

[9] Bhushan B, editor. Springer handbook of nanotechnology. Berlin: Springer-Verlag; 2004.

[10] Roco MC, Bainbridge WS, editors. Societal implications of nanoscience and nanotechnology. Report of the Subcommittee on Nanoscale Science, Engineering and Technology Workshop. Arlington (VA): National Science Foundation/Kluwer Academic Publishers; 2001.

[11] Barber DJ, Freestone IC. An investigation of the origin of the colour of the Lycurgus cup by analytical transmission electron microscopy. Archaeometry 1990;32:33.

[12] Boyle R. Sceptical Chymist. London: Henry Hall, 1661.

[13] Faraday M. The Bakerian lecture: Experimental Relations of Gold (and other Metals) to Light. Philosophical Transactions of the Royal Society, London: Richard Taylor and William Francis; 147, 1847, Part I, 145.

[14] Hornyak GL. Characterization and optical theory of nanometal/porous alumina composite membranes [PhD dissertation UMI number 3064440]. Fort Collins (CO): Colorado State University; 1997.

[15] Ledoux G, Ehbrecht M, Guillois O, et al. Silicon as a candidate carrier for ERE. Astronomy and Astrophysics 1998;333:L39–42.

[16] Witt AN, Gordon KD, Furton DG. "Silicon nanoparticlces: source of extended red emission. The Astrophysical Journal 1998;501:L111–5.

[17] Salata OV. Applications of nanoparticles in biology and medicine. J Nanobiotechnology 2004;2:3.

[18] Hirsch LR, Stafford RJ, Bankson JA, et al. Targeted photothermal tumor therapy using metal nanoshells. In: Proceedings of the Second Joint Engineering in Medicine and Biology Society/Biomedical engineering Society Conference. Houston (TX): 2002;1:530.

[19] Oldenberg S, Averitt R, Westcott S, et al. Nanoengineering of optical resonances. Chem Phys Lett 1998;28:243.

[20] Oldenberg S, Averitt R, Westcott S, et al. Surface enhanced Raman scattering in the near infrared using metal nanoshell substrates. J Chem Phys 1999;111:4729.

[21] Feynman R. There's plenty of room at the bottom, California Institute of Technology. Engineering & Science Magazine 1960;23:22.

[22] Uldrich J, Newberry D. The next big thing is really small: how nanotechnology will change the future of your business. New York: Crown Business; 2003.

[23] Eigler DM, Lutz CP, Rudge WE. An atomic switch realized with the scanning tunneling microscope. Nature 1991;352:600.

[24] Drexler KE. Engines of creation. New York: Random House; 1986.

[25] Cao G. Nanostructures and nanomaterials: synthesis, properties and applications. London: Imperial College Press; 2004.

[26] Shih HD, Jona F, Jepsen DW, et al. Atomic underlayer formation during the reaction of Ti{0001} with nitrogen. Surface Science 1976;60:445.

[27] Bradley JS, Schmid G. Noble metal nanoparticles. In: Schmid G, editor. Nanoparticles. Weinheim, Germany: Wiley-VCH; 2004. p. 270.

[28] Poole CP, Owens FJ. Introduction to nanotechnology. New York: John Wiley & Sons; 2003.

[29] Yoshida M, Muneyuki E, Hisabori T. ATP-synthase–a marvelous rotary engine of the cell. Nature Rev Mol Cell Biol 2001;2:669.

[30] Darst SA. Bacterial RNA polymerase. Curr Op Struct Biol 2001;11:155.

[31] Ban N, Nissen P, Hansen J, et al. The complete atomic structure of the large ribosomal subunit at 2.4 Å resolution. Science 2000;289:905.

[32] Staehelin LA. Chloroplast structure: from chlorophyll granules to supra-molecular architecture of thylakoid membranes. Photosynth Res 2003;76:185.

[33] Li J, Lindsey JS. Synthesis of multi-porphyrin-pthalocyanine light-harvesting arrays. Presented at the National Meeting of the American Chemical Society. Anaheim, CA. March, 1999.

[34] Kuhr W. Integration of molecular components into silicon electronic devices. Presented at the University of Denver, Denver (CO). February 11, 2004.

[35] Drain CM, Batteas JD, Flynn GW, et al. Self-assembly of supramolecular porphyrin arrays that self-organize into nanoscale optical and magnetic materials. Proc Natl Acad Sci U S A 2002;99:6498–502.

[36] Pickles T. Using DNA as a template material for nanomaterials synthesis. Rensselaer Polytechnic Institute, 1998. Available at: http://www.rpi.edu/dept/materials/COURSES/NANO/pickles/.

[37] Liu X, Farmerle W, Schuster S, et al. Molecular beacons for DNA biosensors with micrometer to submicrometer dimensions. Anal Biochem 2000;283:56.

[38] Liu D, Park SH, Reif JH, et al. DNA nanotubes self-assembled from triple-crossover tiles as templates for conductive nanowires. Proc Natl Acad Sci U S A 2004;101:717.

[39] Thurmond KB, Remsen EE, Kowalewski T, et al. Packaging of DNA by shell crosslinked nanoparticles. Nucleic Acids Res 1999;27:2966.

[40] Schultz S, Smith DR, Mock JJ, et al. Single-target molecule detection with non-bleaching multicolor optical immunolabels. Proc Natl Acad Sci U S A 2000;97:996.

[41] Cognet L, Tardin C, Boyer D, et al. Single metal nanoparticle imaging for protein detection in cells. Proc Natl Acad Sci U S A 2003;100:11350.

[42] Sarikaya M. biomimetics materials fabrication through biology. Proc Natl Acad Sci U S A 1999;96:14183.

[43] Liu G-Y, Amro NA. Positioning protein molecules on surfaces: nanoengineering approach to supramolecular chemistry. Proc Natl Acad Sci U S A 2002;99:5165.

[44] Atwood JL, Lehn JM, Gokel GW, et al. Comprehensive supramolecular chemistry. New York: Pergamon; 1996.

[45] Arzt E, Gorb S, Spolenak R. From micro to nano contacts in biological attachment devices. Proc Natl Acad Sci U S A 2003;100:10603.

[46] Lerner EJ. Biomimetic nanotechnology: researchers mimic biology to form nanoscale devices. The Industrial Physicist 2004;10(4):18.

[47] Freitas RA Jr. Nanomedicine. Georgetown (TX): Landes Bioscience; 1999.

[48] Baughman RH, Cui C, Zakhidov AA, et al. Carbon nanotube artificial muscles. Nanotube-99 Workshop. East Lansing, Michigan. July 24-27, 1999.

[49] National Institutes of Health. Roadmap. Available at: http://nihroadmap.nih.gov/nano medicine/index.asp.

[50] National Aeronautics and Space Agency/National Institutes of Health. Available at: http. nasa-nci.arc.nasa.gov.

[51] Wu A, Kolla H, Samudra N, et al. Molecular therapeutics: synthesis of poly (butylcyanoacrylate) nanoparticles for drug delivery [abstract]. ACS 2004.

[52] Lockman PR, Mumper RJ, Khan MA, et al. Nanoparticle technology for drug delivery across the blood-brain barrier. Drug Dev Ind Pharm 2002;28:1.

[53] Cancer nanotechnology plan: a strategic initiative to transform clinical oncology and basic research through the directed application of nanotechnology National Institutes of Health and the National Cancer Institute; 2004. US Department of Health and Human Services.

[54] Gao X, Cui Y, Levinson RM, et al. In vivo cancer targeting and imaging with semiconductor quantum dots. Nat Biotechnol 2004;22:969.

[55] Jain RK, Stroh M. Zooming in and out with quantum dots. Nat. Biotechnol 2004;22959.

[56] Jain RK, Munn LL, Fukumura D. Dissecting tumor pathophysiology using intravital microscopy. Nat Rev Cancer 2002;2:266.

[57] Jaiswal JK, Mattoussi H, Mauro JM, et al. Long-term multiple color imaging of live cells using quantum dot bioconjugates. Nat Biotechnol 2003;21:47.

[58] Ackerman ME, Chan WCW, Laakkonen P, et al. Nanocrystal targeting in vivo. Proc Natl Acad Sci U S A 2002;99:12617.

[59] Chan WCW, Nie SM. Quantum dot bioconjugates using an engineered recombinant protein. Science 1998;281:2016.

[60] Dormer KJ. Available at: http://w3.ouhsc.edu/gpibs/GPiBS04/Biosketches/Dormer%202004.pdf.

[61] Dormer KJ, Seeney CE, Lewelling K, et al. Internalization of nanoparticles in middle ear epithelium and response to external magnetic field. Biomaterials, in press.

[62] Gan RZ, Dyer RK, Wood MW, et al. Mass loading on ossicles and middle ear function. Ann Otol Rhinol Layngol 2001;110(5):478.

[63] Hirsch LR, Stafford RJ, Bankson JA, et al. Nanoshell-mediated near infrared thermal therapy of tumors under magnetic resonance guidance. Proc Natl Acad Sci U S A 2003;100: 13549.

[64] Restrepo D, Finch DS, Zane R, et al. CEMS-based chronic brain implants. Available at: http://cems.colorado.edu/resources.

[65] Ma J, Wong H, Kong LB, et al. Biomimetic processing of nanocrystallite bioactive apatite coating on titanium. Nanotechnology 2003;14:619.

[66] Schatzlein AG. Targeting of synthetic gene delivery systems. J Biomed Biotechnol 2003; 2:149.

[67] Mao C, Flynn CE, Hayhurst A, et al. Viral assembly of oriented quantum dot nanowires. Proc Natl Acad Sci U S A 2003;100:6946.

[68] Ricca E, Cutting SM. Emerging applications of bacterial spores in nanobiotechnology. J Nanobiotechnology 2003;1:6.

[69] Chemla YR, Grossman HL, Poon Y, et al. Ultrasensitive magnetic biosensor for homogeneous immunoassay. Proc Natl Acad Sci U S A 2000;97:14268.

[70] Seeman NC, Belcher AM. Emulating biology: building nanostructures from the bottom up. Proc Natl Acad Sci U S A 2002;99:6451.

[71] Tsapis T, Bennet D, Jackson B, et al. Trojan particles: large porous carriers of nanoparticles for drug delivery. Proc Natl Acad Sci U S A 2002;99:12001.

[72] Moll D, Huber C, Schlegel B, et al. S-layer-streptavidin fusion as template for nanopatterned molecular arrays. Proc Natl Acad Sci U S A 2002;99:14646.

[73] Fischer NO, McIntosh CM, Simard JM, et al. Inhibition of chymotrypsin through surface binding using nanoparticle-based receptors. Proc Natl Acad Sci U S A 2002;99:5018.

[74] Inayatullah S. Presentation at the Conference of the Australia Divisions of General Practice. Brisbane, Australia, November 22, 2003.

ELSEVIER
SAUNDERS

Otolaryngol Clin N Am
38 (2005) 295–305

OTOLARYNGOLOGIC
CLINICS
OF NORTH AMERICA

Progress Towards Seamless Tissue Fusion for Wound Closure

Stephen T. Flock, PhD*, Kevin S. Marchitto, PhD

Rocky Mountain Biosystems, 2207 Jackson Street, Golden, CO, 80401, USA

The most basic wound closure techniques, including mechanical (eg, plant thorns, ant jaws) and thermal (eg, hot liquids, burning applicators) methods, date back thousands of years and. Modern devices and materials for connecting or sealing tissues have increased in sophistication. However, most rely on the same fundamental principals as in the past. Mechanical closures have progressed to include natural and synthetic sutures, staples, tapes, and adhesive compounds, whereas modern thermal closure is achieved by relatively controlled cauterization with electronic devices. Despite the use of advanced materials and technology, some fundamental problems remain, including leakage, dehiscence, infection, and iatrogenic related trauma.

The ideal closure would restore the original integrity of the tissue. The seal would be physiologically and mechanically seamless, be fluid- and air-tight, and have a tensile strength and degree of elasticity suited to the tissue. Additionally, it would be aesthetically acceptable, inexpensive to achieve, and easy to apply even in minimally invasive surgeries. This paper reviews tissue fusion devices and techniques that may one day provide us with such biologically invisible wound closures.

Traditional closures

Arguably, modern closures, such as sutures and staples, ultimately provide a seamless closure once the tissue heals. This is particularly so in the case where absorbable materials and good technique are used [1]. The

---

This work was supported in part by Grant No. 1 R43 HL075886-01A1 from the National Institutes of Health.

* Corresponding author.

E-mail address: stflock@biofusionary.com (S.T. Flock).

0030-6665/05/$ - see front matter © 2005 Elsevier Inc. All rights reserved.
doi:10.1016/j.otc.2004.10.029
oto.theclinics.com

current research in traditional closures revolves around a search for new applicators, materials, and techniques. For example, suture-mediated closure devices have been successfully introduced for arterial access closure [2,3]. New materials include natural (eg, polylactic acid) and synthetic polymers that are often absorbable and have superior biocompatibility. For example, degradable thermoplastic polymers have recently been developed and tested that are able to change their shape after they are heated [4]. Their shape-memory capability enables bulky implants to be placed in the body through small incisions and induce complex tissue deformations. A smart degradable suture has been developed to illustrate the potential of these shape-memory thermoplastics in biomedical applications.

Although traditional suturing remains a popular method for effectuating wound closure, the use of staples and staplers as a closure technique has become increasingly popular, mostly because they are easy to use and reduce procedural time. However, staples are expensive and inelastic.

Modern adhesives

In recent years, synthetic and natural adhesives have been introduced as wound closure products that promise to achieve better and faster wound closure [5]. The concept of using glues for tissue fixation is not new [6]; the use of fibrin glues dates back almost 100 years.

Cyanoacrylates

Over the past two decades, the use of cyanoacrylate (generically referred to as *super glue*) as a tissue adhesive has been varied and widespread among the surgical specialties. The kind of super glue one finds at the local hardware store consists of methyl or ethyl 2-cyanoacrylate. This formulation was studied extensively for its potential medical uses, but has been discarded as a result of toxicity [7].

However, based on the finding that the substitution of longer carbon chains on the molecule reduced toxicity and improved elasticity in the final product, a series of adhesives have since been developed, such as isobutyl-cyanoacrylate, 2-cyano-butyl-acrylate, and, recently, 2-octyl cyanoacrylate which has been introduced to the market as Dermabond (Ethicon Inc., Closure Medical Corp., Raleigh, NC) and is the only super glue approved in the United States for use in humans. Toriumi et al [8] have published a useful review on the use of 2-octyl cyanoacrylate in wound closure.

When used for skin closure in facial plastic surgery, it was also found that 2-octyl cyanoacrylate resulted in a statistically significant, superior cosmetic outcome and a greater degree of patient satisfaction at 1 year when compared with sutures [8]. In another study involving closure of head and neck incisions, the adhesive provided faster skin closure and there were no differences in complications when compared with the suture control group [9].

In addition to its surgical adhesive indication, Dermabond was granted approval by the Food and Drug Administration (FDA) in January 2001 for use as a barrier against common bacterial microbes, including certain Staphylococci, pseudomonads, and *Escherichia coli*. In a seminal study, contaminated wounds closed with sutures had higher infection rates compared with those sealed with topical tissue adhesive [10].

There are some limitations in using cyanoacrylates. For instance, leakage of the glue into the wound prevents adequate approximation and results in a widening of the scar, as opposed to the fine line scar that results from traditional sutures. Furthermore, the glue does not provide the mechanism for wound edge eversion, which is one of the basic axioms of wound closure technique. Care must be taken not to touch the glue while it polymerizes, and one of the shortcomings of this product is the potential adherence of foreign materials, including the fingertips. This rapid curing further limits the ability of the worker to re-appose gaping wounds. Tensile strength has been an issue in some types of glued wounds, but there is some recent evidence that the acute tensile strength of a cyanoacrylate bond may be increased by providing a polymer "scaffold," which seems to ease tissue alignment and reduces problems associated with adhesive flow [11].

Fibrin

The hemostatic protein fibrin can be used to seal wound sites where traditional closure methods cannot control bleeding. It is also being developed for use in conjunction with sutures or tape to promote optimal wound integrity. Clinically, studies using fibrin sealant have shown a low rate of infection and enhanced healing [12]. Commercial preparations available in the United States, such as FDA-approved Tisseel (Tisseel Baxter Corp., Baxter International, Deerfield, IL), and others under development, such as Hemaseel HMN (Haemacure Corporation, Sarasota, FL), are fibrin tissue adhesives made from pooled blood sources [13]. In contrast, sealants from autologous donation, such as CoStasis (Angiotech Pharmaceuticals, Vancouver, British Colombia), do not have the ability to act as glues because of their relatively low fibrin concentration and are therefore only used as a hemostatic agent.

Tissues bonded with fibrin cannot be subjected to even moderate tensile stress without rupturing the bond [14]. It takes about 3 to 10 minutes for an initial bond to develop, but requires about 30 minutes to several hours for full strength to develop. Although skin wounds closed with fibrin do not have sufficient tensile strength, fibrin tissue adhesives can be used to fixate skin grafts and seal cerebrospinal fluid leaks, and has utility in maxillofacial surgery [15]. Because there is evidence that the bond strength may decrease over time [16], the strength may be augmented by the addition of growth factors. Depending on the application, the product may resorb too quickly.

Fibrin glues derived from heterologous (ie, human and animal) serum may provoke undesirable immune responses and expose the patient to the potential risk of viral infection. Autologous fibrin glues may be impractical to obtain, might not be concentrated enough for tissue fixation, and could compromise patient safety.

Other adhesives and sealants

Collagen-based devices have recently been introduced for the purpose of sealing arterial access site wounds. These devices use a biodegradable bovine collagen plug to form a coagulum at the access site [17]. The two approved devices are the VasoSeal (Datascope Corp., Montvale, NJ) and Angio-Seal (St. Jude Medical, St. Paul, MN). The Duett device (Vascular Solutions, Minneapolis, MN) is marketed for sealing vascular access sites, but uses a thrombin-collagen mixture. Sealing success rates using collagen plugs range from 88% to 100%, with an average success rate of 97% [18]. Data on complications are mixed, with several studies showing minor complications comparable to compression [19], but an increase in major complications that require surgical repair [20].

Elastin has also been used experimentally as a wound-closure agent, and shows some promise [21]. Very recently, the FDA granted marketing approval for the SureStat (Sub-Q, San Clemente, CA) extravascular arterial closure system that, as distinct from collagen-based devices, delivers a thrombin-impregnated resorbing gelatin sponge over the vascular puncture to stop bleeding. Other tissue adhesives combine natural proteins, such as collagen or albumin, with aldehyde cross-linking agents. The FDA approved one such product, BioGlue (Cryolife, Atlanta, GA), in 2001 for use as an adjunct to sutures and staples in open surgical repair of large vessels [22]. The glutaraldehyde molecules in BioGlue covalently bond (cross-link) bovine serum albumin molecules to each other and to the tissue proteins at the repair site, creating a flexible mechanical seal within about 2 minutes. Other commercially available or experimental tissue adhesive or sealant products include collagen [23], bovine thrombin [24], albumin cross-linked with glutaraldehyde [25], and hydrogel [26], all having particular advantages and disadvantages.

Energy-based wound closure methods

An alternative to traditional methods and adhesives for sealing wounds is to use compositions suitable for the joining of tissue where an energy source is used to excite biomolecular components in a tissue, or in a glue applied to tissue, thus activating the components to form an immediate bond or seal in or between tissue [27,28].

Photochemical activation

A photochemical sealing method is one in which light absorption is used to initiate a chemical reaction in a target material. Upon activation, the material, which is sometimes referred to as a tissue "solder," undergoes polymerization and subsequent bonding with tissue proteins. One of the bonding mechanisms is believed to occur through the formation of covalent cross-links between tissue proteins.

An FDA-approved surgical sealant called FocalSeal-L (Genzyme Corp., Cambridge, MA), is a water-soluble polyethylene-glycol-lactide hydrogel that is applied and photopolymerized by irradiation with a special xenon light source [29]. The method has potential to prevent anastomotic bleeding and to seal closures in other tissues, such as dura, pancreatic stumps, or open wounds.

Another photochemical approach involves the application of chitosan, a hemostatic agent that is then photoactivated by a light source to cross-link to tissue proteins for the purpose of attaching host tissues together with each other or with implants [30].

Photodynamic sensitizers that generate singlet oxygen on activation have also been used. Related sensitizers are more commonly used in photodynamic therapies where activation results in the generation of singlet oxygen radicals that are toxic to cancer cells. In photochemical tissue fusion, the oxygen radicals act as strong oxidants that mediate cross-linking of tissue proteins, thereby forming a bond. Photochemical activation for attachment of cartilage has provided a viable method for repair of sclera [31] and effective repair of damaged articular surfaces [32]. In another study, repair of tendon was accomplished [33] using this method, suggesting it may be an alternative to sutures, barbs, or fibrin glues for initial fixation.

Laser tissue welding

Lasers have been intensely studied for more than 20 years as a potential means to weld tissue. Tissues are considered to be welded when the actual tissue is fused together. That is, the tissue components actually combine with one another or with an intermediary to form a bond or seal. Often a dye (eg, indocyanine green, fluorescein isothiocyanate) may be mixed into the solder for more efficient absorption of laser radiant energy [34]. The heat produced on irradiation of the solder diffuses out into the tissues to be welded. Purportedly, the heat causes thermal denaturation of the solder and tissue proteins that, when cooled, intertwine and renature to form a bond [35,36]. Thermal denaturation in the solder and tissue requires temperatures to be greater than about 65°C.

Laser welding has some potential advantages over fibrin and cyanoacrylate adhesives, such as enabling wet or dry wounds to be sealed, providing immediate significant tensile strength, and creating good tissue biocompatibility of the solders. The laser-induced welds have proven more effective than suture closures in some applications because the weld offers an immediate watertight tissue closure, reduced iatrogenic trauma, and elimination of foreign body reaction to sutures and clips. It also offers a decreased procedural time, especially when used in microsurgical or laparoscopic applications.

A number of studies testing albumin solders [27,37,38] for laser tissue welding have demonstrated clinically acceptable tensile strength and integrity. Laser procedures have been further enhanced with the use of more complex protein solders [39,40] and strengthening structures [41], and through the addition of growth factors in the solder [42].

The use of lasers for tissue welding appears very promising [27,37,39], however, the technique does have certain limitations. The laser energy must be manually directed by the surgeon, resulting in operator variability, and lasers are expensive and can be hazardous to use. Perhaps of greatest importance, precise control over energy deposition can be difficult to achieve. Laser-generated radiant energy is not dispersed evenly through the tissue; the high energy at the focal point may result in local burns, and the heating effect drops off rapidly at a small distance from the focal point. Furthermore, the operator must rely on highly subjective visual endpoints used to determine when a successful weld has occurred, without burning tissue. These factors make a reproducible laser closure difficult to achieve and control. Methods of automatically controlling temperature during tissue fusion are currently being evaluated [43–45], but because of these limitations, laser tissue welding has been slow to gain acceptance.

Nonlaser heat-mediated fusion

The basis for the bonding that occurs during thermal tissue fusion has not been clearly elucidated, but it is widely accepted that thermal denaturation and cross-linking of proteins play a central role. Because laser tissue fusion results from the conversion of light to thermal energy, it is likely that alternate methods of providing heat externally to a bonding reaction, or a method of generating heat from within the solder, would be desirable, particularly if the heating could be accurately controlled.

In one study, hemostasis in the traumatized liver was achieved by thermally denaturing topically applied albumin using an argon-beam coagulator [46]. In the study, two layers of solder, denatured with the argon-beam coagulator, provided for a balance of usability, strength, and matching of mechanical properties with those of intact liver tissue.

Another study examined the capability of high-frequency electrical diathermy to create effective tissue fusion with limited collateral thermal damage [47]. Using an electrical diathermy device with up to 14 W output power at 13.56 MHz, the cystic ducts of freshly harvested canine gallbladders were fused shut. This study is interesting in that a relatively low power device was used.

These studies have demonstrated that alternative energy sources are useful in achieving heat-mediated tissue fusion. The studies warrant further investigation as some related devices may provide greater control than may be accomplished with lasers.

Inductive tissue fusion: Biofusionary

Clues on how to obtain seamless wound closure may lie in radio-frequency and microwave energy research where tissues are either heated directly, or with the use of target "susceptors." Susceptors comprise any material that improves the efficiency of energy absorption and subsequent heat deposition. In the case of laser welding, the susceptor is a dye that absorbs the laser's radiant energy. The use of a susceptor also allows one to more finely control and localize the heating effect. An interesting example of using energy to heat susceptors concerns experimental hyperthermia of tumors, where implanted susceptors, or thermal "seeds," are heated using a high-frequency, alternating magnetic field generated from a coil external to the body [48]. The temperatures produced in hyperthermia are only about 45°C and the heating times may be hours. However, the process provides some evidence that use of susceptors with high-frequency magnetic or electric fields to fuse tissue may be a possibility. Additionally, if one could configure power supplies to generate sufficient heat in a short period of time, the process would be controllable.

An experimental inductive tissue fusion technique pioneered by the authors and Rocky Mountain Biosystems offers such an alternative. Inductive heating is a noncontact process whereby electrical currents are induced in susceptors by a time-varying magnetic field. Basically, radiofrequency power is coupled to a coil, which establishes a magnetic field of a particular magnitude and geometry [49,50]. The electrical currents induced in the susceptors result in heat production.

In this inductive form of tissue fusion, which is referred to as Biofusionary (Rocky Mountain Biosystems, Golden, Colorado), the susceptors are metals or ionic species impregnated in a biocompatible adhesive, the solder equivalent. In pilot experiments, the adhesive was primarily composed of albumin, with a susceptor of fine particles of stainless steel or sodium chloride. Magnetization of the particles in a high-frequency alternating field (eg, 13.6 MHz) results in the formation of electrical currents in the particles or adhesive, which in turn operate against the electrical resistance of the adhesive to create heat. The resulting heat diffuses from the susceptors into the immediately surrounding volume, resulting in a localized melting of the adhesive and tissue in contact with the material. Seconds later, the adhesive cools, and the tissue and adhesive are tightly bonded to one another.

Tissues have been sealed or anastomosed in our laboratory, using the induction approach, resulting in excellent tensile strength (unpublished data). In an early series of experiments, albumin-based adhesives with stainless steel or nickel particle (approximately 50–100 μm) susceptors were evaluated. In one series of experiments, ex vivo ovine arteries were dissected, the adhesive formulations were sandwiched between the vessel walls, and the ends of the vessels were placed in contact and positioned within the coil. In these experiments, tissue fusion was visually apparent after a few seconds of activation. The tissues anastomosed seamlessly, and it became difficult to tease apart the two sections with forceps. Histologically, a tight seal was apparent and there was no evidence of thermal damage to the vessel walls.

In another experiment, fresh ovine lung tissue was sliced into sections approximately 1.25 cm long and 0.45 cm thick, clamped securely in place between a digital force meter and stationary support, severed medially, then rejoined using Biofusionary tissue adhesive. In this experiment, fused lung samples had tensile strength (1.51 kg/cm^2) equivalent to intact lung tissue (1.46 kg/cm^2).

In separate experiments, it was further demonstrated that punctured lung could be effectively sealed with Biofusionary tissue adhesive, withstanding pressures exceeding 1330 mm Hg.

Biofusionary overcomes many of the inherent disadvantages of using lasers and other forms of energy to fuse tissue. Tissue or adhesive contact is not required with Biofusionary, and the equipment used is inexpensive and can be configured to fit in tight spaces. During inductive heating, a large volume of the adhesive is heated uniformly, thus avoiding the spot welding that is associated with the use of lasers. Furthermore, temperature control in certain Biofusionary formulations is self-limiting. Because of the nature of the inductive heating process, formulations may be created that reach a desired temperature, and then shut off, thus preventing excess drying or burning. This occurs either through the use of ferromagnetic particles that have a Curie point where they become nonmagnetic, or through the use of salt-based formulations that limit the induced flow of currents when they reach a cured state.

Summary

Tissue fusion shows great promise in creating the ideal wound closure; however devices and materials are still at an early stage of development. Energy-based closure methods, such as laser tissue welding, have proven that a thermal-mediated tissue fusion can result in a closure that is physiologically and mechanically seamless, and has sufficient tensile strength. However, the techniques are not easily reproducible and are not cost effective, and therefore they are not gaining wide acceptance. Nevertheless, the work of the scientists who have been exploring tissue welding has laid the foundation for more rapid development of new systems that can deliver energy more efficiently and with greater control. Some additional energy-based systems are available or are being developed that show great promise; however, clinical efficacy has yet to be demonstrated.

References

[1] Moy RL, Waldman B, Hein DW. A review of sutures and suturing techniques. J Dermatol Surg Oncol 1992;18(9):785–95.
[2] Carey D, Martin JR, Moore CA, et al. Complications of femoral artery closure devices. Catheter Cardiovasc Interv 2001;52(1):3–7.
[3] Kahn ZM, Kumar M, Hollander G, et al. Safety and efficacy of the Perclose suture-mediated closure device after diagnostic and interventional catheterizations in a large consecutive population. Catheter Cardiovasc Interv 2002;55(1):8–13.
[4] Lendlein A, Langer R. Biodegradable, elastic shape-memory polymers for potential biomedical applications. Science 2002;296(5573):1673–6.
[5] Reece TB, Maxey TS, Kron IL. A prospectus on tissue adhesives. Am J Surg 2001;182(2 Suppl):S40–4.
[6] Gosain AK, Lyon VB. The current status of tissue glues: part II. For adhesion of soft tissues. Plast Reconstr Surg 2002;110(6):1581–4.
[7] Ronis ML, Harwick JD, Fung R, et al. Review of cyanoacrylate tissue glues with emphasis on their otorhinolaryngological applications. Laryngoscope 1984;94:210–3.
[8] Toriumi DM, O'Grady K, Desai D, et al. Use of octyl-2-cyanoacrylate for skin closure in facial plastic surgery. Plast Reconstr Surg 1998;102(6):2209–19.
[9] Maw JL, Quinn JV, Wells GA, et al. A prospective comparison of octylcyanoacrylate tissue adhesive and suture for the closure of head and neck incisions. J Otolaryngol 1997;26(1):26–30.
[10] Quinn J, Maw J, Ramotar K, et al. Octylcyanoacrylate tissue adhesive versus suture wound repair in a contaminated wound model. Surgery 1997;122(1):69–72.
[11] McNally-Heintzelman KM, Riley JN, Heintzelman DL. Scaffold-enhanced albumin and n-butyl-cyanoacrylate adhesives for tissue repair: ex vivo evaluation in a porcine model. Biomed Sci Instrum 2003;39:312–7.
[12] Spotnitz WD, Falstrom JK, Rodeheaver GT. The role of sutures and fibrin sealant in wound healing. Surg Clin North Am 1997;77(3):651–69.
[13] Anderson KW, Baker SR. Advances in facial rejuvenation surgery. Curr Opin Otolaryngol Head Neck Surg 2003;11(4):256–60.
[14] Shekarriz B, Stoller ML. The use of fibrin sealant in urology. J Urol 2002;167(3):1218–25.
[15] Davis BR, Sandor GK. Use of fibrin glue in maxillofacial surgery. J Otolaryngol 1998;27(2):107–12.
[16] Petratos PB, Felsen D, Trierweiler G, et al. Transforming growth factor-beta2 (TGF-beta2) reverses the inhibitory effects of fibrin sealant on cutaneous wound repair in the pig. Wound Repair Regen 2002;10(4):252–8.
[17] Gwechenberger M, Katzenschlager R, Heinz G, et al. Use of a collagen plug versus manual compression for sealing arterial puncture site after cardiac catheterization. Angiology 1997;48(2):121–6.
[18] Silber S. Rapid hemostasis of arterial puncture sites with collagen in patients undergoing diagnostic and interventional cardiac catheterization. Clin Cardiol 1997;20(12):981–92.
[19] Kussmaul WG 3rd, Buchbinder M, Whitlow PL, et al. Rapid arterial hemostasis and decreased access site complications after cardiac catheterization and angioplasty: results of randomized trial of a novel hemostatic device. J Am Coll Cardiol 1995;25(7):1685–92.

[20] Dangas G, Mehran R, Kokolis S, et al. Vascular complications after percutaneous coronary interventions following hemostasis with manual compression versus arteriotomy closure devices. J Am Coll Cardiol 2001;38(3):638–41.

[21] Kajitani M, Wadia Y, Hinds MT, et al. Successful repair of esophageal injury using an elastin based biomaterial patch. ASAIO J 2001;47(4):342–5.

[22] Coselli JS, Bavaria JE, Fehrenbacher J, et al. Prospective randomized study of a protein-based tissue adhesive used as a hemostatic and structural adjunct in cardiac and vascular anastomotic repair procedures. J Am Coll Surg 2003;197(2):243–52.

[23] Wise PE, Wudel LJ Jr, Belous AE, et al. Biliary reconstruction is enhanced with a collagen-polyethylene glycol sealant. Am Surg 2002;68(6):553–61.

[24] Frost-Arner L, Spotnitz WD, Rodeheaver GT, et al. Comparison of the thrombogenicity of internationally available fibrin sealants in an established microsurgical model. Plast Reconstr Surg 2001;108(6):1655–60.

[25] Menon NG, Downing S, Goldberg NH, et al. Seroma prevention using an albumin-glutaraldehyde-based tissue adhesive in the rat mastectomy model. Ann Plast Surg 2003; 50(6):639–43.

[26] Sung HW, Huang DM, Chang WH, et al. Evaluation of gelatin hydrogel crosslinked with various crosslinking agents as bioadhesives: in vitro study. J Biomed Mater Res 1999;46(4): 520–30.

[27] Bass LS, Treat MR. Laser tissue welding: a comprehensive review of current and future clinical applications. Lasers Surg Med 1995;17(4):315–49.

[28] Talmor M, Bleustein CB, Poppas DP. Laser tissue welding: a biotechnological advance for the future. Arch Facial Plast Surg 2001;3(3):207–13.

[29] Torchiana DF. Polyethylene glycol based synthetic sealants: potential uses in cardiac surgery. J Card Surg 2003;18(6):504–6.

[30] Ono K, Ishihara M, Ozeki Y, et al. Experimental evaluation of photocrosslinkable chitosan as a biologic adhesive with surgical applications. Surgery 2001;130(5):844–50.

[31] Khadem J, Veloso AA, Tolentino F, et al. Photodynamic tissue adhesion with chlorin(e6) protein conjugates. Invest Ophthalmol Vis Sci 1999;40:3132–7.

[32] Sitterle VB, Roberts DW. Photoactivated methods for enabling cartilage-to-cartilage tissue fixation. In: Lasers in surgery: advanced characterization, therapeutics, and systems XIII. Proc. SPIE Vol. 4949; 2003. p. 162–73.

[33] Givens RS, Timberlake GT, Conrad PG, et al. A photoactivated diazopyruvoyl cross-linking agent for bonding tissue containing type-I collagen. Photochem Photobiol 2003; 78(1):23–9.

[34] Hodges DE, McNally KM, Welch AJ. Surgical adhesives for laser-assisted wound closure. J Biomed Opt 2001;6(4):427–31.

[35] Tang J, Zeng F, Evans JM, et al. A comparison of Cunyite and Fosterite NIR tunable laser tissue welding using native collagen fluorescence imaging. J Clin Laser Med Surg 2000;18(3): 117–23.

[36] Bass LS, Moazami N, Pocsidio J, et al. Changes in type I collagen following laser welding. Lasers Surg Med 1992;12(5):500–5.

[37] Jain KK, Gorisch W. Repair of small blood vessels with the neodymium-YAG laser: A preliminary report. Surgery 1979;85(6):684–8.

[38] Fried NM, Walsh JT Jr. Laser skin welding: in vivo tensile strength and wound healing results. Lasers Surg Med 2000;27(1):55–65.

[39] Sorg BS, McNally KM, Welch AJ. Biodegradable polymer film reinforcement of an indocyanine green-doped liquid albumin solder for laser-assisted incision closure. Lasers Surg Med 2000;27(1):73–81.

[40] Alfano RR, Tang J, Evans JM, et al. Gelatin based and power-gel as solders for CR4+ laser tissue welding and sealing of lung air leak and fistulas in organs. United States Patent Application Publication 20020198517. Available at: http://www.uspto.gov. Accessed December 26, 2002.

[41] Sorg BS, Welch AJ. Laser-tissue soldering with biodegradable polymer films in vitro: film surface morphology and hydration effects. Lasers Surg Med 2001;28(4):297–306.

[42] Poppas DP, Massicotte JM, Stewart RB, et al. Human albumin solder supplemented with TGF-beta 1 accelerates healing following laser welded wound closure. Lasers Surg Med 1996;19(3):360–8.

[43] Poppas DP, Stewart RB, Massicotte JM, et al. Temperature-controlled laser photocoagulation of soft tissue: in vivo evaluation using a tissue welding model. Lasers Surg Med 1996; 18(4):335–44.

[44] Pohl D, Bass LS, Stewart R, et al. Effect of optical temperature feedback control on patency in laser-soldered microvascular anastomosis. J Reconstr Microsurg 1998;14(1):23–9.

[45] Cilesiz I, Thomsen S, Welch AJ, et al. Controlled temperature tissue fusion: Ho:YAG laser welding of rat intestine in vivo. Part two. Lasers Surg Med 1997;21(3):278–86.

[46] Moffitt TP, Baker DA, Kirkpatrick SJ, et al. Mechanical properties of coagulated albumin and failure mechanisms of liver repaired with the use of an argon-beam coagulator with albumin. J Biomed Mater Res 2002;63(6):722–8.

[47] Bass LS, Popp HW, Oz MC, et al. Anastomosis of biliary tissue with high-frequency electrical diathermy. Surg Endosc 1990;4(2):94–6.

[48] Stauffer PR, Cetas TC, Jones RC. Magnetic induction heating of ferromagnetic implants for inducing localized hyperthermia in deep-seated tumors. IEEE Trans Biomed Eng 1984;31: 235–51.

[49] Stauffer PR, Sneed PK, Hashemi H, et al. Practical induction heating coil designs for clinical hyperthermia with ferromagnetic implants. IEEE Trans Biomed Eng 1994;41:17–28.

[50] Zinn S. Coil design and fabrication: basic design and modifications. In: Zinn S, Semiatin SL, editors. Elements of induction heating: design, control, and applications. Palo Alto (CA): Electric Power Research Institute; 1988. p. 32–41.

ELSEVIER
SAUNDERS

Otolaryngol Clin N Am
38 (2005) 307–319

OTOLARYNGOLOGIC
CLINICS
OF NORTH AMERICA

Advances in Head and Neck Imaging

Kenneth J. McCabe, MD[a], David Rubinstein, MD[b],*

[a]*Neuroradiology Section, Mallinckrodt Institute of Radiology, Box 8131, 510 South
Kingshighway Boulevard, St. Louis, MO 63110, USA*
[b]*Department of Radiology, University of Colorado Health Sciences Center,
4200 East Ninth Avenue, Denver, CO 80262, USA*

The discovery of the X-ray in 1895 by Wilhelm Conrad Roentgen began the age of diagnostic imaging of the human body with all of its subspecialties, including that of head and neck radiology. Numerous eponymic projections were subsequently created to evaluate the skeleton and the overlying soft tissues. Several of those projections, such as the Water's view and Caldwell view, continue to be performed today in the evaluation of the head and neck with plain-film radiography. Fluoroscopy was introduced by the turn of the century and has continued to be the primary tool of functional evaluation of the upper pharynx, hypopharynx, and esophagus.

Linear tomography was introduced in the 1930s and allowed evaluation of deeper tissues with detail not available by conventional radiography. Circular, elliptic, and hypocycloidal tomographic tube motions were introduced to evaluate different regions of the head and neck. Polytomography was especially helpful in the detailed evaluation of the temporal bones. CT and MRI were introduced in the 1970s and 1980s, respectively, and improved the capability of diagnostic radiology [1]. Additional progress in head and neck imaging has been made in the field of nuclear medicine.

The advances in radiologic capability are used most often for the staging of primary head and neck carcinomas. Specifically, in squamous cell carcinoma, patient management is dependent on tumor staging, which relates to prognosis. New diagnostic capabilities can result in better patient outcomes related to the ability to select the most appropriate treatment protocol. Newer modalities have also made the diagnosis of infections and traumatic injuries easier and faster. The clinically important advances in head and neck radiology increase the sensitivity and specificity in the

---

* Corresponding author.
E-mail address: David.rubenstein@uchsc.edu (D. Rubinstein).

0030-6665/05/$ - see front matter © 2005 Elsevier Inc. All rights reserved.
doi:10.1016/j.otc.2004.10.006
oto.theclinics.com

evaluation of neoplastic, inflammatory, and traumatic processes in the soft tissues of the head and neck.

CT

CT had its infancy in the 1970s with individual image acquisition times requiring approximately 4.5 minutes of scanning time and 1.5 minutes of reconstruction time. The first application was in head scanning. CT evolved into faster axial scanning, and now helical multidetector CT (MDCT) scanning enjoys a wider variety of radiographic uses and indications. Although MDCT is most often used for thoracic and abdominal scanning, the new technology also has advantages for head and neck imaging.

MDCT is rapidly becoming the new standard in CT imaging. In helical mode, MDCT uses pitch, collimation, and reconstruction thickness as parameters to make an image. Pitch describes the amount of movement of the table through the gantry (machine opening) during one revolution of the detectors. Collimation describes the width of the detector elements in the direction perpendicular to the gantry. For example, using a 1.0-second scanner with a table movement of 6 mm/s and 1-mm collimation, the pitch would be 6 (6 mm/1 mm). The multiple detectors allow the acquisition of several (up to the number of detectors) images at once. The information from multiple detectors can also be combined to produce thicker sections. The images can be obtained with the table moving in helical mode or with the stable stationary. The faster scanning techniques and image reconstruction times allow the rapid acquisition of numerous thin axial images. The thinner sections have improved special resolution and can be used to make reformatted images in any plane. Thin collimation and high-definition algorithms have decreased bony and other artifacts in the evaluation of the head and neck including the base of the skull.

These advantages are particularly important in imaging the temporal bone, where CT is mainly used to diagnose and stage external- and middle-ear pathologies. The evaluation of dehiscence and the extent of disease are important in two planes. This evaluation can be accomplished by MDCT with one examination by obtaining thin axial sections and subsequent multiplanar reformations (Fig. 1). Klingebiel and Bauknecht [2] compared virtual examinations with intraoperative correlation in consecutive patients with 95% correct correlation.

MDCT is also useful for evaluating trauma and complex facial fractures. High-impact trauma and polytrauma exclude direct coronal imaging as a diagnostic tool because of positioning limitations resulting from spine trauma and other injuries. Coronal reformatted images of the facial bones can be obtained if the initial axial head CT evaluation of intracranial traumatic injury uses thin collimation. Philipp et al [3] found that with four-detector MDCT, obtaining four 1-mm collimated axial images in one revolution of the X-ray tube is sufficient to make reformatted images that

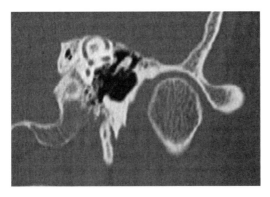

Fig. 1. Coronal reformatted images from thin axial images obtained on a multidetector CT scanner demonstrate dehiscence of the bone overlying the superior semicircular canal.

are adequate for detecting facial fractures. They found 0.5-mm or 1-mm reformatted images with 0.5-mm or 1-mm increments were the best for diagnosing fractures. Sixteen-detector MDCT is now the industry standard, which allows 0.5-mm × 0.25-mm reformations using 120 mA and high-resolution bone algorithms, potentially making CT an even more accurate imaging technique for the detection of facial fractures (Fig. 2).

MDCT has also improved the performance of CT angiograms and dynamic contrast and maneuver imaging. Using peak contrast bolus times, MDCT angiography is used to delineate the great vessels and provide information about the exact location of neoplasm, lymphadenopathy, and infiltration or spread of disease involving the vasculature. CT angiography typically uses 1.5-mm to 3-mm slices with a short delay. MDCT has also allowed faster scanning in the head and neck so dynamic maneuvers can be performed to evaluate mucosal tumor extent. Dynamic maneuvers including the puffed-cheek technique and the modified Valsalva maneuver can be used to evaluate closely opposing mucosal surfaces. The puffed cheek technique uses open pursed-lip exhalation, and the modified Valsalva technique uses closed pursed-lip exhalation to increase the air pressure in the oral cavity, oropharynx, and hypopharynx, respectively, to separate the mucosal surfaces. Phonation, in which the patient says "E" throughout the scan of 10 seconds, may allow better demonstration of small lesions of vocal cords, more precise anatomic localization, and possibly the demonstration of cord paralysis. The open-mouth technique uses a 50-mL syringe in the patient's open mouth to separate the opposing dental amalgam and can allow demonstration of lesions obscured by the dental amalgam artifacts in the soft palate, tongue, and cheeks [4]. These techniques typically use 0.75-mm collimation with a 4:6 pitch, 150 mA, and contrast enhancement of 2 mL/kg at 2 mL/s with a scan delay of 50 to 70 seconds. Examinations using these techniques typically extend from 4 to 5 cm above the area of interest to 4 to 5 cm below the area of interest.

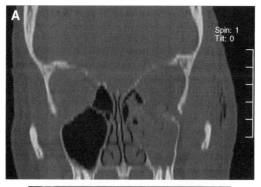

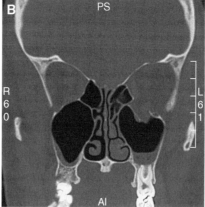

Fig. 2. (*A*) Coronal 1.0-mm reformations from 1.25-mm axial images were created at the time of trauma. (*B*) Direct 2.0-mm coronal images were obtained 2 weeks after trauma. Both images show the left orbital floor fracture and the inferior rectus muscle protruding into the fracture defect.

MRI

Nuclear magnetic resonance (MR) was first used in the 1940s as an analytic tool in chemistry and biochemistry. The proposal to use magnetic field gradients to evaluate the human body began in the 1970s, with clinical applications developing in the 1980s.

Direct imaging of multiple planes within the head and neck for the evaluation of neoplastic and inflammatory lesions has been the mainstay of head and neck MRI for the last 20 years. Multiple new MR techniques have joined T1- and T2-weighted imaging in the evaluation of head and neck diseases. Some of the new techniques in development are inversion recovery MRI, dynamic contrast-enhanced MRI, MR spectroscopy, the use of iron oxide particles for functional MRI to characterize adenopathy, and apparent diffusion coefficient mapping (ADC) of the parotid gland.

Inversion recovery MRI can help delineate tumors and lymphadenopathy for easier identification and measurement. Size criteria still pertain when evaluating for pathologic enlargement. One technique used with coronal imaging, for example, uses high TR-low TE (6000/29) with the inversion time at 189 milliseconds and the flip angle of 180°, 5-mm-thick images at a field of view of 180 mm, and a 154 × 256 matrix. The inversion time is selected to accentuate the lymphadenopathy. The grayscale can then inverted to produce the images shown in Fig. 3. This type of examination sequence needs to be individually programmed for each MR magnet because of subtle differences in each magnet (personal communication, Mark Bahn, MD, St. Louis, MO).

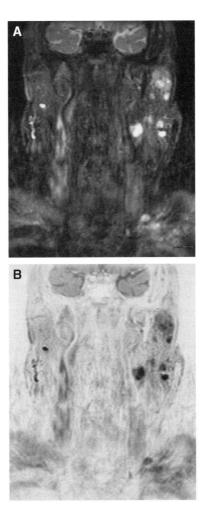

Fig. 3. Coronal inversion recovery images demonstrate adenopathy. (*A*) Original image as scanned using inversion recovery technique. (*B*) Same image with windowing inverted so that lymph nodes appear low intensity. The enlarged low-intensity lymph nodes were pathologic at biopsy.

Dynamic contrast-enhanced MRI uses several properties of malignant tumors to evaluate their spread both locally and to lymph nodes of the head and neck. The basic technique of dynamic contrast-enhanced MRI scans the area of interest, usually a primary tumor or lymphadenopathy, multiple times starting with the noncontrast phase, continuing through the peak contrast phase, and ending with the postcontrast phase for a total of three to four scanning sequences over a period of approximately 2 to 5 minutes. To delineate dysplastic from normal tissue, dynamic imaging takes advantage of the characteristics of a tumor or metastatic lymph node that accelerate growth and metabolic activity. Overall enhancement of a specific tissue depends on numerous factors including the vascularity, permeability of capillaries, and composition of the tissue matrix (intracellular and extracellular fluid) [5]. Primary and secondary neoplasms typically have increased microvascular permeability, increased flow and overall blood volume, increased tissue metabolism, and frequently increased extracellular space. When larger or more aggressive tumors show areas of fibrosis, enhancement is typically both delayed and persistent, secondary to decreased washout of contrast. The dynamic scans can be evaluated in a qualitative or quantitative manner.

Escott et al [6] demonstrated that dynamic contrast-enhanced gradient-echo MRI is superior to conventional contrast-enhanced spin-echo imaging for delineating margins and extent of tumors visually (Fig. 4). In 77% of their 23 cases, the dynamic sequence was judged superior to the conventional spin-echo sequences.

Signal intensity as a function of time can be plotted and used to evaluate both primary and metastatic disease quantitatively. Hoskin et al [7] used this technique to evaluate the response of advanced head and neck cancers to accelerated radiotherapy. They demonstrated that tumors with diminished perfusion at the end of radiotherapy were more likely to respond to radiation.

Several studies have evaluated lymphadenopathy with dynamic contrast-enhanced MRI with the hope of distinguishing metastatic nodes from reactive or lymphomatous nodes. Noworolski et al [5] used multiple factors, including peak time and peak enhancement, in 21 patients with squamous cell carcinoma of the head and neck to demonstrate that tumor nodes were heterogeneous in their contrast enhancement, whereas the nontumor nodes were homogeneous with dynamic imaging. Their technique used a gradient-echo gadolinium-enhanced sequence. Using a similar technique, Fischbein et al [8] showed that tumor involved nodes had a longer time to peak enhancement and lower peak enhancement than reactive lymph nodes. Asaumi et al [9] found greater and faster peak enhancement in lymph nodes involved with squamous cell carcinoma than in nodes involved with lymphoma.

Dynamic contrast-enhanced MRI has also been used to evaluate pleomorphic adenomas and other neoplasms of the salivary glands.

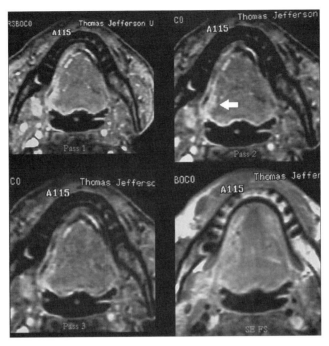

Fig. 4. A squamous cell carcinoma of the tongue is evaluated with dynamic imaging. The first two passes of the dynamic gradient-echo sequence demonstrate the right tongue base carcinoma (*arrow*) better than the fat-saturated T1-weighted image. (Courtesy of Edward J. Escott, MD, Pittsburgh, PA.)

Pleomorphic adenoma is the most common salivary gland tumor, and complete surgical excision is typically curative. With incomplete surgical treatment, recurrence and malignant transformation have been reported. Typical MRI demonstrates a predilection for intermediate signal intensity on T1-weighted images, heterogeneous signal intensity on T2-weighted images, and heterogeneous enhancement. These findings are secondary to the pleomorphic pathologic appearances including the chondroid, myxomatous, or contrary tissue interspersed with epithelial cells. The contrast index enhancement curves typically demonstrate gradually increased enhancement with the maximum index at 135 to 300 seconds [10]. Warthin's tumor, on the other hand, tends to enhance rapidly in the early phase from 30 to 45 seconds with a rapid decrease 30 seconds later and gradual washout thereafter [11]. Malignant tumors such as mucoepidermoid carcinoma and adenoid cystic carcinoma typically have a rapid increase, with the plateau at 90 to 135 seconds and subsequent decrease. The exceptions are typically in recurrent cases of pleomorphic adenomas as well as malignant transformation [10,11].

MRI using iron oxide particles to evaluate the body has been of interest during the past decade. Currently, iron-based MR contrast agents are useful in imaging the liver, spleen, and gastrointestinal system. Ultra-small superparamagnetic iron oxide (USPIO) particles are covered with a low molecular weight dextran and administered intravenously. The USPIO particles are concentrated in the reticuloendothelial system by functioning histiocytes in normal lymph nodes. These normal lymph nodes demonstrate reduced signal intensity on T2*-weighted gradient-echo and T2-weighted MR images. Lymph nodes that have been replaced or invaded by malignant cells do not take up the USPIO particles and consequently keep their precontrast signal intensity. These changes are progressive over 6 to 24 hours after administration of the contrast agent. Typical criteria for CT evaluation of lymph nodes include overall nodal dimensions, heterogeneity of nodal signal intensity, enhancement pattern, shape, and grouping of lymph nodes [12]. Distinguishing reactive lymphadenopathy from metastatic disease is the diagnostic challenge. Metastatic lymph nodes may be missed with CT and MRI when only size criteria are used. Lymph node metastasis in the head and neck region can be less than 10 mm and sometimes less than 5 mm in size [13]. MRI with USPIO particles increases the sensitivity and specificity for detecting metastatic nodes [12,13].

Diffusion-weighted imaging (DWI) is typically used for the evaluation of cerebral vascular ischemia, but it has also been used to investigate neck lesions. Wang et al [14] used DWI to characterize lesions in the head and neck. They found that the apparent diffusion coefficient (ADC) values were different for different types of lesions. Benign cystic lesions had the highest ADC, and benign solid lesions had a higher ADC than squamous cell carcinoma or lymphoma. Sumi et al [15] found that DWI may also help in the evaluation of lymphadenopathy. ADC values were moderately helpful for differentiating between benign and metastatic adenopathy. ADC values were also higher for nodes of well-differentiated carcinomas than for nodes of poorly differentiated carcinomas.

Salivary glands have also been investigated using DWI. Different ADC values are seen in sialoadenitis than in abscess, and different ADC values are seen in parotid glands affected by different stages of Sjögren's disease [16].

Current MR scanners can perform MR spectroscopy, a technique that echoes back to the original use of nuclear MR to evaluate chemical and biochemical properties. In comparing normal tissue to primary head and neck tumors and metastatic lymph nodes, understanding the resonance peaks of choline and creatine may increase the sensitivity and specificity of head and neck tumor evaluation.

Abnormal choline–creatine ratios have been shown to be an MR spectroscopy marker that can distinguish squamous cell carcinoma from normal musculature [17]. The abnormal ratios have been found in both in vitro and in vivo studies [17–20]. The increased ratios are primarily caused by a decline in the creatine peak rather than an elevation in the choline peak. The reduced creatine peak most likely reflects increased energy metabolism within the tumors, whereas the higher choline peak is believed to be caused by increased cell proliferation and biosynthesis [18]. In vivo MR spectroscopy is fraught with difficulty because of artifacts from the air containing structures and bone. Additionally, the voxels used for spectra are usually on the order of 1 cm^3, so smaller lesions cannot be evaluated.

An abnormal choline–creatine ratio is not specific for squamous cell carcinoma and has been demonstrated in other various tumors, including benign neoplasms such as adenomas, schwannomas, and papillomas. An abnormal ratio may differentiate recurrent tumor from typical posttreatment changes, which may be difficult to delineate using routine MRI. Elevation of the choline–creatine ratio in indeterminate masses is indicative of recurrent tumor, whereas a low ratio is suggestive of posttreatment changes [21]. Currently, MRI evaluation of response after radiation treatment is performed at about 4 months, whereas MR spectroscopy may be able to evaluate for tumor response earlier in the treatment.

Most MRI is done using magnets with a magnetic field of 1.5 T or less. Newer magnets may have field strengths of 3.0 T. Imaging at 3.0 T has been used for intracranial imaging and has demonstrated increased signal-to-noise ratio, improved resolution from higher-matrix scanning, faster imaging acquisition times, and improved T1 signal. MR spectroscopy is also improved at 3.0 T [22]. These improvements may benefit MRI for the head and neck.

Nuclear medicine

The role of nuclear medicine in head and neck tumors continues to develop with the reinvention of time-honored techniques used elsewhere in the body as well as newer techniques.

Filtered sulfur colloid has been used in the past primarily for melanoma of the head and neck to evaluate for the sentinel node of drainage. The filtered sulfur colloid of up to 1 micron is injected at the cardinal points around the melanoma and then is taken up in the lymphatics, which drain to the lymph nodes. The first lymph node to appear is considered the sentinel node and can be surgically removed to evaluate for metastasis. If other nodes in other drainage patterns appear simultaneously, those lymph nodes can also be surgically biopsied to evaluate for metastasis. The rationale for the use of this technique is to evaluate the early lymphatic drainage of the neoplasm to a specific nodal chain. This technique has also been used to evaluate squamous cell carcinoma in the head and neck. By injecting the tissue within 2 mm surrounding the primary tumor margin, the sentinel nodes can be evaluated by surgical biopsy at the initial surgery [23].

Positron emission tomography (PET) scanning with [18]fluorodeoxyglu-cose (18FDG) can be used for staging and evaluation of recurrence for multiple primary head and neck tumors. CT and MRI for evaluation of primary and recurrent neoplasms use criteria typically related to tumor or lymph node size. PET is based on the metabolism of the neoplasm, whether primary or recurrent, and is more sensitive than CT or MRI alone for T1-staged lesions [24]. PET is performed by injecting the radiopharmaceutical when the patient is in a quiet room and then placing the patient in the coincidence scanner. A positron particle is emitted from the patient, travels a short distance, and then annihilates into two daughter photons that strike the scanner in opposite directions at the same time (coincidence). An algorithm is then used to project the point of origin in the body. Changes in tumor size and morphology are most likely to occur in the first year after treatment and can vary greatly depending on the initial size, morphology, and treatment used. Enlargement over serial CT or MRI scans may occur as normal postradiation therapy changes and can increase the false-positive rate of these studies. Single-photon emission computed tomography and

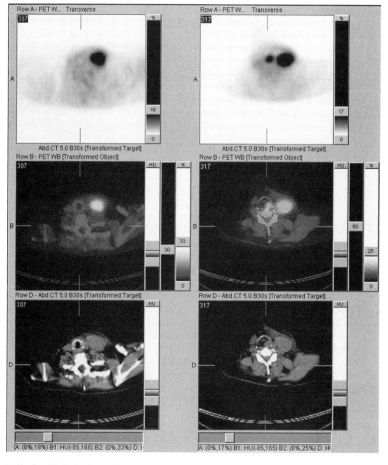

Fig. 5. Fusion PET-CT imaging demonstrates a laryngeal cancer and nodal metastasis. The top row shows the PET images, and the bottom row shows the CT images performed on the hybrid scanner. The middle row shows the fusion images.

PET have poor spatial resolution and can be combined with CT scanning of the head and neck to increase accuracy (89%–97%) over CT alone (69%–75%) [25]. Fusion, the combination of the CT and PET techniques, can also be performed to facilitate better-directed biopsies for more accurate sampling of tissue, a concern in evaluating for tumor. Currently, the most common procedure is to fuse images from a CT examination of the area of interest without contrast with an 18FDG-PET image with the aid of a computer program. Alternatively, new PET-CT fusion machines are available that allow the two examinations to be performed without having to move the patient. The PET-CT scanners provide much better anatomic correlation of the two imaging modalities because the patient is not moved between scans, as is necessary when separate scanners are used for PET and CT and the images are then fused (Fig. 5).

PET imaging or PET-CT imaging can be used for an abundance of head and neck tumors; the most common application is staging of squamous cell carcinoma and lymphoma. Launbacher et al [24] found that PET demonstrated the correct staging of squamous carcinoma in 15 of 17 patients, whereas MRI was correct in 4 of 17 patients. The sensitivity and specificity of PET for detecting individual lymph node involvement were 90% and 96%, respectively, significantly higher than with MRI (78% and 71%, respectively). PET can also be useful in the evaluation of recurrent thyroid cancer.

Typically, recurrence of thyroid cancer is evaluated by a rising thyroglobulin level, with additional imaging performed with radioactive Iodine (1-131) scanning that may localize recurrence in 50% to 67% of patients with papillary and follicular carcinoma respectively [26]. PET can be useful for evaluating the patient with differentiated thyroid cancer, elevated thyroglobulin, and a negative I-131 scan (Fig. 6) [27].

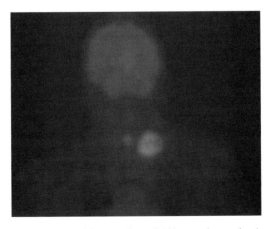

Fig. 6. PET used to evaluate thyroid cancer in an I-131–negative study. An area of increased uptake in the left thyroid is consistent with recurrent tumor.

Contrast-enhanced CT, however, has variable sensitivity because of normal postsurgical changes and can interfere with I-131 scans and treatment. PET is less sensitive in detecting small tumors (<1.0 cm) and tumors of low metabolism and has lower spatial resolution. PET-CT fusion can increase the spatial resolution and provide directed biopsy information. Zimmer et al [28] found that the elevated levels of thyroglobulin were indicative of the PET-CT sensitivity, increasing from 50% to 93% with marked elevation.

Neuroradiology is advancing rapidly with attempts to use modifications of an established imaging modality to solve clinical questions more efficiently and to allow improved patient care. Some of the techniques discussed are being used in clinical practice today to answer practical clinical questions regarding therapeutic and treatment recommendations. Further advances in MDCT and MRI will allow improved evaluation of neoplastic and inflammatory lesions with greater specificity, allowing less invasive and more accurate staging and posttreatment evaluation. The future of head and neck radiology is exciting indeed.

References

[1] Weber AL. History of head and neck radiology: past, present, and future. Radiology 2001; 218:15–24.

[2] Klingebiel R, Bauknecht HC, Freigang B, et al. Virtual endoscopy of the tympanic cavity based on high resolution multislice computed tomographic data. Otol Neurotol 2001;22: 803–80.

[3] Philipp MO, Funovics MA, Mann FA, et al. Four-channel multidetector CT in facial fractures: do we need 2 × 0.5 mm collimation? AJR Am J Roentgenol 2003;180:1707–13.

[4] Henrot P, Blum A, Toussaint B, et al. Dynamic maneuvers in local staging of head and neck malignancies with current imaging techniques: principles and clinical applications. Radio-graphics 2003;23:1201–13.

[5] Noworolski SM, Fischbein NJ, Kaplan MJ, et al. Challenges in dynamic contrast-enhanced MRI imaging of cervical lymph nodes to detect metastatic disease. J Magn Reson Imaging 2003;17:455–62.

[6] Escott EJ, Rao VM, Ko WD. Comparison of dynamic contrast-enhanced gradient-echo and spin-echo sequences in MR of head and neck neoplasms. AJNR Am J Neuroradiol 1997; 8:1411–9.

[7] Hoskin PJ, Saunders MI, Goodchild K, et al. Dynamic contrast enhanced magnetic resonance scanning as a predictor of response to accelerated radiotherapy for advanced head and neck cancer. Br J Radiol 1999;72:1093–8.

[8] Fischbein NJ, Noworolski SM, Henry RG, et al., Assessment of metastatic cervical lymphadenopathy using dynamic contrast-enhanced MR imaging. AJNR Am J Neuroradiol 24;301–11.

[9] Asaumi J, Yanagi Y, Hisatomi M, et al. The value of dynamic contrast-enhanced MRI in diagnosis of malignant lymphoma of the head and neck. Eur J Radiol 2003;48:183–7.

[10] Hisatomi M, Asaumi J, Yanagi Y, et al. Assessment of pleomorphic adenomas using MRI and dynamic contrast enhanced MRI. Oral Oncol 2003;39:574–9.

[11] Hisatomi M, Asaumi J, Konouchi H, et al. Assessment of dynamic MRI of Warthin's tumors arising as multiple lesions in the parotid glands. Oral Oncol 2002;38:369–72.

[12] Anzai Y, Piccoli CW, Outwater EK, et al. Evaluation of neck and body metastases to nodes with ferumoxtran 10-enhanced MR imaging: phase III safety and efficacy study. Radiology 2003;228:777–88.

[13] Mack MG, Balzer JO, Straub R, et al. Superparamagnetic iron oxide-enhanced MR imaging of head and neck nodes. Radiology 2002;222:239–44.

[14] Wang J, Takashima S, Takayama F, et al. Head and neck lesions: characterization with diffusion-weighted echo-planar imaging. Radiology 2001;220:621–30.

[15] Sumi M, Sakihama N, Sumi T, et al. Discrimination of metastatic cervical lymph nodes with diffusion-weighted MR imaging in patients with head and neck cancer. AJNR Am J Neroradiol 2003;24:1627–34.

[16] Sumi M, Takagi Y, Uetani M, et al. Diffusion-weighted echoplanar MR imaging of the salivary glands. AJR Am J Roentgenol 2002;178:959–65.

[17] Mukherji SK, Schiro S, Castillo M, et al. Proton MR spectroscopy of squamous cell carcinoma of the upper aerodigestive tract: in vitro characteristics. AJNR Am J Neuroradiol 1998;17:1485–90.

[18] El-Sayed S, Bezabeh T, Odlum O, et al. An ex-vivo study exploring the diagnostic potential of 1H magnetic resonance spectroscopy in squamous cell carcinoma of the head and neck region. Head Neck 2002;24:766–72.

[19] Mukherji SK, Schiro S, Castillo M, et al. Proton MR spectroscopy of squamous cell carcinoma of the extracranial head and neck: in vitro and in vivo studies. AJNR Am J Neuroradiol 1997;18:1057–72.

[20] King AD, Yeung DK, Ahuja AT, et al. In vivo proton MR spectroscopy of primary and nodal nasopharyngeal carcinoma. AJNR Am J Neuroradiol 2004;25:484–90.

[21] Shah GV, Fischbein NJ, Patel R, et al. Newer MR imaging techniques for head and neck. Magn Reson Imaging Clin N Am 2003;11:449–69.

[22] Scarabino T, Nemore F, Giannatempo GM, et al. 3.0 T magnetic resonance in neuroradiology. Eur J Radiol 2003;48:154–64.

[23] Taylor RJ, Wahl RL, Sharma PK, et al. Sentinel node localization in oral cavity and oropharynx squamous cell cancer. Arch Otol Head Neck Surg 2001;127:970–4.

[24] Laubenbacher C, Saumweber D, Wagner-Manslau C, et al. Comparison of fluorine-18-fluorodeoxyglucose PET, MRI and endoscopy for staging head and neck squamous-cell carcinomas. J Nucl Med 1995;36:1747–57.

[25] Fukui MB, Blodgett TM, Meltzer CC. PET/CT imaging in recurrent head and neck cancer. Semin Ultrasound. CT MRI 2003;24:157–63.

[26] Lubin E, Mechlis-Frish S, Zatz S, et al. Serum thyroglobulin and iodine-131 whole-body scan in the diagnosis and assessment of treatment for metastatic differentiated thyroid carcinoma. J Nucl Med 1994;35:257–62.

[27] Schluter B, Bohuslavizki KH, Beyer W, et al. Impact of FDG PET on patients with differentiated thyroid cancer who present with elevated thyroglobulin and negative 131I scan. J Nucl Med 2001;42:71–6.

[28] Zimmer LA, McCook B, Meltzer C, et al. Combined positron emission tomography/computed tomography imaging of recurrent thyroid cancer. Otolaryngol Head Neck Surg 2003;128:178–84.

ELSEVIER
SAUNDERS

Otolaryngol Clin N Am
38 (2005) 321–332

OTOLARYNGOLOGIC
CLINICS
OF NORTH AMERICA

Bioinformatics in Otolaryngology

Farzin Imani, MD, PhD

University of Colorado Health Sciences Center, UCHSC at Fitzsimons,
P.O. Box 6226, Aurora, CO 80045, USA

The remarkable landmark event of the sequencing of the entire human genome has initiated a new era in the understanding and practice of medicine. The Human Genome Project, which was started in the mid-1980s, was an effort to encourage and coordinate many research groups to sequence the entire human genome. Fifty years after the historic publication of the double-helix structure of DNA by Watson and Crick [1], the Human Genome Project was completed in 2003. Along with high-throughput sequencing of the genome, new tools were required to elaborate the functions and complex interactions of thousands of newly discovered gene sequences. Conventional techniques such as RNA Northern blot hybridization and ribonuclease protection assays are performed on only one gene at a time [2]. More sophisticated methods, such as differential display by polymerase chain reaction (PCR) [3] and serial analysis of gene expression [4] were developed to analyze multiple transcripts simultaneously. The participation of bioengineers and chemists in the Human Genome Project brought forth the use of novel ideas, crucial to the development of microarrays.

An innovative technique was developed that has the capability to analyze the expression level of thousands of genes quantitatively in a single experiment. This technique has been applied to create a library of cDNA on a high-density Cartesian coordinate array, called a "gene microarray" [5,6]. Thus microarrays were born. The cDNA library is typically composed of both defined genes and expression sequence tags (ESTs) [7]. With microarray technology it is possible to study the expression of the entire human genome of approximately 30,000 genes in a single microarray experiment. This revolutionary technique has proved to be a valuable tool for the analysis of complex biochemical pathways and the study of carcinogenesis. This article reviews the recent literature on microarray analysis,

E-mail address: Farzin.Imani@gmail.com

bioinformatics techniques, and genomics in relation to the study of carcinogenesis of head and neck cancers.

Microarray technology

In 1995, the first biologic application of DNA microarrays was published. This microarray was designed with 45 *Arabidopsis* gene probes [5]. A typical current DNA microarray now consists of several hundred to tens of thousands unique probes. These probes are packed at high density in a two-dimensional array. Each probe contains thousands to millions of copies of a given oligonucleotide or cDNA. The oligonucleotide for each probe is a selected fragment that is unique and specific to the gene of interest. Thus each probe detects only its specific target and can be used to determine the mRNA expression by that gene. Currently two main fabrication techniques are used to produce microarrays [8]. In the first technique, probes are synthesized separately using PCR for constructing cDNA or synthetic pathways for building oligonucleotides. The presynthe-sized probes are then placed in an organized fashion into a small grid on the microarray. The substrate for the microarray can be quartz, plastic, or even nylon membranes. The presynthesized probes are delivered onto the surface of the microarray either by mechanical micro-spotting, using computer-controlled robots [5], or by ink-jet ejection, similar to the bubble jet technology used in commercial printers [8,9]. The probes are then covalently attached to the surface of the substrate to ensure stability and repro-ducibility of target detection.

In the second manufacturing technique, all cDNA probes are synthesized simultaneously on the surface of the microarray using a technology combining photolithography and combinatorial chemistry (Fig. 1) [10,11]. Photolithography is a process used in the semiconductor industry for manufacturing microelectronic chips. With this technique, it is possible to produce microarrays with tens of thousands of different probes packed at high density in a small area of less than 2 cm^2. In this method, each probe consists of a 25-base oligonucleotide specifically selected to hybridize with a target gene or an EST [7]. For each probe designed to hybridize perfectly with the target sequence, another probe is synthesized that is identical except for a single-base mismatch at the center. The mismatch probe provides a quantitative measure for nonspecific cross-hybridization and background noise.

To measure the gene expression levels of a particular cell type (eg, tumor cells), several micrograms of mRNA are extracted from the cells. Then the mRNA is reverse-transcribed to double-stranded DNA. This DNA is used to produce biotinylated RNA or DNA fragments referred to as the "target." The microarray is exposed to a solution containing these targets, and hybridization occurs between matching probes and targets. The hybridized probes are amplified with secondary biotinylated antibodies and then

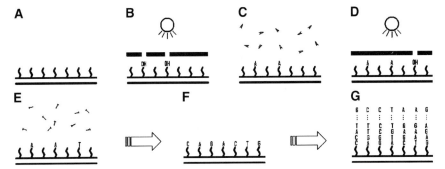

Fig. 1. Photolithographic technique for manufacturing oligonucleotide microarrays. (*A*) Linker molecules are attached on a quartz chip. (*B*) A selected set of linkers is activated by exposure to ultraviolet light through a photomask filter. (*C*) A solution containing a single type of deoxynucleotide (A) is flushed over the chip. The nucleotides attach to the activated linkers. (*D*) A second set of linkers is exposed to ultraviolet light. (*E*) A solution containing nucleotide corresponding to this set is flushed over the chip. (*F*) This process is performed for four different nucleotides to synthesis the first layer. (*G*) The following layers are synthesized similarly to create a microarray of oligonucleotides.

stained with streptavidin phycoerythrin conjugate. A laser confocal fluorescence scanner measures the reflected signals from each spot on the probe array. These signals are proportional to the concentration of hybridized oligonucleotides and reflect the level of gene expression for each specific probe. The results are recorded and used in bioinformatic analysis.

Bioinformatic techniques for microarray analysis

The massive amounts of data generated by microarrays require sophisticated methods of analysis. Multiple analytical algorithms have been developed to explore the data and extract information. Microarray analysis experiments typically evaluate gene expression in two or more phenotypically different populations of cells to discover the underlying genotypic differences. First, the acquired data from the DNA microarray hybridization experiments are normalized, and the ratios of gene expressions are calculated against that of a reference cell. If the differences in expression ratios are significant, this elementary analysis provides valuable information that can be used to identify genes that are tumor markers or are involved in carcinogenesis. A common method to identify significant changes in gene expression is based on fold-changes of expression ratio. For example, a threefold change in the expression level can be selected to separate genes with significantly different expression levels. This method is appropriate for experiments with only a few samples because it does not take into consideration the interexperimental variance of gene expression. An alternative method that requires more samples calculates the threshold level using the *t* test with Bayesian statistical analysis. This method separates genes with significant changes in their expression based on the statistically more appropriate *P* value rather than fold-changes.

Further analysis by cluster algorithms can reveal patterns of expression, allowing genes to be organized according to their similarities. Clustering algorithms use a distance measure to compare similarities of expression values of every gene with all other genes. When the distance is sufficiently small, two genes can be grouped together. A large variety of distance calculations are used for similarity measurements, including Euclidian distance, Manhattan distance, analysis of variance, Pearson correlation coefficient, Spearman rank-order correlation, averaged dot product, Kendall's tau, and mutual information. The paired measurement of similarities is used in various clustering algorithms. These algorithms allow the genes to be organized into groups according to their calculated distances. Various clustering algorithms have been developed, such as hierarchical clustering, k-means, self-organizing maps, principle component analysis, and support vector machines. Because microarray analysis is a new technology, it is particularly important to assess different methods of analyzing microarray data critically and to determine which are most useful in different contexts.

Several recent experiments have shown that clustering of cells based on their genotypic pattern can be used to group together phenotypically similar cells efficiently and also to subclassify cells that are otherwise histopathologically indistinguishable from each other [12–15]. Microarray analysis is a powerful tool that can provide much more specific information than the histopathologic classification of tumors. This information will certainly play an important role in both revealing molecular mechanisms of cancers and in therapeutic decision-making.

Microarray technology in otolaryngology

Head and neck cancer is the sixth most common cancer in North America [16]. More than 90% of head and neck cancers are squamous cell carcinomas [17], of which more than 60% derive from the oral cavity and pharynx [18]. More than 40% of patients with squamous cell carcinoma of the oropharynx have lymph node metastasis at the time of diagnosis [19,20]. Current treatment modalities in head and neck cancers have not greatly improved the survival rate over the past 2 decades. The overall 5-year survival rate for patients diagnosed with head and neck cancer is estimated to be about 50% [20,21]. Screening for early detection in the population at risk has been proposed to decrease the morbidity and mortality associated with oropharyngeal cancer [22]. Unfortunately early detection of epithelial dysplasia and premalignant cells has not been very successful. Histologic criteria for diagnosis are subjective, and even experienced pathologists differ in their diagnosis of dysplasia [23]. Diagnostic methods based on histopathologic classification have a poor correlation with the ultimate outcome. In a prospective study only 11% of the dysplastic oral lesions progressed to malignant lesions [24]. To overcome the diagnostic and therapeutic shortcomings, a comprehensive understanding of genetic changes associated with carcinogenesis is essential.

According to an established model of cancer by Hanahan and Weinberg [25], tumorigenesis is a manifestation of a multistep genetic process. A cancer cell must to acquire six biologic alterations to dictate malignant growth: self-sufficiency in growth signals, insensitivity to antigrowth signals, evasion of apoptosis, limitless replicative potential, sustained angiogenesis, and tissue invasion and metastasis. Although head and neck cancers are thought to result from similar accumulations of genetic lesions [26–28], the precise genes and pathways are still unclear. A global pattern analysis of gene expression is required to discover genes involved in the tumorigenesis process. cDNA microarray analysis has provided a unique opportunity to measure the whole genome expression quantitatively and to elucidate alterations in gene expression patterns leading to cancer. Genomic profiling has been used to identify distinct gene expression patterns and potential tumor markers that can distinguish cancerous lesions and predict prognosis of various neoplasms, including carcinoma of colon [29], breast [30–32], and lung [33] and B-cell lymphomas [12]. DNA microarray analysis has also been recently applied to tumors of the head and neck. Several microarray studies have been performed to identify distinct genetic patterns and potential tumor markers of squamous cell cancers of head and neck (HNSSCs) at different neoplastic stages [13,14,34–40]. These studies have compared genetic expression profiles of metastatic tumors with those of normal epithelial cells and with those of malignant cells in a preinvasive state to discover genetic transformations and alterations in biochemical pathways that regulate proliferation, invasiveness, and metastasis of squamous cell carcinomas. These distinct genetic profiles can be considered as the molecular fingerprint of the cell at each stage of progression to malignancy.

Gene expression profiling of tumors can be performed by using the RNA extract from appropriate cell lines, bulk tumor tissues, or isolated pure tumor cells. Sequence information from cultured cell lines often demonstrates genetic mutations similar to the original tumor cells, but expression patterns are highly influenced by the particular culture conditions, which are likely to be different from natural conditions. The clinical behavior of a particular tumor depends on both the characteristics of tumor cells and the stromal tissue. Although bulk tumor study would provide some information pertinent to the gene expression in the whole tumor, this approach reduces the specificity and rate of gene discovery. With this type of study, the actual cell type of origin for each transcript also remains uncertain. With the new technique of laser capture microdissection, it is now possible to isolate a pure population of tumor cells [41,42]. This approach is essential in identifying distinctive gene expression profiles and unique tumor markers, which may serve as potential targets for pharmacologic intervention [43] and the development of a cancer vaccine.

Leethanakul et al [35], compared the pattern of expression of HNSCC-related genes with matching nonmalignant epithelial cells from the same patients. Laser capture microdissection was used to obtain pure cell populations from frozen samples of cancerous and normal epithelial tissues [42,44]. The mRNA was extracted from the isolated cells and reverse-transcribed to cDNA. The generated cDNAs were amplified, radioactively labeled, and then hybridized to a microarray of 588 known human cancer genes. The authors used fold-changes in expression levels to identify differentially expressed genes. A twofold change in gene expression levels in at least three of the four cancer tissue samples was considered to be of biologic significance. According to this criterion, 59 genes were differentially expressed. The microarray data demonstrated a decrease in the expression of differentiation markers such as cytokeratins and an increase in several signal-transducing and cell cycle regulatory molecules. There was also an increase in the expression of growth factors, angiogenic factors, and tissue-degrading proteases, which was consistent with the nature of the cancer. This study also showed an increase in the expression of members of the wineglass (wnt) and notch growth pathways, which suggests the involvement of these pathways in pathogenesis of HNSCCs.

In another study by Sok et al [13], tumor tissues from nine patients with histologically confirmed HNSCCs were compared with corresponding normal mucosal tissues. The mRNA was extracted from rapidly frozen surgical specimens of malignant and adjacent nonmalignant epithelial tissues. The mRNA was reverse-transcribed to construct a cDNA library. Biotinylated RNA was transcribed from the cDNA library and was hybridized to a high-density microarray with approximately 12,000 human genes. After scanning the microarray, the data were analyzed using the combined t-test and Bayesian statistical analysis. Two hundred twenty-seven genes were identified ($P < 0.001$) with either overexpressed or underexpressed mRNA in HNSCCs compared with normal epithelial tissue of the same patient. Eight of nine cancerous tissues were clustered together, using the hierarchical clustering analysis of genomic data sets with similarity metrics based on the Pearson correlation. The single sample that did not cluster close to other tumor samples was a recurrent case of HNSCC in a patient with a history of previous chemoradiation. The cluster-analysis algorithm also confirmed this case to be separate from other tumor samples, indicating this sample had a genetic expression profile different from the samples. More studies are required to identify the genetic profile of recurrent HNSCCs and tumors resistant to chemoradiotherapy.

In a similar study by Al Moustafa et al [38], HNSCC samples were compared with matched normal epithelial tissue biopsy from the same patient. Using microarray chips with 12,530 human genes, 213 genes were identified that had significantly different expression levels in malignant versus nonmalignant epithelial cells. Ninety-one overexpressed and 122 underexpressed genes were identified. In this study, a 2.5-fold difference in expression levels was defined as significant. In general, most of the genes that were overexpressed in HNSCC encode for growth factors and cell structure, whereas the genes that were underexpressed are involved in cell–cell adhesion and motility, apoptosis, and metabolism. The authors further studied differentially expressed genes from the cell–cell interaction and motility groups because of their considerable function in carcinogenesis and tumor invasion. The expression levels of nine genes were validated by Western blot assay or reverse-transcription PCR. These results confirmed the microarray data: wnt-5a, N-cadherin, and fibronectin were overexpressed, whereas claudin-7, E-cadherin, alpha-catenin, beta-catenin, gamma-catenin, and connexin 31.1 were underexpressed in cancer versus matched normal cells.

A large amount of gene expression data has been generated by individual laboratories using microarrays of partial and full-length gene sequences and ESTs. The National Institute of Health has initiated an elaborate database project, the Cancer Genome Anatomy Project (CGAP), to centralize the generated data and provide a comprehensive molecular characterization of normal, premalignant, and malignant tumor cells [45]. This database is easily accessible through the World Wide Web (http://cgap.nci.nih.gov) and provides a wealth of information freely available to the scientific community. The CGAP efforts were initially focused on the five most prevalent tumor types: breast, colon, lung, prostate, and ovarian, and they were later extended to other cancers, including HNSCCs. The CGAP has classified a large number of mutations that are directly or indirectly active in tumorigenesis [46,47]. Extensive research on these genes and on the biochemical pathways identified by these mutations has led to the understanding of the molecular details underlying tumorigenesis. The remarkable success of some newly introduced cancer drugs, such as imatinib mesylate (Gleevec, Novartis Pharmaceuticals Corp., East Hanover, NJ), trastuzumab (Herceptin, Genentech Inc., South San Francisco, CA), and gefitinib (Iressa, AstraZeneca Pharmaceuticals LP, Wilmington, DE), the development of which was based on these studies, proves that these pathways are legitimate targets for therapy.

In addition to profiling tumor-specific gene expression, microarray analysis can identify potential tumor markers. An ideal tumor marker would be one that is specific and reproducible in both malignant and nonmalignant cells. Microarray DNA hybridization analysis has suggested several tumor markers, including plasminogen activator inhibitor-2 (*PAI-2*) [48], human collagen type XI alpha1 (*COL11A1*) [13,49], and a new gene called head and neck squamous carcinoma-associated gene (*HSCA-1*) [13].

In a microarray study by Hasina et al [48] normal and immortalized cultured keratinocytes as well as normal and dysplastic oral mucosa showed significant expression of *PAI-2*, whereas invasive HNSCC cells showed markedly reduced expression levels. Reduction in *PAI-2* expression has also been shown to be associated with tumor invasion and poor prognosis in lung [50,51] and ovarian cancers [52]. The inverse correlation between *PAI-2* expression and prognosis is consistent with the biology of the gene. The plasminogen cascade is involved in extracellular matrix (ECM) degradation during the tumor invasion process. The activated urokinase type plasminogen activator (u-PA) converts plasminogen to plasmin, which degrades ECM by proteolysis and activation of other matrix metalloproteinases. *PAI-2* inhibits u-PA–mediated proteolysis and is inversely correlated with tumor progression. Comparison of metastatic and nonmetastatic HNSCC cells by Zhang et al [53] also revealed several significant alterations in the expression of metastasis-related genes, including increased expression of the urokinase-type plasminogen activator receptor, integrin beta1, and membrane type 1-matrix metalloproteinase and decreased expression of protease-activated receptor-1. In a similar study, using microarray technology and cluster analysis with principal component analysis and *t* test, Schmalbach et al [49] identified significant overexpression of tissue inhibitor of metalloproteinase 1 (*TIMP-1*) in metastatic tumors. In the same study *COL11A1* had the greatest differential gene expression between metastatic and nonmetastatic tumors. *COL11A1* encodes for collagen type XI alpha1, which is an important structural component of ECM. Molecular details and the role of collagen XI in malignancy are not clear. Sok et al [13] also suggested *COL11A1* and a new gene as potential tumor markers for HNSCCs. Significant expression levels of both tumor markers were observed in all studied cancer cells; however, they were undetectable in normal epithelial cells adjacent to the tumors. The second suggested gene was not related to any previously identified genes. The authors named this gene head and neck squamous carcinoma-associated gene (*HSCA-1*). Again, the biologic significance of this gene in malignancy remains unclear.

These data suggest that certain alterations of metastasis-related gene expression favor invasion of tumor cells, and genes encoding cell surface proteins and extracellular matrices may play major roles in metastasis.

Summary and future prospects

Rapid extensive advances in high-throughput sequencing of the human genome in conjunction with the ability to obtain quantitative information from whole-genome expression profile and the development of powerful analytical algorithms have revolutionized the investigation of the complexity of the tumorigenesis process. The completion of the Human Genome Project in 2003, the invention of DNA microarray technology, and advances in bioinformatics have made these achievements possible.

The pattern of gene expression is the principle element governing cell differentiation and phenotypic characterization. Numerous recent studies confirm that tumorigenesis is a multistep genetic process and that specific patterns of genes are expressed as the transforming cells pass through different stages. Microarray analysis in combination with laser capture microdissection technique to isolate a pure population of cells can capture a snapshot of the activity pattern of thousands of genes simultaneously. This pattern is like a fingerprint that can identify the original cell type and the stage of tumorigenesis. A centralized database such as the Cancer Genome Anatomy Project at National Institute of Health is a valuable asset for storing these expression profiles and for research and development of more accurate pattern-recognition algorithms.

An effort is under way to perform single-cell microarray analysis to obtain more specific expression profiles [54]. This method provides more precise gene expression patterns that would otherwise not be found because of intercellular diversities in multicellular samples. In addition to improvements in DNA microarray technology, several groups are currently developing protein microarrays [55,56]. Protein microarrays are one step closer to studying biochemical pathways and would provide additional information because certain transcripts do not encode bioactive proteins, and others encode more than one protein.

Expansion of databases such as the Cancer Genome Anatomy Project and improvement in pattern-recognition algorithms can provide specific targets for interceptive therapeutics. Vigorous analysis of microarray data can define a minimum number of DNA probes in a microarray required for diagnosis of certain malignancies. The development of these tumor-specific microarrays can eliminate diagnostic uncertainties, aid treatment decisions-making, and improve prognosis greatly.

Acknowledgments

The author thanks S. Dilmaghanian, PhD, for review of manuscript and A. Meyers, MD, for providing this opportunity.

References

[1] Watson JD, Crick FH. Molecular structure of nucleic acids: a structure for deoxyribose nucleic acid. Nature 1953;171(4356):737–8.
[2] Maxam AM, Gilbert W. A new method for sequencing DNA. Proc Natl Acad Sci U S A 1977;74(2):560–4.
[3] Liang P, Pardee AB. Differential display of eukaryotic messenger RNA by means of the polymerase chain reaction. Science 1992;257(5072):967–71.
[4] Velculescu VE, Zhang L, Vogelstein B, et al. Serial analysis of gene expression. Science 1995; 270(5235):484–7.
[5] Schena M, Shalon D, Davis RW, et al. Quantitative monitoring of gene expression patterns with a complementary DNA microarray. Science 1995;270(5235):467–70.
[6] Schena M, Shalon D, Heller R, et al. Parallel human genome analysis: microarray-based expression monitoring of 1000 genes. Proc Natl Acad Sci U S A 1996;93(20):10614–9.
[7] Adams MD, Kelley JM, Gocayne JD, et al. Complementary DNA sequencing: expressed sequence tags and human genome project. Science 1991;252(5013):1651–6.

[8] Schena M, Heller RA, Theriault TP, et al. Microarrays: biotechnology's discovery platform for functional genomics. Trends Biotechnol 1998;16(7):301–6.

[9] Okamoto T, Suzuki T, Yamamoto N. Microarray fabrication with covalent attachment of DNA using bubble jet technology. Nat Biotechnol 2000;18(4):438–41.

[10] Sambrook J, Fritsch EF, Maniatis T. Molecular cloning: a laboratory manual, vol. 1. Cold Spring Harbor (NY): Cold Spring Harbor Laboratory Press; 1989.

[11] Lipshutz RJ, Fodor SP, Gingeras TR, et al. High density synthetic oligonucleotide arrays. Nat Genet 1999;21(1 Suppl):20–4.

[12] Alizadeh AA, Eisen MB, Davis RE, et al. Distinct types of diffuse large B-cell lymphoma identified by gene expression profiling. Nature 2000;403(6769):503–11.

[13] Sok JC, Kuriakose MA, Mahajan VB, et al. Tissue-specific gene expression of head and neck squamous cell carcinoma in vivo by complementary DNA microarray analysis. Arch Otolaryngol Head Neck Surg 2003;129(7):760–70.

[14] Ha PK, Benoit NE, Yochem R, et al. A transcriptional progression model for head and neck cancer. Clin Cancer Res 2003;9(8):3058–64.

[15] Selaru FM, Yin J, Olaru A, et al. An unsupervised approach to identify molecular phenotypic components influencing breast cancer features. Cancer Res 2004;64(5): 1584–8.

[16] Vokes EE, Weichselbaum RR, Lippman SM, et al. Head and neck cancer. N Engl J Med 1993;328(3):184–94.

[17] Wong DT, Todd R, Tsuji T, et al. Molecular biology of human oral cancer. Crit Rev Oral Biol Med 1996;7(4):319–28.

[18] Greenlee RT, Hill-Harmon MB, Murray T, et al. Cancer statistics, 2001. CA Cancer J Clin 2001;51(1):15–36.

[19] Som PM. Detection of metastasis in cervical lymph nodes: CT and MR criteria and differential diagnosis. AJR Am J Roentgenol 1992;158(5):961–9.

[20] Society AC. Cancer facts and figures 2004. Atlanta (GA): American Cancer Society. 2004.

[21] Reid BC, Winn DM, Morse DE, et al. Head and neck in situ carcinoma: incidence, trends, and survival. Oral Oncol 2000;36(5):414–20.

[22] Silverman S. Early diagnosis of oral cancer. Cancer 1988;62:1796–9.

[23] Abbey LM, Kaugars GE, Gunsolley JC, et al. Intraexaminer and interexaminer reliability in the diagnosis of oral epithelial dysplasia. Oral Surg Oral Med Oral Pathol Oral Radiol Endod 1995;80(2):188–91.

[24] Mincer HH, Coleman SA, Hopkins KP. Observations on the clinical characteristics of oral lesions showing histologic epithelial dysplasia. Oral Surg Oral Med Oral Pathol 1972;33(3): 389–99.

[25] Hanahan D, Weinberg RA. The hallmarks of cancer. Cell 2000;100(1):57–70.

[26] Mao EJ, Schwartz SM, Daling JR, et al. Loss of heterozygosity at 5q21–22 (adenomatous polyposis coli gene region) in oral squamous cell carcinoma is common and correlated with advanced disease. J Oral Pathol Med 1998;27(7):297–302.

[27] Kinzler KW, Vogelstein B. Lessons from hereditary colorectal cancer. Cell 1996;87(2): 159–70.

[28] Vogelstein B, Kinzler KW. The multistep nature of cancer. Trends Genet 1993;9(4):138–41.

[29] Alon U, Barkai N, Notterman DA, et al. Broad patterns of gene expression revealed by clustering analysis of tumor and normal colon tissues probed by oligonucleotide arrays. Proc Natl Acad Sci U S A 1999;96(12):6745–50.

[30] Sgroi DC, Teng S, Robinson G, et al. In vivo gene expression profile analysis of human breast cancer progression. Cancer Res 1999;59(22):5656–61.

[31] Sorlie T, Perou CM, Tibshirani R, et al. Gene expression patterns of breast carcinomas distinguish tumor subclasses with clinical implications. Proc Natl Acad Sci U S A 2001; 98(19):10869–74.

[32] van't Veer LJ, Dai H, van de Vijver MJ, et al. Gene expression profiling predicts clinical outcome of breast cancer. Nature 2002;415(6871):530–6.

[33] Sugita M, Geraci M, Gao B, et al. Combined use of oligonucleotide and tissue microarrays identifies cancer/testis antigens as biomarkers in lung carcinoma. Cancer Res 2002;62(14): 3971–9.

[34] Villaret DB, Wang T, Dillon D, et al. Identification of genes overexpressed in head and neck squamous cell carcinoma using a combination of complementary DNA subtraction and microarray analysis. Laryngoscope 2000;110(3 Pt 1):374–81.

[35] Leethanakul C, Patel V, Gillespie J, et al. Distinct pattern of expression of differentiation and growth-related genes in squamous cell carcinomas of the head and neck revealed by the use of laser capture microdissection and cDNA arrays. Oncogene 2000;19(28):3220–4.

[36] Hanna E, Shrieve DC, Ratanatharathorn V, et al. A novel alternative approach for prediction of radiation response of squamous cell carcinoma of head and neck. Cancer Res 2001;61(6):2376–80.

[37] Belbin TJ, Singh B, Barber I, et al. Molecular classification of head and neck squamous cell carcinoma using cDNA microarrays. Cancer Res 2002;62(4):1184–90.

[38] Al Moustafa AE, Alaoui-Jamali MA, Batist G, et al. Identification of genes associated with head and neck carcinogenesis by cDNA microarray comparison between matched primary normal epithelial and squamous carcinoma cells. Oncogene 2002;21(17):2634–40.

[39] Gonzalez HE, Gujrati M, Frederick M, et al. Identification of 9 genes differentially expressed in head and neck squamous cell carcinoma. Arch Otolaryngol Head Neck Surg 2003;129(7): 754–9.

[40] Frierson HF Jr, El-Naggar AK, Welsh JB, et al. Large scale molecular analysis identifies genes with altered expression in salivary adenoid cystic carcinoma. Am J Pathol 2002;161(4): 1315–23.

[41] Alevizos I, Mahadevappa M, Zhang X, et al. Oral cancer in vivo gene expression profiling assisted by laser capture microdissection and microarray analysis. Oncogene 2001;20(43): 6196–204.

[42] Bonner RF, Emmert-Buck M, Cole K, et al. Laser capture microdissection: molecular analysis of tissue. Science 1997;278(5342):1481–3.

[43] Sugiyama Y, Sugiyama K, Hirai Y, et al. Microdissection is essential for gene expression profiling of clinically resected cancer tissues. Am J Clin Pathol 2002;117(1):109–16.

[44] Simone NL, Bonner RF, Gillespie JW, et al. Laser-capture microdissection: opening the microscopic frontier to molecular analysis. Trends Genet 1998;14(7):272–6.

[45] Strausberg RL, Dahl CA, Klausner RD. New opportunities for uncovering the molecular basis of cancer. Nat Genet 1997;15(Spec No):415–6.

[46] Strausberg RL. The Cancer Genome Anatomy Project: new resources for reading the molecular signatures of cancer. J Pathol 2001;195(1):31–40.

[47] Strausberg RL, Buetow KH, Greenhut SF, et al. The Cancer Genome Anatomy Project: online resources to reveal the molecular signatures of cancer. Cancer Invest 2002;20(7–8): 1038–50.

[48] Hasina R, Hulett K, Bicciato S, et al. Plasminogen activator inhibitor-2: a molecular biomarker for head and neck cancer progression. Cancer Res 2003;63(3):555–9.

[49] Schmalbach CE, Chepeha DB, Giordano TJ, et al. Molecular profiling and the identification of genes associated with metastatic oral cavity/pharynx squamous cell carcinoma. Arch Otolaryngol Head Neck Surg 2004;130(3):295–302.

[50] Yoshino H, Endo Y, Watanabe Y, et al. Significance of plasminogen activator inhibitor 2 as a prognostic marker in primary lung cancer: association of decreased plasminogen activator inhibitor 2 with lymph node metastasis. Br J Cancer 1998;78(6):833–9.

[51] Robert C, Bolon I, Gazzeri S, Veyrenc S, et al. Expression of plasminogen activator inhibitors 1 and 2 in lung cancer and their role in tumor progression. Clin Cancer Res 1999; 5(8):2094–102.

[52] Chambers SK, Ivins CM, Carcangiu ML. Plasminogen activator inhibitor-1 is an independent poor prognostic factor for survival in advanced stage epithelial ovarian cancer patients. Int J Cancer 1998;79(5):449–54.

[53] Zhang X, Liu Y, Gilcrease MZ, et al. A lymph node metastatic mouse model reveals alterations of metastasis-related gene expression in metastatic human oral carcinoma sublines selected from a poorly metastatic parental cell line. Cancer 2002;95(8):1663–72.

[54] Kamme F, Salunga R, Yu J, et al. Single-cell microarray analysis in hippocampus CA1: demonstration and validation of cellular heterogeneity. J Neurosci 2003;23(9):3607–15.

[55] Lueking A, Horn M, Eickhoff H, et al. Protein microarrays for gene expression and antibody screening. Anal Biochem 1999;270(1):103–11.

[56] Bussow K, Konthur Z, Lueking A, et al. Protein array technology. Potential use in medical diagnostics. Am J Pharmacogenomics 2001;1(1):37–43.

ELSEVIER
SAUNDERS

Otolaryngol Clin N Am
38 (2005) 333–359

OTOLARYNGOLOGIC
CLINICS
OF NORTH AMERICA

Distraction Osteogenesis in the Craniofacial Skeleton

Randolph C. Robinson, MD, DDS[a,b,*], Terry R. Knapp, MD[b]

[a]Private Practice, Oral and Maxillofacial Surgery, 7430 E Park Meadows Drive, Lone Tree, CO 80124, USA
[b]OrthoNetx, Inc., 7451 North 63rd Street, Superior, CO 80503, USA

Overview

Distraction osteogenesis (DO) is a surgically induced process in which a bone of endochondral (long bone of an extremity) or membranous (skull, face) origin is subject to corticotomy (osteotomy through cortical bone, respecting cancellous bone and periosteal blood supply), then mechanically separated at a precise daily rate and rhythm. The result is the predictable production of healthy, permanent new bone in the distraction gap. The effective lengthening of bone, when properly planned and applied, may successfully correct congenital and acquired length discrepancies and deformities in limbs, jaws, facial bones, and the skull.

The term "distraction osteogenesis," however descriptive, does not tell the whole story. More precisely, tensile stress across cut bone ends to elongate or reshape a skeletal member necessarily forces remodeling and adaptive growth of surrounding soft tissues. From a clinical perspective, the better term for the process of tissue generation by application of tensile stress may be "mechanically induced growth" (MIG).

The induced growth of soft tissue alone (skin, muscle, blood vessels, and nerves) is broadly used in reconstructive surgery under the rubric of tissue expansion. MIG using silicone or polyurethane balloons progressively distended with saline has enabled expanded composite tissue flap coverage of defects throughout the body. Bone-based MIG is truly pansomatic, and the clinician who adopts this viewpoint is more likely to avoid many of the

The authors are stockholders and employees of OrthoNetx, Inc.
* Corresponding author. Suite 300, 7430 E Park Meadows Drive, Lone Tree, CO 80124.
E-mail address: RCRobR@cs.com (R.C. Robinson).

soft tissue complications that may accompany the process. These complications can include compromised blood supply with skin and soft tissue necrosis, compartment syndromes, paresthesias and paralysis, and secondary musculoskeletal injury and deformity resulting from overly tight fascia and ligament structures.

MIG based on DO was described exactly 100 years ago, in June, 1904, by A. Cordivilla of Bologna, Italy, at the eighteenth meeting of the American Association of Orthopaedic Surgeons, where he presented a paper entitled, "On the means of lengthening, in the lower limbs, the muscles and tissues which are shortened through deformity." Cordivilla described 26 cases in which he inserted transosseous nails through the calcaneus or tibia, enclosed them in plaster, and used them to distract the lower leg against a pelvic stop to lengthen the bone and soft tissues of the femoral or tibia/fibula regions after having created an osteotomy at the desired site of lengthening. He was able to straighten and lengthen affected limbs by 3 to 8 cm. His use of skeletal traction evolved specifically to avoid pressure necrosis and other complications that resulted from generating tensile forces through the soft tissues alone.

Cordivilla's early work was reinforced by Abbott [1] in a formal report in 1927. DO was substantially advanced by Gavriel Ilizarov [2], who in the 1950s at the Kurgan (USSR) Institute for Experimental Orthopaedics and Traumatology began to use skeletal distraction systematically across planned osteotomies to "regulate the genesis and growth of tissues in arms and legs through the application of tensile stress." He described a "universal apparatus" consisting of percutaneous transosseous pins proximal and distal to a planned osteotomy, with the pins fixed to ringlike external halos encircling the extremity. The rings were connected by extensible rods to enable precise, gradual elongation of the distance between the proximal and distal bone fragments [2]. The Ilizarov external fixation apparatus and its variants are to this day the most frequently employed mechanical devices for DO.

In 1972, Clifford Snyder and his colleagues [3] demonstrated that canine mandibles, previously foreshortened by surgical means, could be restored to normal length by DO. In 1989, using an external fixation device for DO, Karp et al [4] at New York University (NYU) confirmed Snyder's work and demonstrated in canine mandibles that distraction osteogenesis as previously applied to endochondral bone is also efficacious for producing membranous bone de novo in the craniofacial skeleton. Several years later, the NYU group reported clinical success using external fixation devices to lengthen mandibles in children [5]. Since then, numerous mechanical devices, both internal and external, have been employed on an ever-increasing basis to correct bone and associated soft tissue deficiencies in the craniomaxillofacial region. This article focuses on the clinical experience, primarily in the mandible, of one of the authors (RCR), and projects future developments in the field of DO and MIG.

Physiology of distraction osteogenesis

In his extensive body of work, Ilizarov [2] elucidated the physiologic factors and variables that he attributed to a "tension-stress" model for mechanically induced growth of new tissue whereby "slow, steady traction of tissues causes them to become metabolically activated, resulting in an increase in the proliferative and biosynthetic functions." Practically, he divided the process of DO into three distinct periods or phases: latency, activation, and consolidation (Fig. 1).

The latency phase is defined as the period of time between the creation of the osteotomy and the initiation of mechanical distraction. Usually this period lasts 5 to 7 days. The biologic events and histologic changes are as one would expect during the initial phases of fracture healing. An initial hematoma, followed by the invasion of inflammatory cells and evidence of bony necrosis at the site of fracture, is swiftly followed by the appearance of osteoprogenitor cells and neovascularization. Fibroblasts and associated collagen deposition become prominent. Soft callus begins to form [6].

The activation phase constitutes the entire time that mechanically induced tensile stress is applied across the osteotomized bone segments.

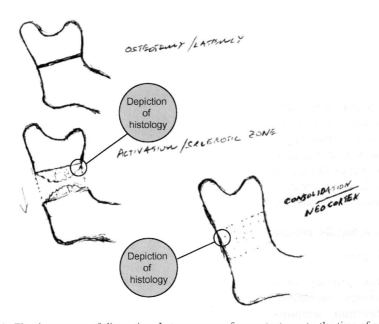

Fig. 1. The three stages of distraction. Latency occurs from osteotomy to the time of active distraction. The activation phase is associated with distinctive radiographic and histologic changes. The neocortex appears during the consolidation phase and is a sign that there is sufficient bone strength to begin functional chewing. The bone across the distraction gap during consolidation is more vascular, and the trabecular pattern is in line with the vector which in most cases is 90° to the fading osteotomy line. (© OrthoNetx, Inc., 2004; with permission.)

Without the longitudinal tension-stress of DO, the osteotomy site would transition from soft to hard callus as ossification, trabecular formation, and calcification take place—to be followed by final remodeling. Activation interrupts this natural sequence and instead induces the creation of three rather distinct zones of activity that are manifest by 5 to 10 days of activation. At the middle of the distraction gap one finds the fibrous interzone (FZ), a radiolucent region of high metabolic activity consisting of spindlelike fibroblasts and collagen bundles aligned along the axis of distraction. The existence of both fibrous and primitive cartilaginous tissue in the FZ suggests that both membranous and endochondral bone formation contribute, regardless of bone of origin. At each end of the FZ, abutting the cut ends of the distracting bone fragments, one finds mineralization zones (MZ). Neovascular activity is paramount in the MZ, as is osteoid formation with increasing histologic and radiographic evidence of trabecular bone formation, speculation, and microtubule formation as osteoid begins to differentiate into maturing bony architecture [7,8].

The rate of distraction during activation is of clinical importance. A rate of distraction that is too slow (< 0.5–1.0 mm/day) may result in premature consolidation of the regenerate and great difficulty in continuing the distraction with potential injury to the regenerate or damage to the distraction device. On the other hand, a rate of distraction that is too aggressive (> 1.5–2.0 mm/day) may outstrip the ability of the regenerate to form new bone, thus creating a fibrous non-union that may require reoperation.

The consolidation phase, beginning when application of continuous tensile force ceases and continuing until removal of the distraction device, is characterized by maturation of soft callus, ossification of the FZ, and the formation of neocortex as evidenced on radiographs. During this period, gradual increase of physiologic stress on the regenerate, such as mastication, is allowed. In the craniofacial area, the consolidation period is usually lasts two to four times as long as the activation phase.

Following removal of the DO device, and with normal activity, additional remodeling of the new bone will continue for up to a year [9].

Distracting the mandible

Indications

The primary indications for mandibular DO include severe bone deficiency, including those with associated malocclusion, masticatory dysfunction, temporomandibular ankylosis, failed costochondral grafts, obstructive apnea, apertognathia, and reflexive facial and maxillary canting with growth restriction. Syndromes and recognized anomalies with these problems can include Treacher-Collins syndrome, Goldenhar's syndrome, hemifacial microsomia, Pierre Robin anomaly, Stickler syndrome, oral-facial-digital syndrome, and others.

DO of the mandible is an important new adjunct to conventional orthognathic surgery. Many mandibular advancements will continue to be accomplished by the Obwegeser sagittal split osteotomy [10]. Although DO has an important place in mandibular defect reconstruction, the authors currently believe that DO is contraindicated in postradiation bone.

DO has proved useful for severe bone deficiencies and deformities of the mandible. Now, DO is being increasingly used to correct more moderate deformities because of its considerable advantages. These advantages include physiologic adaptation of associated soft tissues and joint structures, functional seating of the temporomandibular joint during correction, improved facial esthetics, and stability of result. DO is emerging as the preferred method of treatment in the growing child. The authors consider DO the preferred method of treatment for mandibular lengthening when there is more than 7 mm of horizontal overjet, when there is an anterior open bite, when there is a history of temporomandibular joint (TMJ) symptoms or instability, or when repeat surgery is indicated for relapse.

Planning the surgery

Planning for DO of the mandible must be predicated on and directed toward three key decisions: (1) the type and placement location of the distraction device; (2) the desired length of distraction; and (3) the summation vector (SV) of distraction. Planning data are derived from clinical examination in the neutral head position, radiographs to evaluate bone volume and relationships, mounted dental study models to check the occlusal relationships, three-dimensional (3D) CT scans to define the bone contours, and stereolithographic models to predefine device placement and osteotomy positions accurately. Not every patient will require all these modalities, but the surgeon should select a combination of these aids depending on the complexity of the deformity and the experience of the surgeon.

The clinical examination must note midline relationships, occlusal canting, mandibular inferior border position and angulation relative to the horizontal position, dental relationships and crowding, and degree of open bite, deep bite, and horizontal overjet. Maxillary position and the overall facial growth pattern are also important elements to understand when projecting the desired final result. Indeed, the ability to visualize and project the final normal facial relationships as differentiated from the preoperative status provides the surgeon with the plan for osteotomy placement, device orientation, and distraction length to achieve the desired long-term result.

The presurgical bone anatomy and the desired permanent postsurgical alterations can be viewed as two sets of points in a 3-D (x, y, and z axis) Cartesian coordinate system (Fig. 2). Component vectors connecting presurgical state to desired postsurgical result serve to derive a summation

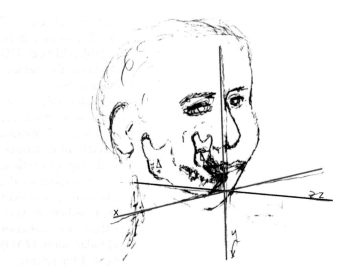

Fig. 2. The Cartesian coordinates for three-dimensional planning of the component vectors that will result in the SV for distraction. The illustration represents a patient with bilateral mandibular ramus deficiency. The planning coordinates intersect at the chin point. The SV is represented as the hypotenuse of a right triangle consisting of the vertical distance for correction (*y* axis) and the desired anterior correction (*z* axis). The osteotomy will be at a right angle (90°) to the SV. (© OrthoNetx, Inc., 2004; with permission.)

vector (SV) that is followed in distraction. In another example (Fig. 3), if the midline (*x*) must move to the left 6 mm, the left mandibular angle (*y*) must come down 7 mm, and the mandibular incisors must advance 10 mm (*z*) to create the angle class I position, then there is an SV in space relative to those three component vectors. The distraction device should be positioned as close as possible to achieve distraction along the SV.

The SV can best be determined by obtaining a lateral cephalometric radiograph head tracing (Fig. 4) or with acrylic models constructed from a 3-D CT scan. Models are advantageous because one may actually cut them at the planned osteotomy site to validate the SV. Some companies that provide models can fabricate the planned osteotomy into the model.

Planning and preparation for mandibular DO also depends on the other factors. If permanent dentition is present, and a final occlusal position is desired, orthodontics and elastics will be necessary during the final phases of distraction. The presurgical orthodontic setup for distraction is the same as for orthognathic surgery. These preparations include correcting dental crowding by alignment of the teeth in the alveolus, removing or stripping teeth and closing spaces, leveling marginal ridges, and removing all dental compensations to reveal the true skeletal deformity. Presurgical orthodontia is critical to most adult, adolescent, and preadolescent distraction.

When mandibular DO is indicated in the infant because of airway obstruction, the final objective must still be to achieve an angle class I

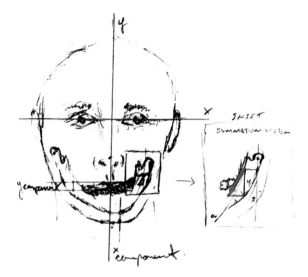

Fig. 3. A unilateral hypoplastic mandible that requires horizontal (x axis) movement as well as vertical (y axis) lengthening. Again, the SV is a composite of the movements, represented as the hypotenuse of the right triangle formed by the desired changes in x and y. The osteotomy is perpendicular to the SV. Because the opposite condyle/TMJ complex represents a fixed point, any change in the anterior-posterior (z axis) position will subtend an arc based on these fixed structures. (© OrthoNetx, Inc., 2004; with permission.)

position. A preoperative 3-D CT scan, obtained under general anesthesia, serves to create a stereolithographic model. The surgeon uses the model to determine where incisive edges of the primary teeth will meet in an edge-to-edge occlusion. Clinically, this final position for the infant will be when the predentate ridges are edge to edge. After 5 months of age the mandibular incisors begin to erupt, serving as useful guides for the final distracted position.

Occasionally, staged DO is indicated. The circumstances dictating this approach include prevention of airway problems and deteriorating facial appearance with degenerating bone or a problem so severe that single-stage DO is insufficient to create a final correction. The goal of the initial stage of staged DO is not a final occlusal position. It is to advance the skeleton to a position for a definitive correction at the final stage.

Choosing a device for distraction osteogenesis

Distraction osteogenesis devices for the craniofacial skeleton can be classified as external or internal (implantable). They may be further subcategorized as unidirectional/uniplanar or multidirectional/multiplanar.

Although the authors do not have experience with multidirectional/multiplanar devices in the mandible, they are available on the market. They offer the option of changing the direction of distraction during the DO

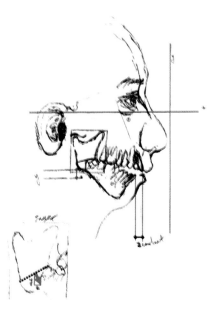

Fig. 4. Bilateral mandibular hypoplasia with high-angle open bite. "High-angle" refers to the mandibular plane relative to the sella nasion line. Y is the vertical line that is perpendicular to the line of sight in the neutral head position. This line may or may not be close to Frankfort horizontal depending on the skull base. The horizontal overjet is the distance from the facial of the lower central incisor to the palatal surface of the maxillary central incisor at a point 2 mm up from its incisive edge. This distance is the amount that can be distracted before edge-to-edge occlusion begins to limit the amount of horizontal distance (z). The chin position at pogonion is not useful except in determining if a sliding genioplasty is needed to help with profile aesthetics and mentalis muscle position. The horizontal overjet is the z component. In the majority of high-angle open bite cases, the osteotomy should be above the angle. (© OrthoNetx, Inc., 2004; with permission.)

process, similar to the Taylor spatial frame used in limb lengthening. The clinical strategy for the long bone, however, is actually the opposite of the multiplanar strategy for the mandible. When long-bone lengthening is employed to correct alignment deformities of rotation, varus, and valgus, the spatial frame (an external device) is used to realign the bone ends into a single column. With multiplanar distraction devices for the mandible, the goal is to create rotation, varus, and valgus of the segment. Therefore, the movements of multiplanar mandibular distraction are to misalign the segments—the exact opposite of the goal in long-bone multiplanar distraction. Consequently, the authors believe that there are several flaws in the logic for using multiplanar mandibular devices.

First, the bone callus microtubules will align according to the SV, not the intermediate component vectors, no matter what adjustments are made. Second, multiplanar and multidirectional DO devices introduce differential distraction rates within the distraction callus, so that one side may be distracted at an unacceptable rate greater than 2 mm per day, and the other side may actually be compressed. This differential may lead to fibrous nonunion on the accelerated side and premature consolidation on the compression side. Third, the frequency and intricacy of adjustment to the multidirectional/multiplanar device is daunting, if not impossible, for the patient or caregiver and introduces a high error potential. Fourth, all three commercially available multiplanar distraction devices are external with the associated stigma, scarring, and snagging potential. For these reasons, the authors cannot recommend multiplanar DO in single-osteotomy surgery.

A case can be made for external distraction when bone stock is inadequate for attachment of an internal device. Nevertheless, external devices require 2-mm half pins set 4 mm apart in each bone segment, with each set of pins 4 mm from the osteotomy site, thus necessitating a substantial amount of required bone. External DO devices may also be preferable to avoid a large area of periosteal stripping when there is a paucity of available bone. Although the osteotomy may be performed with a closed technique, an open approach usually is required to position the pins properly and to complete the osteotomy. Vector planning for an external device is the same as for an internal device, except that the external device must be distracted a greater distance because some bending of the pins is caused by the moment arm when the force of distraction is applied at a distance from the bone surface.

There are several commercially available implantable DO devices, all of which are activated by a pin or shaft protruding through the skin or oral mucosa. Most may be implanted through intraoral incisions for mandibular DO. All but one are unidirectional. The LOGI device (OsteoMed Corp., Addison, TX) creates a curvilinear (multidirectional) distraction vector.

Surgical technique

The major surgical steps for DO of the mandible include (1) access, (2) osteotomy and vector transfer, (3) partial osteotomy or corticotomy, (4) device placement, (5) completion of osteotomy, (6) activation testing, and (7) wound closure. Although the authors' experience and illustrative cases are largely based on using the GenerOs CF internal device (OrthoNetx, Inc., Niwot, Colorado), which was designed and developed by the author (RCR), the principles described apply to all devices for mandibular distraction.

With the addition of a few specialized instruments, surgical set-up and instrumentation for mandibular DO are similar to those for most major operations on the mandible. A nasal endotracheal tube or a low-profile tracheostomy is essential for airway management.

Proper preparation and draping of the patient assures that the ear lobules, clavicles, and midface are in clear view. Eye protection, throat pack, and injection of local anesthesia with epinephrine for hemostasis at the surgical site are standard.

342   ROBINSON & KNAPP

The approach to the mandible is through incision in the retromolar area extending into the mandibular vestibule. Sufficiently elevate the periosteum along the lateral ramus and mandibular body to allow insertion of the DO device. Then dissect the anterior ramus by elevating and reflecting the anterior fibers of the temporalis muscle superiorly. With a ramus clamp (a specially modified Kocher clamp), grasp the ramus and retract the tissues superiorly. Elevate the periosteum on the medial surface of the ramus over the internal oblique ridge. The same exposure can be achieved through an extraoral approach using a submandibular incision with the protection of the marginal mandibular nerve.

Prepare to transfer the osteotomy and vector position to the lateral surface of the mandible with a marking pen. The important consideration for osteotomy location, based on planning, is whether the mandibular deficiency is primarily of ramus origin or of mandibular body origin. The osteotomy should be above the angle of the mandible for the former and anterior to the angle for the latter. Avoid making the osteotomy through the angle, because doing so will cause it to become blunted. Next, choose an observable reference integral to the mandible that is consistent whether the mouth is open or closed. The consistent reference may be the occlusal plane, the orthodontic arch wire, or the inferior border of the mandible. Mark the osteotomy and SV with a marking pen.

Initiate the osteotomy with a reciprocating saw (Fig. 5) and abundant irrigation to prevent friction heat injury of the bone. Make sure the cut is

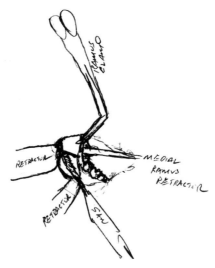

Fig. 5. Creating the osteotomy. A reciprocating saw is used to cut completely through the posterior border but only through the external oblique ridge on the anterior border. The central portion of the cut is only through the cortex, and the inferior alveolar nerve is spared. (© OrthoNetx, Inc., 2004; with permission.)

complete through the posterior border and the inferior border, because these areas are difficult to access once the DO device is mounted. The central portion of the osteotomy should be cut through cortex only, to avoid the inferior alveolar nerve. In higher ramus osteotomies, a short sagittal step can be made. The anterior or superior part of the osteotomy should be completed through the external oblique ridge but not through the internal ridge initially. The key point for the incomplete osteotomy is a cut sufficient to allow the mandible to fracture easily after the DO device is applied but stable enough beforehand to allow device placement without a flail segment of bone. The same principle holds for extraoral DO device placement.

Tooth buds or erupting teeth in the path of the osteotomy should be removed if possible, although they may be removed later if necessary. With infants, an expectant position must be taken, but chances are significant that the patient will have some permanent damage to the molars. This tooth loss can be restored later in life with dental implants.

Next, assemble or modify the device so that it fits the particular positioning on the mandible as dictated by the osteotomy and SV. It may be necessary to remove redundant fixation points, adjust plate contours, or temporarily remove the activation pin (Fig. 6). Then position the device along the SV of distraction. Secure the device to the proximal bone fragment with at least two bone screws and drill two indexing holes nearest to the osteotomy on the distal fragment. Do not place the distal screws until after the osteotomy is complete. Drilling of the pilot holes and the placement of screws is usually performed through a transcutaneous trochar when an intraoral approach is employed (Fig. 7).

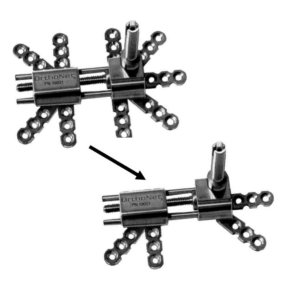

Fig. 6. The device can be modified to fit the anatomic demands of the site. (© OrthoNetx, Inc., 2004; with permission.)

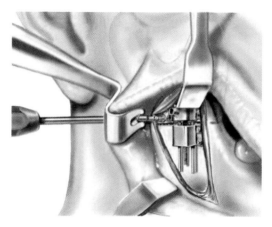

Fig. 7. Fixation of the device to the bone segments with transbuccal screws placed using a trocar. (© OrthoNetx, Inc., 2001; with permission.)

Then begin completion of the osteotomy by cutting the internal oblique ridge with the reciprocating saw. Use an osteotome to complete the cut without cutting the nerve. Usually, this maneuver simply involves a twisting motion after the osteotome is inserted into the anterior aspect of the bone cut. Make sure not to bend or deform the guide rods or the drive shaft on the selected DO device.

Once the osteotomy is completed, replace the distal screws, reinsert the activation pin of the DO device, and open the device approximately 4 mm (Fig. 8). This procedure confirms the functioning of the device and the completion of the osteotomy. This step is important because it is possible to

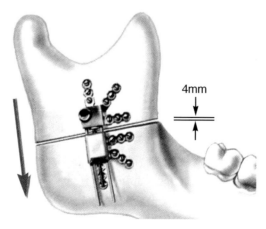

Fig. 8. Once the device is secured, it is important to activate it to assure completeness of the osteotomy. Return the device to the starting (closed) position before wound closure. (© OrthoNetx, Inc., 2001; with permission.)

create an incomplete greenstick fracture of the mandible in young patients and not recognize the problem until 2 weeks after surgery, when the patient encounters difficulty during activation because one side of the osteotomy is not opening. In this situation, reoperation may be necessary to complete the osteotomy and insert a new device.

Next, close the device to its original position. Forcible compression of the osteotomy to speed callus formation is not necessary and could damage the device.

Irrigate and close the surgical site in typical fashion. If there is a transcutaneous pin site, it should not be closed. The pin incision, if performed correctly, should not be more than 6 mm in length and should be parallel the regional relaxed skin tension lines. Place the pin cap (Fig. 9) and a sterile dressing over the pin site to capture residual drainage. If the patient has a presurgical history of airway obstruction, careful monitoring will be require in the early postoperative period.

Aftercare

Transcutaneous pin care requires daily cleaning and dressing changes during the latency and activation phases. Place the patient on a soft, non-chew diet to avoid excessive forces on the mandible. Once activation begins, an activation schedule and calendar should be updated at each activation session. Typically, two to four activation sessions per day are optimal to create the desired 1 mm per day of distraction (Fig. 10). See the patient on a regular basis to evaluate the distraction process. Take periodic radiographs to determine device and bone changes. Track the occlusal relationship while approaching the terminal position. Begin using elastics to guide the occlusion and adjust the midlines. In the cases of severe deformities

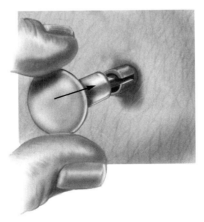

Fig. 9. Protect the protruding activation pin with the supplied cap. (© OrthoNetx, Inc., 2004; with permission.)

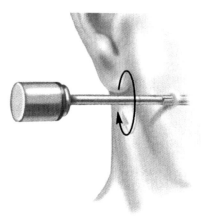

Fig. 10. Activation is accomplished by using the activation tool to rotate the activation pin one full turn (360° = .25 mm) four times daily, to achieve 1.0 mm of daily distraction. (© OrthoNetx, Inc., 2001; with permission.)

causing airway obstruction in infants, completion of activation can be judged by a trial of plugging the tracheostomy tube and examining the airway.

At the end of the activation period, the activation pin may be removed, and a small adhesive strip may be placed over the skin incision to re-approximate the margins. The patient should continue on a soft diet and elastics during most of the consolidation period. Monitor the patient for rebound swelling that may indicate an infection, which may be treated with antibiotics or by reopening of the pin tract.

As a rule, the consolidation period lasts two to three times longer than the activation period. For example, if the activation distance is 12 mm, then the activation period would approximate 12 days, and the consolidation period would be 24 to 36 days thereafter. A good indication of proper consolidation is a visible cortical outline on radiographs. Once consolidation is complete, the DO device may be removed. There is no urgency to remove an implanted DO device unless there are signs of infection or the device is palpable and an irritation.

Usually removal of an internal DO device requires an intraoral incision under a general anesthesia. The distracted device is dimensionally larger than the original device and may occasionally be difficult to remove. Stainless steel devices tend to promote fibrous capsules, which dissect easily; titanium devices tend to promote tissue adherence. There have been verbal reports of bone growing onto titanium devices, necessitating drilling away the hypertrophic bone. Sometimes cutting through the drive shafts and guide rods, thus dividing the DO device into two segments, aids removal. At device removal, one may confirm complete consolidation. Usually there is a striated appearance to the new bone along the vector of distraction. The new bone often feels solid but may have a few softer areas. The authors have seen one case of device removal in which good bone callus was present, but the segments were slightly mobile. In this case, a single 2-mm bone plate was placed across the callus, and the patient remained on a soft diet and in elastics for 3 more weeks. Two years after surgery she has excellent occlusion, normal bone architecture, and stability. The authors have taken many biopsies of various cases at the time of device removal, which demonstrate normal bone.

Case studies

Case 1

K.B. is a 16-year-old female with mandibular ramus hypoplasia, skeletal apertognathia, and TMJ pain and dysfunction (Fig. 11A, B). She was referred for surgical evaluation when 6 years of orthodontics failed to correct the unrecognized skeletal deformities and her joint symptoms were becoming worse. On examination, she had 8 mm of horizontal overjet and 6 mm of open bite. Her TMJs were tender with popping and crepitus. Her maxilla was in good position, and her smile line was even. Treatment of the mandible alone was required.

Mandibular DO was selected because of the predominance of ramus deficiency contributing to her open bite (as contrasted with posterior vertical maxillary excess). TMJ symptomatology suggested that the lower forces of DO would be beneficial compared with acute changes and forces on the joints associated with sliding osteotomy. The overall tendency for instability of large counterclockwise rotation advancements of the hypoplastic

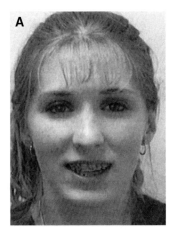
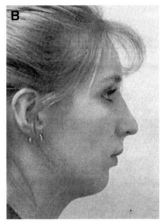

Fig. 11. (*A, B*) Patient K.B with bilateral mandibular ramus hypoplasia. Preoperative anterior and lateral facial views.

mandible in open-bite cases also favored DO. Also, addressing the mandible, the root of the problem, rather than impacting the posterior maxilla avoids leaving the patient with a steep mandibular plane angle and a telltale facial contour that looks "operated."

Clinical examination showed that the midline landmarks were normal, and the mandibular angle could be dropped lower to improve the inferior border with the facial plane. Orthopantomogram and lateral cephalometric radiographs facilitated vector planning with a predictive tracing used to gauge the angulation of the vector based on the occlusal plane as a reference (Fig. 12A, B). Dental study models showed that final class I occlusion was possible.

Bilateral internal DO devices were place across the rami about 1 cm above the mandibular angle. Third molars were removed at the time of osteotomy.

A 7-day latency period was followed by approximately 12 mm of distraction on one side and 14 mm of distraction on the other (Fig. 13A, B). She had excellent consolidation, but device removal was delayed until she completed her cheerleading obligations. Elastics and finishing orthodontics gave a final class I occlusion.

Now, 6 years post surgery, she has no TMJ symptoms, no limitation of opening, and no relapse of her open bite. Pin scars are barely discernible (Figs. 14A, B; 15; 16).

Case 2

K.N. is a 14-year-old female with congenital otomandibular syndrome consisting of mandibular hypoplasia, limited mandibular opening, skeletal open bite, class I occlusion, high mandibular and occlusal plane angles,

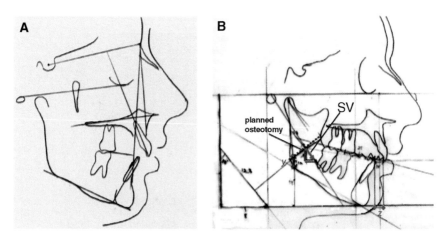

Fig. 12. Patient K.B. (*A*) Preoperative cephalometric tracing. (*B*) Calculated SV based on planned anterior (*z* axis) movement and vertical (*y* axis) ramus lengthening. Planned osteotomy is at right angles to SV.

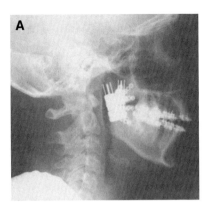
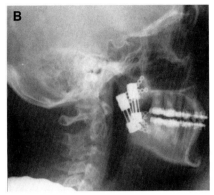

Fig. 13. Patient K.B. (*A*) Distraction devices in place before activation phase. (*B*) Completion of activation and onset of consolidation phase.

malar deficiency, dorsal nasal deformity, microtia, and impacted third molars (Fig. 17A, B). Midline landmarks were aligned, and the maxillary smile line was normal. For comprehensive correction of facial deformities (except the microtia) at a single intervention, the author (RCR) decided to perform bilateral mandibular DO, along with passive Le Fort I maxillary distraction, removal of the third molars, malar implant augmentation, sliding genioplasty, and rhinoplasty.

Planning and vector design were based on the lateral cephalometric radiograph (Fig. 18A, B). The authors decided to hinge the maxilla at the Le Fort I level by placing interosseous stainless steel wires at the pyriform aperture bilaterally. A submental endotracheal tube passage was made to

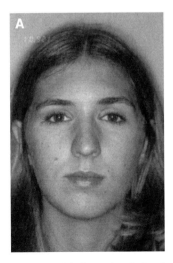
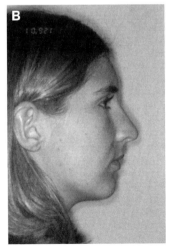

Fig. 14. Patient K.B. (*A*) distraction devices in place before activation phase. (*B*) Completion of activation and onset of consolidation phase.

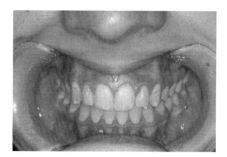

Fig. 15. Patient K.B. Stable class I postoperative occlusion.

allow for the rhinoplasty without having to change the tube position during the procedure. Ramus osteotomies were made above the angle, and a vertical orientation of the internal DO devices was chosen to "disimpact" the posterior face. Elastics were used during the activation to bring the maxilla along with the mandible. Twelve millimeters of distraction bilaterally was completed before the activation pin was removed (Fig. 19). The DO devices were later removed.

After 2 years her occlusion and function have remained stable (Figs. 20A. B; 21A, B). There is no sign of relapse or joint degeneration, and she is awaiting total ear reconstruction.

Case 3

J.K. is an infant with Stickler syndrome (Pierre Robin syndrome variant) with associated mandibular hypoplasia, cleft palate, airway obstruction, and

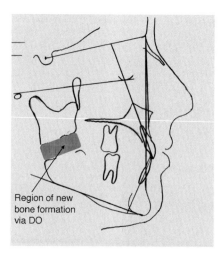

Fig. 16. Patient K.B. Long-term postoperative cephalometric tracing of final position of bony landmarks.

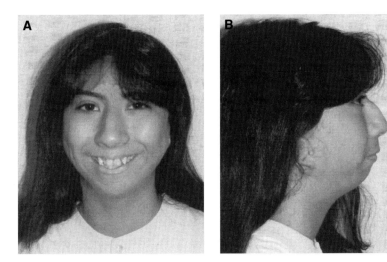

Fig. 17. (*A, B*) Patient K.N. with otomandibular syndrome, including mandibular hypoplasia, steep mandibular plane angle, vertical posterior maxillary deficiency, malar retrusion, limited jaw opening, nasal deformity, and bilateral microtia.

retinal degeneration. At birth, she experienced acute airway obstruction requiring intubation, then tracheostomy at 3 days of age (Fig. 22A, B). Bilateral internal mandibular DO was performed at 3 months of age. SV and osteotomies were planned from a stereolithographic model (Fig. 23). DO device placement was performed through intraoral incisions with

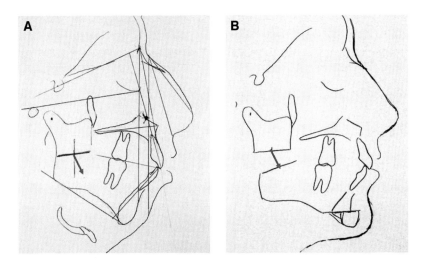

Fig. 18. (*A, B*) Patient K.N. Preoperative cephalometric tracings showing SV. Maxilla to undergo LeFort I osteotomy and pivot around wires at pyriform aperture during mandibular distraction. Planned sliding genioplasty.

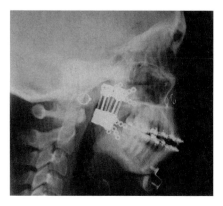

Fig. 19. Patient K.N. Lateral radiograph in consolidation phase after completion of device activation. Note sliding genioplasty.

transcutaneous activation pins. Once 15 mm of bilateral DO was obtained, the tracheostomy tube was capped for a trial period. She was able to maintain her own airway. Tracheostomy tube and the activation pins were removed in the operating room to allow direct laryngoscopy (Fig. 24). The final mandibular position was an edge-to-edge relationship of the predentate maxillary and mandibular alveolar ridges (Fig. 25). Her cleft was repaired at age 11 months of age without airway problems. She was growing normally 2 years after the operation (Fig. 26A, B). Now age 4 years, she has class I occlusion in primary dentition, normal speech, and no residual airway obstruction. Pin scars have faded, and there is only mild dysesthesia of the lips.

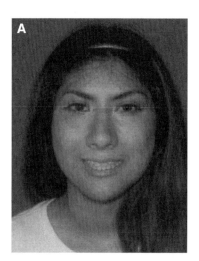
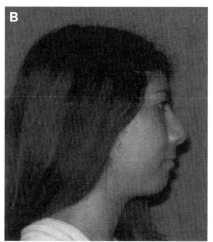

Fig. 20. (*A, B*) Patient K.N. Posttreatment results, frontal and lateral.

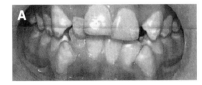 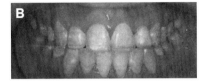

Fig. 21. Patient K.N. Dental occlusion and alignment. (*A*) Pretreatment. (*B*) Posttreatment.

Distraction osteogenesis of the maxilla and the cranium

DO of the maxilla may be successfully performed at all three Le Fort osteotomy levels. The cranium may be distracted at the various suture lines to correct variants of craniosynostosis. The orbits and frontal bone may also be distracted using the frontofacial monoblock advancement described by Tessier [11] and others. Because of space, discussion here is limited to external distraction of maxilla.

DO at the Le Fort I and II levels is best performed by an external halo because no predictable internal device is yet available. For Le Fort III facial advancement, distraction may be performed with either a halo device or an internal device because fixation at the zygoma or the temporal bone serves as a platform for device attachment. Maxillary DO seems to be most efficacious for movements of more than 6 mm in cases of cleft palate surgery and for movements of more than 10 mm in cases of synostosis. Although a high degree of relapse is associated with advancement of the maxilla because of scarring in patients with cleft palate, the authors have found that advancement of the maxilla in cleft palate patients is more stable using DO than with conventional surgery and bone grafting.

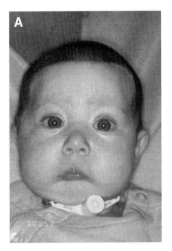 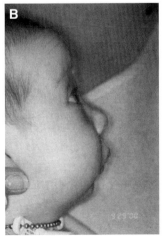

Fig. 22. (*A, B*) Patient J. K. at age 3 months. Stickler syndrome with severe Pierre Robin anomaly required tracheostomy and feeding gastrostomy at age 3 days.

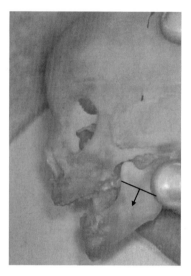

Fig. 23. Patient J. K. Stereolithography model with planned osteotomy and SV for distraction.

By performing model surgery and fabricating a maxillary distraction splint, predictable final occlusion can be achieved. For external (halo) devices, the splint is made by indexing the mandibular dentition on the inferior surface and imbedding 0.045-inch round distraction wires into the splint. The wires are bent so that they do not impinge the lips and may be stepped to achieve the best vector. These wires are attached to the halo frame by means of 24-gauge stainless steel wires.

The osteotomy of the maxilla, regardless of level, is usually preformed in an open standard fashion with just enough mobilization to assure that all osteotomies are complete, especially at the pterygomaxillary suture. Relying

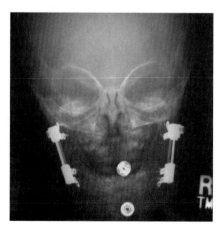

Fig. 24. Patient J. K. Radiograph during consolidation phase.

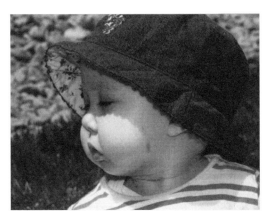

Fig. 25. Patient J. K. at age 9 months. No tracheostomy; no gastrostomy; DO devices removed.

on the force of distraction to fracture incomplete osteotomies will usually fail and require reoperation. Wire the splint to the orthodontic appliances on the maxillary teeth. Any intermediate palatal osteotomies or segmentation with bone grafting can be performed at this time. Be sure the attachment wires do not impinge the lips.

Attachment and alignment of the halo is important because its position will affect the distraction vector. Assure that the vertical strut is in the facial midline and far enough away to accommodate the length of the splint attachment wires. Set the transverse bar and the angulation of the distraction screws to the desired vector. Attach the distraction screws to the 0.045-inch attachment wires with an intermediate 24-gauge wire.

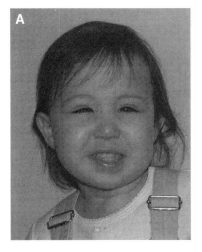
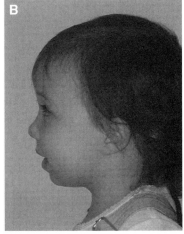

Fig. 26. (*A, B*) Patient J. K. 2 years after completion of DO. Mandibular growth and occlusion have remained normal.

Activate the screws to take up any slack, but do not distract until the latency phase is complete. The authors believe that the latency phase is important in the maxilla because the bones are thinner, and the greater mobilization and separation required at the time of surgery may delay callus formation.

After a 7-day latency period, distract at 1 mm per day and begin using class III elastics to the mandible to help keep the maxilla aligned and level. Once the maxilla is advanced to the desired degree, begin using vertical elastics to bring about proper occlusion. Maintain the halo and tension on the wires for 6 weeks during consolidation. At this point the halo and splint may be removed, and elastics may be placed to guide the final occlusion. If a palatal expansion was performed at the same time as the distraction osteotomies, be sure to use cross-arch elastics from the palatal surface of the maxillary first molars to the buccal surface of the mandibular first molars, or place a transpalatal orthodontic wire.

At this time it is beneficial for the patient to begin using a reverse-pull facemask to help support the maxilla in the final position. These facemasks, which hook to the first molars with elastic orthodontic tubes, are designed with a forehead support and a chin cup to hold the maxilla forward. The authors usually have the patient wear them at night for about 2 months. If it seems that the final advanced position is not complete at the time of halo and splint removal, the face mask should be worn at all times with stronger elastics.

Goals of internal DO at the Le Fort III (or monoblock) level include correction of posterior upper airway obstruction, exorbitism, and the initial stages of synostotic and syndrome-related malocclusion. Frontofacial monoblock DO does not usually serve as the definitive surgery to correct malocclusion and should be regarded as an initial stage. The advantage of distraction at this level is diminution of relapse and avoidance of major bone grafting. Reported problems include difficult device removal and difficulty with device attachment to the deficient zygomas. Complete bony mobilization is important here also.

Case study

S.A. is a 15-year-old female with a bilateral cleft lip and palate, severe midface deficiency, and mandibular hyperplasia with pronounced class III dental occlusion (Figs. 27A, B; 28). She has had previous bone grafting, palatal surgery, and lip repair. There is a residual whistle deformity of the lip and decrease nasal tip projection.

The plan was to advance the maxilla to a favorable position but to delay mandibular set back until growth was complete. Therefore, no attempt was made to correct the occlusion to a class I with the first surgery. The second surgery would correct the final occlusion with tertiary surgery to include rhinoplasty and an Abbe flap for final lip contouring.

At Le Fort I osteotomy, the maxilla was mobilized and placed back into its original position. A halo distractor was positioned over the cranium and

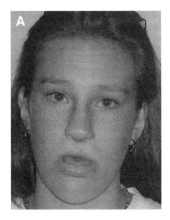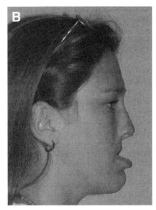

Fig. 27. (*A, B*) Patient S. Severe hypoplasia of the maxilla secondary to bilateral cleft lip and palate deformity.

secured so that it was parallel to Frankfort horizontal, with the vertical central bar in the midline. Wires and the splint were attached as described previously (Fig. 29A, B). Following a 7-day latency period, activation advanced the maxilla 8 mm. Then the mandible was indexed into the splint. After 6 weeks the halo was removed, and elastics were used for 6 more weeks to help hold the position, which remained stable.

Two years later, the patient, then 17 years old, underwent a mandibular set back and rhinoplasty. Thereafter, final-phase orthodontics and Abbe flap lip reconstruction were completed. The maxillary position has remained stable 4 years after maxillary DO (Fig. 30A, B). She retains a slight class III occlusal tendency, but it is deemed acceptable.

Osteoplastic surgery and the future of distraction osteogenesis

Osteoplastic surgery, literally the forming and molding of bone, is made possible by DO. The experience of many pioneers, both in characterizing the

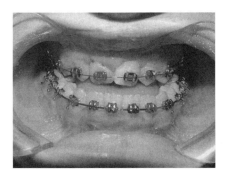

Fig. 28. Patient S. Preoperative class III occlusion.

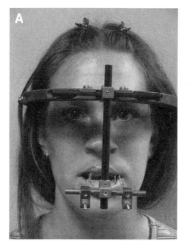
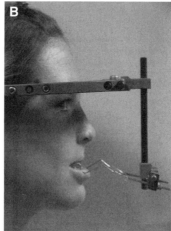

Fig. 29. (*A, B*) Patient S. Postoperative Le Fort I maxillary osteotomy with halo placement to allow DO.

physiology and methodology of the clinical process and in developing the devices that generate mechanically induced growth, leads the authors to believe that DO and the resulting pansomatic growth is applicable throughout the body when a bone-based center of new growth is desirable to correct a clinical condition.

The authors' experience alone has seen remarkable success with DO in lengthening limbs in both upper and lower extremities and in generating dental alveolar bone with concurrent, integrated dental implant functionality. Although indications to date have centered on congenital and acquired deformities with associated bone loss, the authors have every reason to

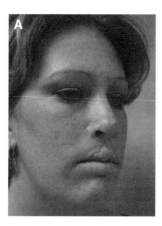
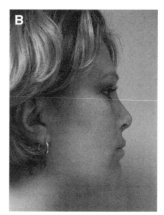

Fig. 30. (*A, B*) Patient S. Postoperataive Le Fort I maxillary osteotomy with DO, followed by final lip/nose repair.

believe that elective DO for appearance and height enhancement will become commonplace. Already, and even with rather crude devices, the demand is growing for height enhancement, both in the United States and worldwide.

With sophisticated devices and approaches that provide the doctor and patient with easily placed, user-friendly, easy-to-manage devices that reduce operative time, pain, and scarring, demand will increase, and new applications will emerge. One can even imagine remote monitoring and control of automated device-in-patient by the treating surgeon. Clearly, DO is an important, proven tool that should reside in every reconstructive surgeon's armamentarium.

References

[1] Abbott LC. The operative lengthening of the tibia and fibula. J Bone Joint Surg 1927;9:128.

[2] Ilizarov GA. The principles of the Ilizarov method. Bull Hosp Joint Dis Orthop Inst 1988; 48:1.

[3] Snyder CC, Levine GA, Swanson HM, et al. Mandibular lengthening by gradual distraction: preliminary report. Plast Reconstr Surg 1973;51(5):506.

[4] Karp NS, Thorne CHM, McCarthy JG, et al. Bone lengthening in the craniofacial skeleton. Ann Plast Surg 1990;24:231.

[5] McCarthy JG, Schreiber J, Karp NS, et al. Lengthening the human mandible by gradual distraction. Plast Reconstr Surg 1992;89(1):1.

[6] Samchukov ML, Cope JB, Cherkashin AM. Biological basis of new bone formation under the influence of tension stress. In: Samchukov ML, Cope JB, Cherkashin AM, editors. Craniofacial distraction osteogenesis. St. Louis (MO): Mosby; 2001. p. 21–36.

[7] Ueda M, Matsuno M, Sakai K, et al. Mechanism of new bone formation during distraction osteogenesis: a preliminary report. In: Samchukov ML, Cope JB, Cherkashin AM, editors. Craniofacial distraction osteogenesis. St. Louis (MO): Mosby; 2001. p. 37–41.

[8] Meyer U, Joos U, Kruse-Losler B, et al. Mechanically induced tissue response during distraction. In: Samchukov ML, Cope JB, Cherkashin AM, editors. Craniofacial distraction osteogenesis. St. Louis (MO): Mosby; 2001. p. 42–52.

[9] Nocini PF, Wangerin K, Albanese M, et al. Histologic evaluation of human bone tissue 1 year after distraction. In: Samchukov ML, Cope JB, Cherkashin AM, editors. Craniofacial distraction osteogenesis. St. Louis (MO): Mosby; 2001. p. 68–71.

[10] Obwegeser H. Indications for surgical correction of mandibular deformity by the sagittal splitting technique. Br J Oral Surg 1964;1:157–68.

[11] Tessier PL. The definitive plastic surgical treatment of the severe facial deformities of craniofacial dysostosis, Crouzon and Apert disease. Plast Reconstr Surg 1971;48:419–42.

ELSEVIER
SAUNDERS

Otolaryngol Clin N Am
38 (2005) 361–369

OTOLARYNGOLOGIC
CLINICS
OF NORTH AMERICA

Soft Tissue Implants and Fillers

Jonathan M. Owens, MD

*Department of Otolaryngology-Head and Neck Surgery, University of Colorado Health
Sciences Center, 4200 East Ninth Avenue, Denver, CO 80262, USA*

The modern cosmetic and reconstructive surgeon encounters many situations requiring augmentation of soft tissue of the head and neck. Most commonly, cosmetic concerns of patients necessitate use of such techniques. With the aging of the baby boomers and an ever-increasing societal pressure encouraging youthful appearance, facial rejuvenation has increased in popularity. Soft tissue augmentation is a critical component of comprehensive facial rejuvenation in areas such as the midface, lips, or areas of static skin lines. Implants have also been important complementary components in other aspects of facial cosmetic surgery, including rhinoplasty, lip augmentation, mentoplasty, and midface enhancement. Implants are used in other areas of otolaryngology, including laryngoplasty, ossiculoplasty, facial reanimation, mucosal grafting, and tympanoplasty.

The ideal implant would be biologically inert, resemble tissue in its texture and pliability, possess longevity, be easily inserted and altered to the desired shape, create minimal morbidity at the insertion site or elsewhere, be minimally visible following placement, and be inexpensive. Such an implant has not been produced to date. To market a product as a medical implant or device in the United States, a manufacturer need not meet these criteria but must receive approval from the Food and Drug Administration (FDA) by filing for premarket approval. This approval simply confirms the safety of the device and its efficacy for the proposed applications. Long-term data regarding the true clinical utility of the device are generally not yet available upon approval for use. This information is attained through the combined experience of practicing clinicians and ultimately allows critical evaluation of the utility and merits of each particular implant. The past 2 decades have witnessed significant advances in the implants and fillers available to surgeons, particularly bioengineered autologous and allogeneic materials. Many different synthetic materials—polytetrafluoroethylene (Gore-Tex),

E-mail address: jonathan.owens@uchsc.edu

silicone rubber (Silastic), silicone, hydroxyapatite—as well as biologic
materials—collagen, hyaluronic acid, allogeneic dermis, autologous dermis,
and collagen—have reached the marketplace. Experience with each type of
implant has highlighted advantages and disadvantages that must be
critically compared with regard to the situation at hand. The two main
classes are solid implants and injectable fillers.

Implants

Autologous implants

The use of autologous implants has been reported for more than 3 centuries, with the first report of calvarial bone grafting in 1670 [1]. Cartilage
from septal, conchal, and costal sources has been used for nasal and
auricular reconstruction. Bone from calvarium, iliac crest, and tibia has
been incorporated in nasal and mandibular repair. Autologous fat has been
used as an injectable implant in the face and in the larynx and for
obliteration of the paranasal sinuses. The major drawback to autologous
implants is the donor-site morbidity.

Silicone

Silicone is the polymer created from dimethylsiloxane subunits that can
be vulcanized to create silicone rubber (Silastic). This product has been used
for decades as a facial implant. Silastic typically has no pores, eliminating
the possibility of fibrous ingrowth and blunting the inflammatory host
response following implantation. Fenestrated implants contain pores that
allow greater fibrous ingrowth, which prevents implant migration. Once in
place, Silastic implants are difficult to palpate. Furthermore, complications
such as bony erosion, infection, seroma, and extrusion, are quite rare.

A wide variety of Silastic facial implants is marketed by many companies.
These implants range from thin, conformable sheets used in middle ear
surgery and for nasal dorsal augmentation to preshaped malar and
mandibular implants. Silastic implants are also easily modified in the
operating room to adapt to the shape desired for such applications as
thyroplasty implants.

Gore-Tex

Gore-Tex is a product manufactured of expanded polytetrafluoroethylene. Gore-Tex, like Silastic, has been used successfully for decades,
primarily for vascular graft implants. This material does possess pores,
averaging approximately 22 μm, which allows limited fibrous ingrowth and
incorporation into the implant while preventing significant inflammatory
responses. The biocompatibility of Gore-Tex is excellent; low complication
rates are associated with its use.

The head and neck applications for which Gore-Tex has been used are similar to those of Silastic, including thyroplasty implants, nasolabial fold fillers, malar implants, and mandibular implants.

AlloDerm

AlloDerm (LifeCell Corp, Branchburg, New Jersey) is an acellular dermal graft product processed from cadaveric human skin. This material is processed by removing epithelial components, leaving the basement membrane intact. Dermal cells are then removed by a series of non-denaturing detergents while matrix degradation is prevented by inhibition of native metalloproteinases. This removal of cells limits the immunogenicity of the product, limiting rejection. The material is then freeze-dried in a manner that prevents damage to the collagen matrix. In the operating room, AlloDerm is rehydrated for 10 to 20 minutes in saline solution before use.

Following implantation, host fibroblasts migrate to the graft and begin native collagen deposition. Angiogenesis also occurs, creating a vascular matrix. This remodeling process continues for up to 180 days as the host incorporates the graft into the healing wound. Volume loss has been noted, with 30% to 50% loss at 1 year reported [2].

The initial application of AlloDerm was in burn surgery, but it has found numerous otolaryngologic applications as well. Its use has been reported in parotidectomy [3] and facial defect repair [4], nasal dorsal augmentation [5], lip augmentation, mucosal grafting [6], tympanoplasty, nasal perforation repair [7], and static facial rehabilitation following facial paralysis [8].

MEDPOR

MEDPOR (Porex, Newnan, Georgia) is an implantable, high-density polyethylene with large pores (>100 μm); the pore volume of the material is greater than 50%. This product is prepared as preformed implants or is available as a thin block that is easily fashioned to the appropriate dimensions in the operating room using standard surgical instruments. MEDPOR is typically placed subperiostially and may be secured in place with titanium screws, when possible, to prevent implant migration.

The large pore size facilitates rapid tissue ingrowth and incorporation within the implant [9]. This incorporation has been reported to be hastened by impregnation of the implant with autologous blood clot before implantation [10].

Applications that have been reported for MEDPOR include orbital reconstruction, rhinoplasty, midfacial skeleton augmentation, cranioplasty, and auricular reconstruction. MEDPOR has also been used for laryngotracheoplasty in animal studies [11]. The complication rate associated with the use of MEDPOR is low, with fracture [12] and infection [13] being reported.

Fillers

Bovine collagen

Bovine collagen has been used as an injectable filler for nearly 30 years [14]. The duration of effect from an injection of bovine collagen is typically less than 6 months. Zyderm (marketed by INAMED Aesthetics, formerly McGhan Medical, Santa Barabara, California) was the original injectable bovine collagen and was introduced in 1981. Zyderm was followed in 1985 by Zyplast, which was developed to provide a longer-lasting effect by cross-linking collagen fibrils with glutaraldehyde. Zyderm is packaged as Zyderm-I, a phosphate-buffered saline solution of 35 mg/mL of collagen with 0.3% lidocaine, and Zyderm-II, a concentration of 65 mg/mL of collagen with 0.3% lidocaine. Zyplast is similarly packaged with a concentration of 35 mg/mL of collagen, also with 0.3% lidocaine.

Skin testing is required before administration of these products, because 3% of the population will display a response to bovine collagen on skin challenge [15,16]. The response is typically a delayed hypersensitivity response, with erythema and wheal occurring 48 to 72 hours following exposure. Some sources even recommend a second skin test following a negative first test before initiating therapy, because 2% of patients will demonstrate hypersensitivity after repeat exposure despite initial nonreactivity [17]. It is also possible to develop hypersensitivity to bovine collagen following repeated injections, which must be monitored.

Overcorrection of collagen to the target tissue is necessary to achieve a desired result, because loss of water from within the injected material occurs. This loss may be as much as 20% to 30%. Degradation and resorption of collagen are also common, so that repeat injections are typically required at 4- to 6-month intervals to maintain the desired effect.

The applications described for bovine collagen injection are many. Correction of deep nasolabial folds, lip augmentation, and leveling of depressed facial scars are among those commonly reported.

Hyaluronic acid

Hyaluronic acid is a component of the proteoglycan portion of mesenchymal tissue. The substance is identical across all species and is therefore poorly immunogenic when used as an injectable filler. Skin testing, as required, for bovine collagen, is not necessary. Hylaform (INAMED, Santa Barbara, California) and Restylane (Q-Medical, Uppsala, Sweden) are two FDA-approved preparations of hyaluronic acid for soft tissue augmentation. Hylaform is produced from rooster combs and is a gel of hyaluronic acid with a small amount of avian protein. Hylaform is packaged in saline solution at a concentration of 5.5 mg/mL. Restylane is produced by bacteria in a biofermentation process and is packaged in a buffered solution at a concentration of 20 mg/mL.

A recent randomized, double-blind comparison of Restylane and Zyplast for correction of nasolabial folds found the effect of Restylane to be more durable at 6 months follow-up, with no difference in the complication rates associated with the two products [18]. Furthermore, hyaluronic acid binds more water than collagen, resulting in less loss of injected volume with hyaluronic acid products than with collagen injections. Thus, the amount of overcorrection required to achieve desired results is less with hyaluronic acid injections than with collagen.

The applications for injectable hyaluronic acid are similar to those of collagen, namely correction of deep facial folds and depressed scars.

Isolagen

Isolagen (Isolagen Technologies, Houston, Texas) is a unique product based on injection of the patient's own cells to correct a dermal defect. Isolagen is an injectable product consisting of autologous fibroblasts generated from a punch biopsy of postauricular skin using tissue culture techniques. The 3-mm punch biopsy is shipped on ice to the company for processing, which includes separation of native fibroblasts from the remainder of the tissue. The cells are then cultured and packaged as 1.0- to 1.5-mL injectable fillers approximately 6 weeks later. Injection is usually performed on three occasions, 2 weeks apart, to correct facial lines, wrinkles, and scars. The fibroblasts generate new collagen in situ, correcting the imperfection of the injected area.

An initial report of Isolagen included 10 patients, 9 of whom showed 60% to 100% improvement of the injected area at 6 months [19]. The authors also performed biopsies of injection sites before and after injection and noted significant increase in the density of dermal collagen [19]. A follow-up study of 94 patients revealed a 92% rate of patient satisfaction at 12 months and 70% satisfaction at 36 to 48 months [20].

Few adverse effects have been reported with Isolagen, because the material is autologous. The company reports a few cases of slight hypersensitivity to injection but no other adverse effects. Isolagen is not currently available in the United States. The FDA previously temporarily halted its review of the product after classifying the product as a medical device. Prospective, multicenter stage III trials are currently underway. The product is available in Europe, Asia, and Australia.

Autologen

Autologen (Collagenesis, Beverly, Massachusetts) is another product prepared from autologous tissue, with the injected product being a suspension of collagen. Autologen is prepared as a standard 4% solution in a phosphate buffer and also as Autologen XL, a 6% solution. Preparation of Autologen requires the harvest of donor skin, which is most commonly done in conjunction with other facial rejuvenation procedures such as blepharoplasty or rhytidectomy. This skin may be frozen for up to 2 weeks before shipment to the manufacturer. One mL of injectable final product can be obtained from 2 square inches of skin.

As with Isolagen, several Autologen injections are often required to achieve the desired result, because a volume loss of 20% to 30% is noted following injection [21]. Loss of correction also occurs over time, with 50% correction noted at 6 months [22].

Autologen has been studied in comparison to injectable bovine collagen. The two products produce similar clinical and histologic results [23]. The autologous nature of Autologen eliminates the necessity of skin testing as required with bovine collagen. The cost and donor site morbidity are major limitations associated with this product.

Dermalogen

Homologous human collagen from banked donor tissue is also available as an injectable filler. Dermalogen (Collagenesis, Beverly, Massachusetts) is prepared similarly to Autologen but with banked donor skin serving as the source of material. The banked tissue is thoroughly screened for infectious contamination before processing. The product is available in 3.5% buffered solutions and is distributed in prepackaged syringes.

The major advantage of homologous human collagen is that skin testing is not necessary as required with bovine collagen. Furthermore, Dermalogen has been shown to persist longer than injected bovine collagen at 12 weeks' follow-up, but more local inflammation was noted with Dermalogen [24]. Overcorrection by 20% to 30% is recommended to achieve desired results given the resorption of the product over time.

Dermalogen has been used as a dermal filler as well as an injected implant in vocal folds [25]. One reported foreign-body granulomatous response has been reported to Dermalogen [26].

Cymetra

Cymetra is a micronized form of Alloderm; Cymetra is dried and packaged in 330-mg samples. The particles are resuspended in 1 mL of lidocaine or saline, depending on whether anesthesia is necessary for the application. The product closely resembles Dermalogen but also contains dermal elements in addition to collagens, including elastins and proteogly-cans. Following injection, host fibroblasts and collagen are noted to infiltrate the implanted material [27].

The longevity of Cymetra has been noted to be greater than that of injected bovine collagen at 1 and 3 months [27]. Cymetra has been used as a dermal filler as well as for injection laryngoplasty [28]. Skin testing is not necessary when using Cymetra, and no adverse effects have been reported.

Hydroxyapatite

Hydroxyapatite, the mineral component of bone, has been engineered into various implant products, including ceramic implants, cement (Bone-Source, Stryker, Kalamazoo, Michigan), and injectable microspheres (Radiesse, formerly Radiance, Bioform, San Mateo, California). Furthermore, otologic implants of hydroxyapatite have been in use for many years.

BoneSource is packaged as a powder that is resuspended in saline to create a putty that can then be formed to the desired configuration. The putty forms a stable shape in 20 minutes and sets completely at 4 to 6 hours. The implant is converted to new bone rather than being resorbed over time, a process termed "osseoconversion" [29].

Radiesse is a product consisting of calcium hydroxyapatite spheres ranging 25 to 45 μm in diameter suspended in an aqueous gel, along with glycerin and sodium carboxycellulose. It may be applied to an open defect or injected into soft tissue. This injectable microsphere formulation has been shown to experience little migration following implantation and has a texture resembling native soft tissue [30].

The biocompatibility of hydroxyapatite products is excellent, with little to no inflammatory response noted at the implant site [29]. Applications for hydroxyapatite include cranioplasty and midface reconstruction, frontal sinus obliteration, soft tissue defect augmentation, laryngoplasty, and ossiculoplasty. The duration of effect of hydroxyapatite implants varies with the use. For cranioplasty the reconstruction is long-lived, with osseoconversion noted; with the injectable form, results are noted to last at least 2 years [30].

Summary

The number and variety of soft tissue implants and fillers at the clinician's disposal continues to increase rapidly as new materials and bioengineering techniques evolve. The ideal implant for all purposes does not yet exist, so the clinician must be familiar with a wide variety of products for each application. Continued advances in synthetic, allogeneic, and autologous products and experience with existing products will further augment the surgeon's armamentarium in the coming years.

References

[1] Van Meekren J. Observation medicohisurgicae. Amsterdam: Henrici and T. Bloom; 1670.
[2] Terion EO. AlloDerm acellular dermal graft: applications in esthetic and reconstructive soft tissue augmentation. In: Klein AW, editor. Tissue augmentation in clinical practice: procedures and techniques. New York: Dekker; 1998. p. 349–77.
[3] Chao C, Freidman C, Alford E, et al. Acellular dermal allograft prevents post-parotidectomy soft tissue defects: a preliminary experience. Journal of Otorhinolaryngology Head and Neck 1999;2:1–6.

[4] Achauer BM, VanderKam VM, Celikoz B, et al. Augmentation of facial soft-tissue defects with AlloDerm dermal graft. Ann Plast Surg 1998;41:503–7.

[5] Jackson IT, Yavuzer R. AlloDerm for dorsal nasal irregularities. Plast Reconstr Surg 2001; 107:553–8.

[6] Rhee PH, Friedman CD, Ridge JA, et al. The use of processed allograft dermal matrix for intraoral resurfacing: an alternative to split-thickness skin grafts. Arch Otolaryngol Head Neck Surg 1998;124:1201–4.

[7] Cohen NA, Mirza N. Acellular human dermal allograft in repair of unilateral partial-thickness and full-thickness nasal septal mucosal defects. Laryngoscope 2000;110:2005–8.

[8] Winslow CP, Wang TD, Wax MK. Static reanimation of the paralyzed face with an acellular dermal allograft sling. Arch Facial Plast Surg 2001;3:55–7.

[9] Niechajev I. Porous polyethylene implants for nasal reconstruction: clinical and histologic studies. Aesthetic Plast Surg 1999;23:395–402.

[10] Sabini P, Sclafani AP, Romo T, et al. Modulation of tissue ingrowth into porous high-density polyethylene implants with basic fibroblast growth factor and autologous blood clot. Arch Facial Plast Surg 2000;2:27–33.

[11] Hashem FK, Al Homsi M, Mahasin ZZ, et al. Laryngotracheoplasty using the Medpor implant: an animal model. J Otolaryngol 2001;30:334–9.

[12] Ozturk S, Sengezer M, Coskun U, et al. An unusual complication of a Medpor implant in nasal reconstruction: a case report. Aesthetic Plast Surg 2002;26:419–22.

[13] You JR, Seo JH, Kim YH, et al. Six cases of bacterial infection in porous orbital implants. Jpn J Ophthalmol 2003;47:512–8.

[14] Knapp TR, Kaplan EN, Daniels JR. Injectable collagen for soft tissue augmentation. Plast Reconstr Surg 1977;60:389–405.

[15] Framer FM, Churukium MM. Clinical use of injectable collagen: a three-year retrospective review. Arch Otolaryngol 1984;110:93–8.

[16] Cooperman LS, Mackinnon V, Bechler G, et al. Injectable collagen: a six-year clinical investigation. Aesthetic Plast Surg 1985;9:145–51.

[17] Stegman S, Chu S, Armstrong R. Adverse reactions to bovine collagen implant: clinical and histologic features. J Dermatol Surg Oncol 1988;14(Suppl):39–48.

[18] Narins RS, Brandt F, Leyden J, et al. A randomized, double-blind, multicenter comparison of the efficacy and tolerability of restylane versus Zyplast for the correction of nasolabial folds. Dermatol Surg 2003;29:588–95.

[19] Watson D, Keller GS, Lacombe V, et al. Autologous fibroblasts for treatment of facial rhytids and dermal depressions. Arch Facial Plast Surg 1999;1:165–70.

[20] Boss WK, Usal H, Fodor PB, et al. Autologous cultured fibroblasts: a protein repair system. Ann Plast Surg 2000;44:536–42.

[21] Fagien S. Facial soft-tissue augmentation with injectable autologous and allogeneic human tissue collagen matrix (Autologen and Dermalogen). Plast Reconstr Surg 2000; 105:362–73.

[22] DeVore DP, Kelman CD, Fagien S, et al. Autologen: autologous, injectable dermal collagen. In: Bosniak S, editor. Principles and practice of ophthalmic plastic and reconstructive surgery. Philadelphia: WB Saunders; 1995. p. 650–75.

[23] Sclafani AP, Romo T, Parker A, et al. Autologous collagen dispersion (Autologen) as a dermal filler: clinical observations and histologic findings. Arch Facial Plast Surg 2000; 2:48–52.

[24] Sclafani AP, Romo T, Parker A, et al. Homologous collagen dispersion (Dermalogen) as a dermal filler: persistence and histology compared with bovine collagen. Ann Plast Surg 2002;49:181–8.

[25] Courey MS. Homologous collagen substances for vocal fold augmentation. Laryngoscope 2001;111:747–58.

[26] Moody BR, Sengelmann RD. Self-limited adverse reaction to human-derived collagen injectable product. Dermatol Surg 2000;26:936–8.

[27] Sclafani AP, Romo T, Jacono AA, et al. Evaluation of acellular dermal graft in sheet (AlloDerm) and injectable (micronized AlloDerm) forms for soft tissue augmentation. Clinical observations and histological analysis. Arch Facial Plast Surg 2000;2:130–6.

[28] Pearl AW, Woo P, Ostrowski R, et al. A preliminary report on micronized AlloDerm injection laryngoplasty. Laryngoscope 2002;112:990–6.

[29] Friedman CD, Costantino PD, Takagi S, et al. BoneSource hydroxyapatite cement: a novel biomaterial for craniofacial skeletal tissue engineering and reconstruction. J Biomed Mater Res 1998;43:428–32.

[30] Tzikas TL. Evaluation of the radiance FN soft tissue filler for facial soft tissue augmentation. Arch Facial Plast Surg 2004;6:234–9.

ELSEVIER
SAUNDERS

Otolaryngol Clin N Am
38 (2005) 371–395

OTOLARYNGOLOGIC
CLINICS
OF NORTH AMERICA

New Radiation Therapy Techniques for the Treatment of Head and Neck Cancer

Meisong Ding, PhD*, Francis Newman, MS,
David Raben, MD

*Department of Radiation Oncology, University of Colorado Health Science Center,
Suite 1032, 1665 North Ursula Street, Aurora, CO 80010, USA*

Radiation therapy, also referred to as radiotherapy or radiation oncology, is one of the three principal treatments for cancer, the other two being surgery and chemotherapy. In many tumor types, surgery is the primary form of treatment, and it leads to good therapeutic results in some early nonmetastatic tumors. Radiotherapy has replaced surgery for the long-term control of many tumors of the head and neck, cervix, bladder, prostate, and skin, in which it often achieves a reasonable probability of tumor control with good cosmetic results. In contrast to other medical specialties that rely mainly on the clinical knowledge and experience of medical specialists, radiotherapy, with its use of ionizing radiation in treatment of cancer, relies heavily on modern technology. There are two main categories of radiotherapy procedures: teletherapy (external beam radiotherapy) and brachytherapy. In external beam radiotherapy, the radiation source is located at a certain distance from the patient, and the target and the tumor volume, delineated by the radiation oncologist, are irradiated with an external radiation beam. In brachytherapy, radiation sources are placed directly into the target volume or onto a target. Most external beam radiotherapy is performed with photon beams from a linear accelerator, some with electron beams, and a very small fraction with more exotic particles, such as protons, neutrons, or heavier ions. The general goal of radiotherapy is to control local tumor growth by delivering a prescribed dose while minimizing damage to healthy tissues.

Traditionally, surgery or radiotherapy alone has been used to treat head and neck cancer. During the past decade, various radiotherapy fractionation

---

* Corresponding author.
E-mail address: Meisong.ding@uchsc.edu (M. Ding).

schedules or a combination of radiotherapy and chemotherapy has been used to increase tumor control and maintain organ integrity [1–5]. To date, success in rehabilitation to circumvent the problems of dysphagia has been modest. Investigations have focused on diagnostic studies and understanding specific events involved in the pathophysiology. Current research has incorporated measures aimed at sparing normal tissue structures from the acute and chronic effects of radiation therapy and has introduced new radiotherapy modalities. Common radiotherapy for treatment of head and neck cancer has been described in many articles in the oncology literature [6–9]. As well as introducing new treatment modalities for different head and neck cancers [7], the literature often gives site-by-site analysis of head and neck treatments [6,8–9]. This article focuses on the development of radiation therapy techniques for the treatment of head and neck cancer and tries to cover the most current radiation treatment modalities and diagnostic techniques in the field.

Interstitial brachytherapy

Permanent implantation of encapsulated radioactive seeds in tumors has widely been used as a primary or adjuvant therapy for treating head and neck cancer [10–12]. Low-dose-rate (LDR) brachytherapy with permanent implants and high-dose-rate (HDR) brachytherapy with remote after-loading devices have equivalent long-term results for treatment of head and neck cancer. With the advantage of eliminating potential radiation exposure to the operators, HDR brachytherapy has started to supplant LDR brachytherapy at some clinics.

At present, seeds that contain the radionuclide of Iodine-125 (^{125}I) or Palladium-103 (^{103}Pd) are routinely used in permanent interstitial implants [13]. The ^{125}I seed has a long decay half-life (59.4 days), whereas the ^{103}Pd seed has a shorter half-life (16.991 days) [14]. ^{103}Pd seeds are generally considered to be more effective for fast-growing tumors, whereas ^{125}I seeds are better for slow-growing tumors [15]. Because tumors may contain both fast- and slow-growing cells, it would seem desirable to use a mixture of radionuclides with short and long half-lives (eg, ^{103}Pd and ^{125}I) in the same tumor volume. Recently interstitial seed implants containing mixtures of seeds with different half-lives have been investigated and used clinically [16–21].

Chen and Nath [16] illustrated the dose delivered as a function of implant time for a ^{125}I and a ^{103}Pd implant, as shown in Fig. 1. As an example, the time required to deliver 80% of dose to full decay differs by a factor of more than three, amounting to about 140 days for ^{125}I implants and about 40 days for ^{103}Pd implants. This difference in the rate of dose delivery can result in different clinical responses for a given total dose when the surviving cells in the irradiated volume are continuously proliferating and the sublethally damaged cells can be repaired during the protracted dose delivery. When seeds of different half-lives are mixed in the same implant, the temporal dose

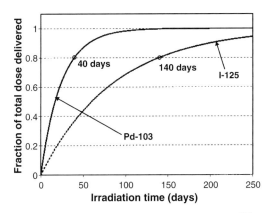

Fig. 1. Accumulative dose delivered as a function of implant time for ^{125}I and ^{103}Pd implants. The vertical axis was plotted as the ratio of delivered dose to the dose to full decay. (*From* Chen Z, Nath R. Biologically effective dose (BED) for interstitial seed implants containing a mixture of radionuclides with different half-lives. Int J Radiat Oncol Biol Phys 2003; 55(3):825–34; with permission.)

delivery pattern to a point within the implant is defined by the decay characteristics of all radionuclides that contribute dose to it.

Using a generalized equation for the biologically effective dose, Chen and Nath [16] examined the effects of cell proliferation and sublethal damage repair and pointed out that an implant containing a mixture of ^{125}I and ^{103}Pd seeds demonstrates that the conventional dose prescription to an isodose surface is not unique for such an implant. When the prescription dose is based on existing clinical experience using ^{125}I seeds alone, mixing ^{103}Pd seeds with ^{125}I seeds increases the cell kill. On the other hand, if the prescription dose is based on existing clinical experience using ^{103}Pd seeds alone, mixing ^{125}I seeds with ^{103}Pd seeds in the same implant creates radiobiologic "cold" spots (ie, an increase in cell survival) at locations where a major portion of the prescription dose is contributed by the ^{125}I seeds. For fast-growing tumors, these "cold" spots can become significant. Chen and Nath [16] concluded that total dose alone is not sufficient for a complete characterization of a permanent seed implant containing a mixture of radionuclides with different half-lives because of the effects of cell proliferation and sublethal damage repair during the protracted dose delivery. When radionuclides of different half-lives are mixed in a permanent implant, using the dose prescription established from existing clinical experience with implants with the longer half-life radionuclide helps avoid radiobiologic "cold" spots.

LDR interstitial brachytherapy (LDRIB) is an effective modality for the treatment of oropharyngeal carcinoma. Excellent local control (65%–89%) has been reported using this modality [17–21]. With LDRIB, however, radiation exposure to medical personnel is unavoidable, even when an afterloading device is used. To eliminate this concern, Nose et al [22] use

HDR interstitial brachytherapy (HDRIB), which consists of implanting plastic tubes in the pharyngeal cavity that subsequently receives ^{192}Ir sources by manual afterloading [23]. Between 1993 and 2003, they used HDRIB plus external beam radiotherapy to treat 83 patients with oropharyngeal squamous cell carcinomas. From their 10-year experience, Nose et al [22] concluded that HDRIB could achieve excellent local control and acceptable rates of complication, equivalent to the results reported for LDRIB series. Because of the advantage of radioprotection, HDRIB may replace LDRIB in the treatment of head and neck cancer.

Hyperfractionation and accelerated fractionation radiotherapy

A variety of fractionation schedules, including standard fractionation, hyperfractionation, accelerated fractionation, and their variants, have been used in the radiotherapy of advanced head and neck cancer. The failure of conventional radiotherapy to control more tumors can be attributed to several biologic and physical factors. Rapid repopulation of surviving clonogenic tumor cells has received much attention as a possible cause of failure, particularly in treatment schedules with a long overall time span [24–25]. During the last 2 decades, accelerated radiotherapy schedules have been investigated with the objective of shortening overall treatment time in head and neck cancer [26–31]. In essence, it is predicted that accelerated fractionation will improve the therapeutic ratio through a differential response of tumors and normal tissues to fractionated radiotherapy. Theoretically, with hyperfractionation, the use of multiple smaller dose fractions makes it possible to increase the total dose, thereby increasing the probability of tumor control, without increasing late complications. Accelerated fractionation, by shortening the overall treatment time, should minimize tumor repopulation during treatment and therefore increase the probability of tumor control with a similar total dose.

The recent Radiation Therapy Oncology Group trial [32] tested the efficacy of hyperfractionation and two types of accelerated fractionation individually against standard fractionation. In this large trial, eligible patients were randomly assigned to receive radiotherapy delivered using

1. Standard fractionation at 2 Gy/fraction/day, 5 days/week, to 70 Gy/35 fractions/7 weeks
2. Hyperfractionation at 1.2 Gy/fraction, twice daily, 6 hours apart, 5 days/week to 81.6 Gy/68 fractions/7 weeks
3. Accelerated fractionation with split at 1.6 Gy/fraction, twice daily, 6 hours apart, 5 days/week, to 67.2 Gy/42 fractions/6 weeks including a 2-week rest after 38.4 Gy
   or
4. Accelerated fractionation with concomitant boost at 1.8 Gy/fraction/day, 5 days/week to large field plus 1.5 Gy/fraction/day to boost field

given 6 hours after treatment of the large field for the last 12 treatment days to a total dose of 72 Gy/42 fractions/6 weeks.

Additional boost doses not exceeding 5.0 Gy through reduced fields to persistent primary tumor or clinically positive nodes were allowed. Neck dissection was allowed for neck nodes larger than 3 cm before radiotherapy at the discretion of the responsible head and neck surgeon and radiation oncologist. Radiotherapy was delivered using linear accelerators or cobalt-60 machines with a source-to-surface or source-to-isocenter distance of 80 cm or more.

Fig. 2 shows the outcome of the trial. The results suggest that both total dose and treatment duration are important in the outcome of radiotherapy. Local-regional control was significantly increased by an increase of the total dose without changing the overall time using hyperfractionation or by a shortening of the overall time while maintaining the same total dose using accelerated fractionation with concomitant boost. Accelerated fractionation with split was not shown to improve local-regional control in this randomized trial.

Although both hyperfractionation and accelerated fractionation with concomitant boost resulted in a gain in local-regional control and disease-free survival, the overall survival did not change significantly in this analysis. Data in the literature suggest that chemotherapy given concurrently with radiotherapy improves the results over radiotherapy alone for locally advanced head and neck cancer [33–36]. The optimal chemotherapy regimen to be combined with radiotherapy remains to be determined.

Intensity-modulated radiation therapy

Although conventional radiation therapy can address the primary tumor site and the adjacent lymphatic drainage, conventional radiation therapy, including three-dimensional conformal radiation therapy (3-D CRT), frequently impairs salivary gland function, causing permanent xerostomia. Recent technologic advances have led to the successful clinical implementation of intensity-modulated radiation therapy (IMRT). IMRT can spare normal tissues that are surrounded by targets with concave surfaces, and this advantage is currently being exploited to escalate tumor dose. Such truly 3-D conformal dose distributions are now possible through the addition of inverse algorithms in treatment planning and the introduction of the multileaf collimator (MLC)-equipped treatment machines capable of delivering intensity-modulated beams. Compensator-based IMRT (also known as solid IMRT) has also been incorporated into clinical practice but is not as common as the MLC-based methods. These new developments involve complex concepts, and it is vital that those who intend to implement IMRT in a clinical program clearly understand the process so that this new modality is safely applied.

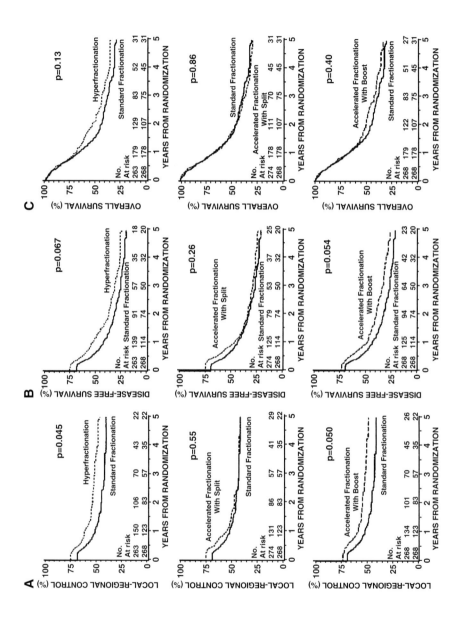

The combined committee of the American Society for Therapeutic Radiation and Oncology and the American Association of Physicists in Medicine [36] points out some differences between IMRT and conventional planning and treatment techniques:

- IMRT dose distributions are often more heterogeneous within the target, so prescribing a dose to a single point is generally unsatisfactory.
- IMRT intensity maps can contain many extremes and are often nonintuitive and unfamiliar to most radiation oncologists, physicists, and dosimetrists. Thus, incorrect placement and orientation of modulated fields may not be obvious to the user, forcing additional burdensome quality assurance (QA) steps.
- Radiation leakage through and between the MLC leaves, as well as through other shielding in the accelerator head, can result in a higher whole-body dose during IMRT, because the accelerator usually gives substantially more monitor units to deliver the desired tumor dose.
- IMRT allows the simultaneous treatment of the primary tumor and regions of subclinical disease. This feature can make it difficult or even impossible to use standard dose fractionation for both volumes.
- Conformal radiation techniques, especially IMRT, often require an acute understanding of radiographic anatomy for definition of both tumor and critical structures.
- The highly conformal nature of IMRT is leading to significant improvements in such areas as detection and control of target and organ motion and in patient immobilization.
- IMRT requires a greatly expanded emphasis on QA procedures to guarantee its proper implementation.

Head and neck cancer is an attractive site for IMRT [37]. In the head and neck, organ motion is practically absent, and only the set-up uncertainties need to be addressed. Many critical and radiation-sensitive organs are in close proximity to the targets. Tight dose gradients around the targets, limiting the doses to the noninvolved tissue, offer the potential for a therapeutic gain.

Inverse-planned treatment system

Inverse treatment planning starts with a treatment objective and obtains the solution by optimizing an objective function. The clinical objectives are usually multifaceted and may be incompatible. A set of importance factors

Fig. 2. Kaplan-Meier estimates of (A) the duration of local-regional control of disease, (B) disease-free survival, and (C) overall survival. (From Fu KK, Pajak TF, Trotti A, et al. A Radiation Therapy Oncology Group (RTOG) phase III randomized study to compare hyperfractionation and two variants of accelerated fractionation to standard fractionation radiotherapy for head and neck squamous cell carcinomas: first report of RTOG 9003. Int J Radiat Oncol Biol Phys 2000;48(1):7–16; with permission.)

is often incorporated in the objective function to parametrize trade-off strategies and to prioritize the dose conformality in different anatomic structures. Whereas the general formalism remains the same, different sets of importance factors characterize plans of obviously different character and thus critically determine the final plan.

The University of California-San Francisco (UCSF) experience can demonstrate the use of IMRT for the treatment of nasopharyngeal carcinoma (NPC) using a commercial inverse treatment planning system [38–40]. Patients with early-stage (T1 and T2) and advanced-stage (T3 and T4) disease were treated consecutively with inverse-planned (IP) IMRT between October 1997 and January 2000 at UCSF. For all NPC patients, the treatment goal was to deliver a dose of 70 Gy (2.12 Gy/fraction) to 95% or more of the gross tumor volume (GTV) and a dose of 59.4 Gy (1.8 Gy/ fraction) to 95% or more of the planning target volume (PTV) simulta- neously, while keeping doses to all adjacent sensitive structures below tolerance. The tolerance doses to sensitive structures are defined as follows:

- The maximum point doses to the spinal cord and the brainstem are to be less than 45 Gy and 54 Gy, respectively.
- The maximum point doses to the optic structures, such as the chiasm and optic nerves, are to be less than 54 Gy.
- The mean dose to either parotid gland is to be less than 26 Gy.
- The maximum point doses to the temporomandibular joints and mandible are to be less than 70 Gy (ie, no more than 1 cm^3 of the volume received a dose greater than 70 Gy).
- The doses to other structures such as the middle and inner ears, brain, tongue, and larynx should be as low as possible.

The IMRT plans are delivered using a conventional MLC and are generated with the CORVUS planning system (NOMOS Corp., Sewickley, Pennsylvania). In the planning system, gantry angles, couch angles, collimator angles, and beam energy are selected manually.

Forward-planned treatment system

Although IP-IMRT is the most ideal treatment technique for patients with head and neck cancer, this technology is not readily available in every radiotherapy clinic, and some patients are not ideal candidates for IP- IMRT because of their inability to remain immobilized for a prolonged time during the course of treatment. Forward-planned IMRT (forward- planned multisegmented technique, FPMS) can improve dose distributions over conventional opposed-lateral fields [41–43]. In forward-planned IMRT, the planning dosimetrist or physicist selects the number, energy, weighting, and angle of beams. The computer then calculates the dose distribution and generates beam's-eye views, along with dose–volume histograms. The plan is optimized by manual iteration or trial and error.

This process is in contrast to IP, in which one first defines the desired dose to the target and the normal tissues, and after multiple iterations a computerized optimization program finds the optimal parameters that will yield the desired dose distribution.

At UCSF, 38 patients with primary head and neck cancer were treated using the FPMS technique between 1995 and 2002 [43]. The primary tumor and the upper neck nodes were treated with seven gantry angles, including an anterior, two lateral, two anterior oblique, and two posterior oblique beams with a total of 13 beam shapes formed by MLCs, called "MLC segments." The shape of each MLC segment was carefully designed, and the associated weights were optimized through manual iterations. The lower neck nodes and the supraclavicular nodes were treated with a split-beam anterior field, matched to the inferior border of the FPMS plan at the isocenter. With an autosequencing delivery system, all fields, including dynamic wedges, can be automatically treated.

Aperture-based treatment system

The IP-IMRT previously described typically divides the beam's-eye view of the tumor into a series of finite-sized beams (beamlets). The beamlet dose distributions are computed, and their corresponding weights are optimized. During the optimization, the quality of the plan is scored based on the predefined treatment goals. After the optimization is complete, a leaf-sequencing algorithm translates the final intensity maps for each beam direction into a set of deliverable beam segments. The resulting MLC leaf sequence often contains a large number of segments, resulting in a large monitor unit-to-cGy ratio. The large number of segments also creates significant uncertainties in leakage, head scatter, and tongue-and-groove effects.

Recently, there has been a growing interest in aperture-based IP (ABIP) for IMRT [44–46]. The attractive features of this approach include faster optimizations, because fewer degrees of freedom are involved, and the avoidance of the degrading segmentation phase inherent in beamlet-based IP. Moreover, if the apertures are related in a useful way to the anatomy of the patient, the treatment verification may be simplified. Even where small fields or small numbers of monitor units are involved, however, the need for additional verifications is not eliminated.

For each beam direction, ABIP generates segments by a multistep procedure. During the initial steps, beam's-eye-view projections of the PTVs and organs at risk (OARs) are generated. These projections are used to make a segmentation grid with negative values across the expanded OAR projections and positive values elsewhere inside the expanded PTV projections. Outside these regions, grid values are set to zero. Subsequent steps transform the positive values of the segmentation grid to increase with decreasing distance to the OAR projections and to increase with longer pathlengths measured along rays from their entrance point through the skin contours to their respective grid point. The final steps involve selection of iso-value lines of the segmentation grid as segment outlines that are transformed to leaf and jaw positions of a MLC. Segment shape approximations, if imposed by MLC constraints, are constructed to minimize overlap between the expanded OAR projections and the segment aperture.

By inferring the segment shapes directly from the geometry of the PTVs and the patient's anatomy, ABIP allows millimeter-precise control of the location of dose gradients in the planned dose distribution. Thus without requiring a dose computation, ABIP is a fast procedure to generate a set of segments during IMRT planning. The plan is finalized by assigning weights to the segments or by further optimization of segment shapes and weights. ABIP avoids the step of translating complicated intensity maps to sequences of segments.

Immobilization in intensity-modulated radiation therapy

To realize the benefit of IMRT, highly precise patient set-up and immobilization are necessary [47–48]. Because IMRT requires greater precision than conventional radiation therapy, there is an increased chance of patient displacement during IMRT treatment. To ensure that patient displacement is within the tolerance margin used in treatment planning, it is essential to have an immobilization system that works effectively for long treatment durations. Immobilization devices can reduce patient movement significantly. How much immobilization systems can reduce intrafraction motion varies from one disease site to another and depends on the type of device used [49].

In IMRT for the treatment of head and neck cancer, a facemask is an immobilization device commonly used to avoid patient movement. Kim et al [50] evaluated the uncertainty of intrafraction patient displacement in head and neck IMRT patients. Immobilization is performed in three steps: (1) the patient is immobilized with a thermoplastic facemask, (2) the patient displacement is monitored using a commercial stereotactic infrared camera (ExacTrac, BrainLab, Westchester, Illinois) during treatment, and (3) repositioning is performed as needed. The displacement data were recorded using the camera system during beam-on time for the entire treatment duration for five patients. As an evaluation tool, Kim et al [50] used the concept of cumulative time versus the patient position uncertainty histogram, referred to as the uncertainty time histogram (UTH). UTH is defined as the relative accumulated time during which a patient stays within a certain displacement uncertainty. Results of the UTH show that for the first five IMRT patients treated with this immobilization system, the patient displacement was kept within 1.5 mm for 95% of the treatment. Analysis indicates that such immobilization procedures for head and neck IMRT patients are quite effective.

Recently, at the University of Florida, the Vac Fix (S & S Par Scientific, Odense, Denmark) mold immobilization procedure has been used for patients who are claustrophobic or cannot tolerate a facemask during IMRT of the head and neck [51]. The immobilization procedure combines the use of the commercial stereotactic infrared ExacTrac camera system for patient set-up and monitoring. The Vac Fix mold is placed on the headrest and is folded up as needed to provide support before the mold is hardened. Although this system causes more frequent interruptions of beam delivery, it is as effective as the mask plus the camera system in immobilizing patients within the tolerance limit.

Extracranial stereotactic radiotherapy

Stereotactic radiosurgery

Stereotactic radiosurgery (SRS) offers the merits of the mechanical accuracy of stereotaxy—high and homogeneous dose distribution within a small target volume, and the rapid dose fall-off in the surrounding normal tissues. SRS has been successful in treating small brain tumors with high accuracy. The gamma knife and linear accelerator are two of the most common machines for photon beam radiosurgery. The same SRS equipment used for intracranial lesions can treat head and neck lesions, as long as the headframe is placed low enough on the skull to permit CT scanning and MRI through both the stereotaxic fiducial device and skull base in at least one axial plane [52–53].

Among the crucial requirements for stereotactic procedures are patient immobilization and precise anatomic localization of the target. These requirements are achieved either by frame-based methods [52–55], using a suitable head-and-neck stereotactic frame, or by frameless means [56]. For frame-based SRS, the Gill-Thomas-Cosman (GTC) frame [54] is commonly used for treatment of intracranial lesions. The GTC frame design incorporates a mouthpiece, an occipital pad, and a head strap for support and immobilization. Kassaee et al [57] modified the GTC frame by lowering it a few centimeters to accommodate lower-lying lesions, including nasopharyngeal and paranasal sinus tumors. Radionics XKNIFE software (Tyco, Burlington, Massachusetts) was used for the treatment planning. CT scanning of the patient is done with the modified frame in the same way as with the original frame. The modification rods do not alter the quality of the CT images and appear in the CT image without introducing artifacts in the treatment area. Treatment planning is performed in the usual manner with both stereotactic cones and a mini-MLC. The modification of the frame with additional pieces allows immobilization of the patient with stereotactic precision. The modification of the frame does not alter the patient tolerance of the device. The modification of the existing commercial intracranial GTC relocatable stereotactic localization frame allows stereotactic radiation therapy of the skull base, nasopharynx, selected paranasal sinus, and upper neck tumors. The advantage of such a device is accurate positioning of the patient with the precision obtainable by stereotactic localization. The accuracy of repositioning showed results similar to those achieved with the original frame [57].

Fractionated stereotactic radiotherapy

Fractionated stereotactic radiation therapy (FSRT) is a modification of SRS. The substantial risk of radiation-induced morbidity of the single high-dose radiation has motivated the development of FSRT technique [58]. FSRT requires the technology of SRS, which includes the sophisticated treatment planning system, the high-energy therapy machine, and the stereotactic immobilization devices. The immobilization devices, however, must be uniquely designed for relocatable daily use; the relocatable stereotactic frame system is the essential component of the FSRT technique. FSRT offers the radiobiologic advantage of conventional fractionation in addition to the mechanical precision achieved by stereotactic devices.

An example of clinical experience using FSRT for extracranial head and neck tumors comes from South Korea [59]. Individualized treatment planning was performed using the XKnife-3 system with a relocatable GCT frame. For some patients FSRT was applied as a boost technique following the two-dimensional conventional external radiation therapy. For the other patients FSRT was the sole radiotherapy modality. The fractionation schedule was five treatments per week, and the fractional doses were 2–3 Gy, depending on the treatment aim and the FSRT volume. The FSRT doses varied depending on the nature of the primary disease. The local tumor response in patients with NPC was excellent compared with retrospective data, and there were no unexpectedly severe complications. FSRT to other regions was well tolerated by the patients and resulted in good to excellent local tumor responses with no unacceptable side effects. FSRT is an effective and safe modality for the treatment of extracranial head and neck tumors.

Neutron radiotherapy

Adenoid cystic carcinomas (ACC) arising in the head and neck are relatively uncommon entities and account for only 1% to 2% of all head and neck malignancies [60]. Historically, surgical resection was the primary mode of treatment. In the 1980s, studies examining the effect of high linear energy transfer radiation were begun on a variety of tumors in an attempt to determine whether with neutron radiotherapy offers any therapeutic benefit [61]. These studies found a radiobiologic effect (RBE) for fractionated neutron radiotherapy of 8 for ACC compared with a RBE of 3 to 3.5 for most late-reacting, normal tissues. Thus fractionated neutron therapy results in a therapeutic gain of approximately 2.5 over conventional photon radiotherapy in salivary gland tumors.

In neutron radiotherapy, patients are usually treated using a high-energy, hospital-based, Scanditronix MC 50 cyclotron (Scanditronix Wellhöfer AB, Uppsala, Sweden) [62]. The cyclotron uses a 50.5 MeV p → Be reaction and is equipped with an isocentric rotating gantry and an MLC system that permits the use of conformal field shaping. Fields are individualized according to the location and extent of the primary tumor and areas at risk for tumor spread. Most patients with major salivary gland tumors are initially treated using a three-field parotid technique to spare the contralateral parotid gland as much as possible [63]. A CT-based, 3-D conformal treatment planning system is used to design the boost fields. Fraction sizes ranged from 1.7 neutron Gy given three times per week to 1.05 neutron Gy given four times a week. The median total dose prescribed to isocenter is 19.2 neutron Gy (range, 15.2–22.55). Recently, the most commonly used fractionation scheme has been 1.2 neutron Gy given four times a week to a total dose of 19.2 Gy.

Douglas et al [64] examined the efficacy of fast neutron radiotherapy for the treatment of locally advanced and recurrent adenoid cystic carcinoma of the head and neck and for identifying prognostic variables associated with local-regional control and survival. They concluded that fast neutron radiotherapy is an effective treatment for locally advanced ACC of the head and neck region in patients with gross residual disease, with 5-year actuarial cause-specific survival and local-regional control rates of 77% and 57%, respectively. Patients not having high-risk factors (eg, base of skull [BOS] involvement, positive lymph nodes, recurrent tumors) at the time of treatment had a 5-year actuarial cause-specific survival rate of 100%. Local-regional control was also good, 80% at 5 years, in patients without BOS invasion who had undergone a surgical debulking. Outcomes in patients with BOS involvement evidently continue to be unsatisfactory, with local-regional control rates of approximately 30% at 5 years.

Electron conformal radiotherapy

Conventional radiotherapy for head and neck cancer uses photon beams, electron beams, or a combination of the two. In the past, photon conformal radiotherapy was the primary method, because there was a lack of accuracy in planning electron treatments and because the large penumbra that developed at the edge of the electron field inhibited the use of electrons as the primary modality. The physics of X-ray energy deposition suggests that the photon beam is not well suited to the treatment of shallow targets. Furthermore, in many cases the slow attenuation of photon beams makes photon conformal therapy a poor choice for some targets with distal critical structures. In contrast, electron beams, with comparatively higher surface doses and more rapid depth–dose fall-off, are well suited to treat superficial target volumes in the head and neck.

The goal of electron conformal radiotherapy is to select optimal conditions to conform a 90% isodose surface to the distal border of a target volume, while simultaneously maintaining as uniform dose within a PTV and as little dose to nearby critical organs and normal tissue as possible. In addition to the irregular surface commonly seen in head and neck patients, the PTV thickness is not usually uniform and may sometimes vary from less than 1 cm to greater than 5 cm. An electron beam with a spatially uniform energy and intensity may irradiate critical underlying structures unnecessarily. The solution to this problem is a beam that has higher energy where more penetration is necessary and lower energy where less penetration is required. This variability can be achieved using electron bolus [65–66] or specially designed electron MLCs [67–68], which provide spatially dependent energy modulation of the electron field, thus compensating for the irregularities.

The use of a custom-shaped electron bolus is not a new concept. Custom-shaped boluses are commonly used in electron therapy for treatment of breast cancer [69–70] and other cancers [71]. Recently, at the M. D. Anderson Cancer Center, Kudchadker et al [65] developed a custom 3-D electron bolus for electron beam radiotherapy for tumors located in the head and neck region. The treatment planning and delivery methods used in their bolus electron conformal therapy include the following concepts:

1. Acquisition of a 3-D model of the patient using CT
2. Development of a treatment plan and approval by the physician
3. Fabrication of the electron bolus and other patient-specific treatment hardware
4. QA to assess the quality of the electron bolus and the plan

The patient's bolus is designed using bolus design tools implemented in their in-house treatment planning system. The bolus is fabricated using a computer-controlled milling machine. After the bolus passes the QA process (to ensure proper fabrication and placement of the bolus), the patient undergoes a second CT scan with the bolus. The final plan is based on the data from the second CT scan. Bolus electron conformal radiotherapy offers a useful method for achieving electron conformal therapy in head and neck cancer, especially when the patient's surface anatomy has surgical defects and when the PTV is near the patient's surface and has a variable thickness.

An electron multileaf collimator (eMLC) has the potential to revolutionize electron radiotherapy just as the photon multileaf collimator (xMLC) has for photon radiotherapy. An eMLC could be useful for shaping irregular fields and allowing intensity-modulated electron therapy, thus making the fabrication of custom blocking and a custom electron bolus unnecessary. Modulated electron radiotherapy using an eMLC is a new electron modality that has been developed to deliver highly conformal doses to shallow targets. Dose conformity in the beam direction can be achieved by energy modulation; lateral uniformity and conformity can be achieved by intensity modulation using eMLC.

One of the earliest proposed applications of an eMLC was in arc therapy. Leavitt et al [72] showed that by dynamically shaping the eMLC as the gantry rotates, a homogeneous dose could be delivered for chest wall irradiation, regardless of the positioning of the isocenter. Recently, Ma et al [67] demonstrated that their prototype manual eMLC could deliver modulated electron radiation therapy (MERT). MERT uses multiple beams of differing electron energies, each beam being intensity modulated by the eMLC, to deliver an optimized dose distribution. Highly conformal treatment plans using MERT have been calculated for the chest wall [67,73]. There are two options for the MERT: the use of the xMLC for electrons or the development of a specific eMLC. Investigators using the xMLC for electron beams having dual scattering foil systems concluded that the width of the resulting penumbra was too great, even when treating at source-surface-distances (SSDs) as small as 65 cm [74–75]. It seems clinically impractical to use current commercial xMLCs in modulated electron radiotherapy. A prototype eMLC has been applied in the clinic at M. D. Anderson Cancer Center as shown in Fig. 3 [68]. In Fig. 3A, the prototype eMLC is attached to a Siemens Primus (Siemens AG, Munich, Germany) X-ray blocking tray. The eMLC does not have its retraction or deployment systems, with only four rods used to fix the position of the eMLC at 90-cm source-collimator-distance (SCD). Fig. 3B shows a top view of the leaf bed. The brass leaves are fabricated using electronic discharge machining to a tolerance of less than 6.35 μm (0.25 mil). The leaves are mounted on an aluminum base plate and ride on rods that keep them tracking properly and allow them to interdigitate. An overhead bar pressed on the leaves prevents them from moving once they are properly positioned. Such an eMLC could be a substitute for the applicator system for fixed-beam therapy.

Imaging and diagnostic techniques

Combined positron emission tomography/CT system

CT and MRI are the standard imaging techniques used for the evaluation of a patient with head and neck cancer. They provide structural information with high spatial resolution and are therefore used routinely in the initial staging of tumors in these patients. A complete range of biochemical events associated with cancer, however, cannot be imaged using anatomic/geometric techniques such as CT and MRI. Positron emission tomography (PET) is a quantitative imaging modality that can assess biologic characteristics of the tissue, including metabolism, proliferation, and blood flow. The information obtained by PET is essentially independent of tumor location and lesion size.

PET has been used in the clinic for the assessment of tumor aggressiveness [76], for treatment evaluation [77], and for detection of

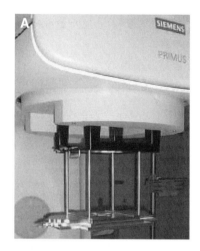

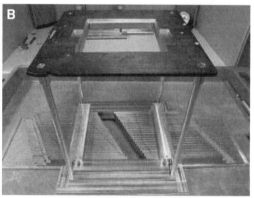

Fig. 3. (*A*) View of eMLC mounted on Siemens Primus accessory tray holder. Note the upper trimmer and lower leaf bed. Rigid rods placed the eMLC leaves 10 cm from the isocenter (90-cm SCD) for the present set of measurements. (*B*) View showing details of 21 leaf pairs. Indices on the leaf bed support and guidance plate are used for the manual positioning of leaves. (*From* Hogstrom K, Boyd RA, Antolak JA, et al. Dosimetry of a prototype retractable eMLC for fixed-beam electron therapy. Med Phys 2004;31(3):443–62; with permission.)

recurrent disease [78] in patients with head and neck cancer. Because of the additional information provided by PET, the current trend in radiotherapy is to incorporate PET imaging data to reduce or to eliminate geographical misses and help guide dose intensification to the most metabolically active areas within the neoplasm. Because of the lack of anatomic detail in the imaging the complex anatomy in the head and neck region, and because a number of normal structures (eg, lymphoid tissue, laryngeal muscle, and salivary glands) demonstrate a wide variety of patterns and intensity of fluorodeoxyglucose (FDG) uptake, PET techniques have not been widely applied in routine radiotherapy for head and neck cancer. Registration of CT and PET data will improve the ability of radiotherapy to treat the tumor adequately when compared with both CT and PET imaging modalities considered individually. Combined PET/CT is a recent imaging technique that permits almost synchronous image acquisition and exact coregistration of anatomic and metabolic data sets [79]. The combined technique has an advantage in the interpretation of PET images in patients with head and neck malignancies [80].

In a recent example of integrated PET/CT applied in radiotherapy for treatment of head and neck cancer comes from Switzerland [81]. CT and a FDG-PET studies in treatment position were obtained using an integrated PET/CT scanner (Discovery LS, GE Medical Systems, Milwaukee, Wisconsin) for 12 patients with head and neck cancer. The PET/CT device combined a GE Advance NXi PET and a multislice helical CT scanner (LightSpeed plus) in one system. The axes of both systems were mechanically aligned to coincide. CT data were acquired first, during shallow breathing. PET images were acquired during free breathing and over multiple respiratory cycles. The PET and CT data sets were acquired in two independent acquisition computer systems that were connected by an interface to transfer CT data to the PET scanner. The CT data set was the primary image set used for dose calculation, and the PET data were used as an overlay. Matching was done simply by hardware coregistration and by the table coordinates. Planning was performed in two steps. First, using CT, the target volume was defined. Second, planning was repeated by the same radiation oncologist with the coregistered PET/CT data being available. The volume was thus delineated using the additional information from the PET data. In this study, with PET/CT the delineation of the GTV was increased by more than 25% in 2 of 12 patients, and the GTV was reduced by more than 25% in 4 of 12 patients. The changes in GTV were 32% ($\pm$11%). The corresponding change in PTV was 20% ($\pm$5%). If the GTV is being scored as macroscopic disease distal from the primary tumor (eg, in a lymph node metastasis in the lower jugular area), a significant alteration of the PTV may result from a small increase in the GTV. Ciernik et al [81] concluded that integrated PET/CT for treatment planning for 3-D conformal radiation therapy improves the standardization of volume delineation compared with that of CT alone. The PET/CT system has the potential of reducing the risk for geographic misses, of minimizing the dose of ionizing radiation applied to nontarget organs, and of changing the current practice in 3-D conformal radiation therapy planning by taking into account the metabolic and biologic features of cancer.

Integrated CT/linear accelerator system

Many patients receiving fractionated radiotherapy for head and neck cancer have marked anatomic changes during their course of treatment, including shrinking primary tumors or nodal masses, resolving post-operative edema, and changes in overall body weight loss [82]. Conventional radiotherapy is planned using a single set of CT scans acquired before the start of treatment. As recommended by the committee of the International Commission on Radiation Units, the treated clinical target volume (CTV) includes a margin around the GTV for potential microscopic spread, and the CTV is enlarged by a further margin to create a PTV [83]. The margin is chosen to include uncertainties resulting from organ motion and from errors in physical set-up to assure consistent dose delivery to the CTV. Studies have shown that there are significant set-up uncertainties in external beam radiation treatments. A significant cause of these errors is the use of external (skin) markers, because they do not accurately represent the current position of the internal target [84,85]. The anatomic changes occurring throughout radiotherapy for head and neck cancer could have significant dosimetric effects in the setting of highly conformal treatment approaches, such as IMRT.

The daily use of target-localization techniques to locate internal structures can reduce these uncertainties and systematic errors. Advanced imaging technologies have already allowed in-room target localization techniques to play an important role in the delivery of highly conformal external beam radiation treatments. Several localization techniques have been used in the clinic. These techniques include ultrasound-based noninvasive techniques for prostate cancer treatment [86,87], implanted fiducial markers for tumor tracking [88–90], video-based surface tracking for patient positioning [91–92], in-room cone-beam CT for image-guided radiation therapy [93], and megavoltage CT imaging for tomotherapy [94]. More recently, with the availability of integrated CT/linear accelerator combinations, internal anatomy can often be imaged with the patient in the treatment position [95–98]. A commercialized CT/linear accelerator system (EXaCT Targeting, Varian Medical Systems, Inc., Palo Alto, California, and PRIMATOM, Siemens Medical Solutions, Iselin, New Jersey) is shown in Fig. 4.

In Fig. 4, the integrated CT/linear accelerator system allows CT imaging at daily radiotherapy sessions while the patient remains immobilized in the treatment position. Barker et al [98] studied the volumetric and geometric changes occurring during fractionated radiotherapy for head and neck cancer using this integrated CT/linear accelerator system at the M. D. Anderson Cancer Center. Eligible patients in the study had to have a pathologic diagnosis of head and neck cancer, be treated with definitive external beam radiotherapy, and have gross primary or cervical nodal disease measuring at least 4 cm in maximal diameter. All patients were treated using the integrated CT/linear accelerator system that allows CT imaging at the daily radiotherapy sessions while the patient remains immobilized in the treatment position. CT scans were acquired three times per week during the entire course of radiotherapy, and both GTV (primary tumor and involved lymph nodes) and normal tissues (parotid glands, spinal canal, mandible, and external contour) were manually contoured on every axial slice. Volumetric and positional changes relative to a central bony

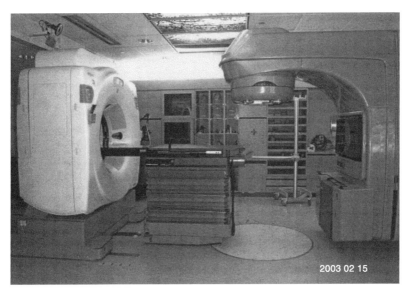

Fig. 4. Integrated CT/linear accelerator system (EXaCT) installed at the M. D. Anderson Cancer Center. (*From* Court L, Rosen I, Mohan R, et al. Evaluation of mechanical precision and alignment uncertainties for an integrated CT/LINAC system. Med Phys 2003;30(6):1198–210, with permission; Barker JL, Garden AS, Ang KK, et al. Quantification of volumetric and geometric changes occurring during fractionated radiotherapy for head-and-neck cancer using an integrated CT/linear accelerator system. Int J Radiat Oncol Biol Phys 2004;59(4):960–70, with permission.)

reference were determined for each structure. Barker et al [98] found that GTV decreased throughout the course of fractionated radiotherapy, at a median rate of 0.2 cm^3 per treatment day (range, 0.01–1.95 cm^3/d). The GTV decreased at a median rate of 1.8% per treatment day (range, 0.2–3.1%/d) as a percentage of the initial volume. On the last day of treatment, this decrease corresponded to a median total relative loss of 69.5% of the initial GTV (range, 9.9%–91.9%). In addition, the center of mass of shrinking tumors changed position with time, indicating that GTV loss is frequently asymmetric. At the end of treatment, the median center of the mass displacement (after corrections for variations in daily set-up) was 3.3 mm (range, 0–17.3 mm). Parotid glands also decreased in volume (median, 0.19 cm^3/d; range, 0.04–0.84 cm^3/d), and shifted medially (median, 3.1 mm; range, 0–9.9 mm) with time. There was a high correlation between the medial displacement of the parotid glands and weight loss during treatment.

An integrated CT/linear accelerator system can quantify the geometric and volumetric changes in anatomy for patients who undergo fractionated external beam radiotherapy for head and neck cancer. Geometric changes in the patient external contour and in target shape and location may result in suboptimal treatment, especially when highly conformal treatment techniques, such as IMRT, are used.

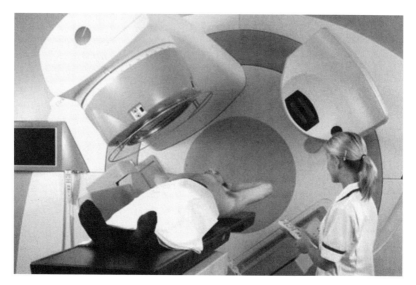

Fig. 5. Combined cone beam tomography and linear accelerator. (*Courtesy of* Elekta Oncology Systems, Inc., Elekta AB, Stockholm, Sweden)

Image-guided radiotherapy

IMRT has compelled the radiotherapy community to pursue greater precision. Although there has not been extensive use of image-guided radiotherapy (IGRT) in head and neck treatment, this modality commands attention for the potential that it promises in localization and reproducibility of patient treatments. The intention of IGRT is to combine patient positioning devices and imaging tools to target the lesion with this enhanced precision. There are several ways to employ IGRT in the clinical setting. The integrated CT/linear accelerator system discussed previously is one example of IGRT. Electronic portal imaging has been explored by Buck et al [99] and as a prospect for IGRT. Another approach attaches X-ray tubes to the linear accelerator gantry and employs cone beam tomography to obtain real-time images of the patient in the treatment position for localization and verification. An example of this technology is shown in Fig. 5 [100] and has been demonstrated effectively in prostate treatments.

References

[1] Kies MS, Haraf DJ, Athanasiadis I, et al. Induction chemotherapy followed by concurrent chemoradiation for advanced head and neck cancer: improved disease control and survival. J Clin Oncol 1998;16(8):2715–21.
[2] Haraf DJ, Kies M, Rademaker AW, et al. Radiation therapy with concomitant hydroxyurea and fluorouracil in stage II and III head and neck cancer. J Clin Oncol 1999;17(2):638–44.

[3] Vokes EE, Kies MS, Haraf DJ, et al. Concomitant chemoradiotherapy as primary therapy for locoregionally advanced head and neck cancer. J Clin Oncol 2000;18(8):1652–61.

[4] Fu KK, Pajak TF, Trotti A, et al. A Radiation Therapy Oncology Group (RTOG) phase III randomized study to compare hyperfractionation to standard fractionation radiotherapy for head-and-neck squamous cell carcinoma: first report of RTOG 9003. Int J Radiat Oncol Biol Phys 2000;48(1):7–16.

[5] Olmi PS, Fallai CC, Torri V, et al. Locoregionally advanced carcinoma of the oropharynx: conventional radiotherapy vs accelerated hyperfractionated radiotherapy vs concomitant radiotherapy and chemotherapy: a multicenter randomized trial. Int J Radiat Oncol Biol Phys 2003;55(1):78–92.

[6] Parsons JT, Mendenhall WM, Bova FJ, et al. Head and neck cancer. In: Levitt SH, Khan FM, Potish RA, editors. Technological basis of radiation therapy: practical clinical applications. 2nd edition. Philadelphia: Lea & Febiger; 1992. p. 203–31.

[7] Sidransky D, Schantz SP, Sessions RB, et al. Cancer of the head and neck. In: DeVita VT, Hellman S, Rosenberg SA, editors. Cancer: principles and practice of oncology. 5th edition. Philadelphia: Lippincott-Raven; 1997. p. 735–848.

[8] Chao KS, Brizel DM, Barker JL, et al. Head and neck tumor. In: Perez CA, Brady LW, Halperin EC, et al, editors. Principles and practice of radiation oncology. 4th edition. Philadelphia: Lippincott Williams & Wilkins; 1998. p. 897–1200.

[9] Shaha AR, Patel S, Shasha D, et al. Head and neck cancer. In: Lenhard RE, Osteen RT, Gansler T, editors. Clinical oncology. Atlanta (GA): The American Cancer Society; 2001. p. 297–330.

[10] Lefebvre JL, Coche-Dequeant B, Castelain B, et al. Interstitial brachytherapy and early tongue squamous cell carcinoma management. Head Neck 1990;12(3):232–6.

[11] Son YH, Sasaki CT. Nonsurgical alternative therapy for bulky advanced head and neck tumors. Arch Otolaryngol Head Neck Surg 1995;121(9):991–3.

[12] Vikram B, Mishra S. Permanent iodine-125 implants in postoperative radiotherapy for head and neck cancer with positive surgical margins. Head Neck 1994;16(2):155–7.

[13] Nath R. New directions in radionuclide sources for brachytherapy. Semin Radiat Oncol 1993;3(4):278–89.

[14] Kinsey RR. The NuDat Program for nuclear data on the web. Nuclear Data Center, Brookhaven National Laboratory (1999). Available at: http://www.nndc.bnl.gov/nudat2/index.jsp.

[15] Ling CC. Permanent implants using Au-198, Pd-103, and I-125: radiobiological considerations based on the linear quadratic model. Int J Radiat Oncol Biol Phys 1992;23(1):81–7.

[16] Chen Z, Nath R. Biologically effective dose (BED) for interstitial seed implants containing a mixture of radionuclides with different half-lives. Int J Radiat Oncol Biol Phys 2003;55(3):825–34.

[17] Pernot M, Malissard L, Hoffstetter S, et al. Influence of tumoral, radiobiological, and general factors on local control and survival of a series of 361 tumors of the velotonsillar area treated by exclusive irradiation (external beam irradiation + brachytherapy or brachytherapy alone). Int J Radiat Oncol Biol Phys 1994;30(5):1051–7.

[18] Pernot M, Malissard L, Taghian A, et al. Velotonsillar squamous cell carcinoma: 277 cases treated by combined external irradiation and brachytherapy—results according to extension, localization, and dose rate. Int J Radiat Oncol Biol Phys 1992;23(4):715–23.

[19] Harrison LB, Lee HJ, Pfister DG, et al. Long term results of primary radiotherapy with/without neck dissection for squamous cell cancer of the base of tongue. Head Neck 1998;20(8):668–73.

[20] Puthawala AA, Syed AMN, Eads DL, et al. Limited external beam and interstitial ^{192}iridium irradiation in the treatment of carcinoma of the base of the tongue: A ten year experience. Int J Radiat Oncol Biol Phys 1988;14(5):839–48.

[21] Puthawala AA, Syed AMN, Eads DL, et al. Limited external irradiation and interstitial ^{192}iridium implant in the treatment of squamous cell carcinoma of the tonsillar region. Int J Radiat Oncol Biol Phys 1985;1(9):1595–602.

[22] Nose T, Koizumi M, Nishiyama K. High-dose-rate interstitial brachytherapy for oropharyngeal carcinoma: results of 83 lesions in 82 patients. Int J Radiat Oncol Biol Phys 2004;59(4):983–91.

[23] Lapeyre M, Peiffert D, Hoffstetter S, et al. Curved angiocatheter metal guide for the implantation in velo-tonsillar carcinomas. Radiother Oncol 2000;55(1):81–3.

[24] Fowler JF, Lindstrom MJ. Loss of local control with prolongation in radiotherapy. Int J Radiat Oncol Biol Phys 1992;23(2):457–67.

[25] Withers HR, Taylor JM, Maciejewski B. The hazard of accelerated tumor clonogen repopulation during radiotherapy. Acta Oncol 1988;27(2):131–46.

[26] Bourhis J, Fortin A, Dupuis O, et al. Very accelerated radiation therapy: preliminary results in locally unresectable head and neck carcinomas. Int J Radiat Oncol Biol Phys 1995;32(3):747–52.

[27] Knee R, Fields RS, Peters LJ. Concomitant boost radiotherapy for advanced squamous cell carcinoma of the head and neck. Radiother Oncol 1985;4(1):1–7.

[28] Lamb DS, Spry NA, Gray AJ, et al. Accelerated fractionation radiotherapy for advanced head and neck cancer. Radiother Oncol 1990;18(2):107–16.

[29] Saunders MI, Dische S, Fowler JF, et al. Radiotherapy employing three fractions on each of twelve consecutive days. Acta Oncol 1988;27(2):163–7.

[30] Fowler JF. How worthwhile are short schedules in radiotherapy? A series of exploratory calculations. Radiother Oncol 1990;18(2):165–81.

[31] Ang KK, Peters LJ, Weber RS, et al. Concomitant boost radiotherapy schedules in the treatment of carcinoma of the oropharynx and nasopharynx. Int J Radiat Oncol Biol Phys 1990;19(6):1339–45.

[32] Fu KK, Pajak TF, Trotti A, et al. A Radiation Therapy Oncology Group (RTOG) phase III randomized study to compare hyperfractionation and two variants of accelerated fractionation to standard fractionation radiotherapy for head and neck squamous cell carcinomas: first report of RTOG 9003. Int J Radiat Oncol Biol Phys 2000;48(1):7–16.

[33] Brizel DM. Radiotherapy and concurrent chemotherapy for the treatment of locally advanced head and neck squamous cell carcinoma. Semin Radiat Oncol 1998;8(4):237–46.

[34] Fu KK. Combined modality therapy for head and neck cancer. Oncology 1997;11(12):1781–96.

[35] Wendt TG, Grabenbauer GG, Rodel CM, et al. Simultaneous radiochemotherapy versus radiotherapy alone in advanced head and neck cancer: a randomized multicenter study. J Clin Oncol 1998;16(4):1318–24.

[36] Galvin JM, Ezzell G, Eisbrauch A, et al. Implementing IMRT in clinical practice: a joint document of the American Society for Therapeutic Radiology and Oncology and the American Association of Physicists in Medicine. Int J Radiat Oncol Biol Phys 2004;58(5):1616–34.

[37] Eisbruch A. Intensity-modulated radiotherapy of head-and-neck cancer: encouraging early results. Int J Radiat Oncol Biol Phys 2002;53(1):1–3.

[38] Xia P, Lee N, Liu Y, Poon I, et al. A study of planning dose constraints for treatment of nasopharyngeal carcinoma using a commercial inverse treatment planning system. Int J Radiat Oncol Biol Phys 2004;59(3):886–96.

[39] Lee N, Xia P, Quivey JM, et al. Intensity-modulated radiotherapy in the treatment of nasopharyngeal carcinoma: an update of the UCSF experience. Int J Radiat Oncol Biol Phys 2002;53(1):12–22.

[40] Xia P, Fu KK, Wong G, et al. Comparison of treatment plans involving intensity-modulated radiotherapy for nasopharyngeal carcinoma. Int J Radiat Oncol Biol Phys 2000;48(2):329–37.

[41] Sultanem K, Shu KK, Xia P, et al. Three-dimensional intensity-modulated radiotherapy in the treatment of nasopharyngeal carcinoma: The University of California-San Francisco experience. Int J Radiat Oncol Biol Phys 2000;48(3):711–22.

[42] van Dieren EB, Nowak PJCM, Wijers O, et al. Beam intensity modulation using tissue compensators or dynamic multileaf collimation in three-dimensional conformal radiotherapy of primary cancers of the oropharynx and larynx, including the elective neck. Int J Radiat Oncol Biol Phys 2000;47(5):1299–309.

[43] Lee N, Akazawa C, Akazawa P, et al. A forward-planned treatment technique using multisegments in the treatment of head-and-neck cancer. Int J Radiat Oncol Biol Phys 2004;59(2):584–94.

[44] De Gersem W, Claus F, De Wagter C, et al. An anatomy-based segmentation tool for intensity-modulated radiation therapy and its application to head-and-neck cancer. Int J Radiat Oncol Biol Phys 2001;51(3):849–59.

[45] Shepard D, Earl M, Li X, et al. Direct aperture optimization: a turnkey solution for step-and-shoot IMRT. Med Phys 2002;29(6):1007–18.

[46] Beaulieu F, Beaulieu L, Tremblay D, et al. Automatic generation of anatomy-based MLC fields in aperture-based IMRT. Med Phys 2004;31(6):1539–45.

[47] Xing L, Lin Z, Donaldson SS, et al. Dosimetric effects of patient displacement and collimator and gantry angle misalignment on intensity modulated radiation therapy. Radioth Oncol 2000;56(1):97–108.

[48] Manning MA, Wu Q, Cardinale RM, et al. The effect of setup uncertainty on normal tissue sparing with IMRT for head-and-neck cancer. Int J Radiat Oncol Biol Phys 2001;51(5):1400–9.

[49] Bentel GC, Marks LB, Hendren K, et al. Comparison of two head and neck immobilization systems. Int J Radiat Oncol Biol Phys 1997;38(4):867–73.

[50] Kim S, Akpati HC, Kielbasa JE, et al. Evaluation of intrafraction patient movement for CNS and head & neck IMRT. Med Phys 2004;31(3):500–6.

[51] Kim S, Akpati HC, Li JG, et al. Improved treatment of pelvis and inguinal nodes using modified segmental boost technique: dosimetric evaluation. Int J Radiat Oncol Biol Phys 2004;59(5):1523–30.

[52] Buatti JM, Friedman WA, Bova FJ, et al. LINAC radiosurgery for locally recurrent nasopharyngeal carcinoma: rationale and technique. Head Neck 1995;17(1):14–9.

[53] Cmelak AJ, Cox RS, Adler JR, et al. Radiosurgery for skull base malignancies and nasopharyngeal carcinoma. Int J Radiat Oncol Biol Phys 1997;37(5):997–1003.

[54] Gill SS, Thomas DGT, Warrington AP, et al. Relocatable frame for stereotactic external beam radiotherapy. Int J Radiat Oncol Biol Phys 1991;20(3):599–603.

[55] Ashamalla H, Addeo D, Ikoro N, et al. Commissioning and clinical results utilizing the Gildenberg-Laitinen adapter device for X-ray in fractionated stereotactic radiotherapy. Int J Radiat Oncol Biol Phys 2003;56(2):592–8.

[56] Bova FJ, Buatti JM, Friedman WA, et al. The University of Florida frameless high-precision stereotactic radiotherapy system. Int J Radiat Oncol Biol Phys 1997;38(4):875–82.

[57] Kassaee A, Das IJ, Tochner Z, et al. Modification of Gill-Thomas-Cosman frame for extracranial head-and-neck stereotactic radiotherapy. Int J Radiat Oncol Biol Phys 2003;57(4):1192–5.

[58] Souhami L, Olivier A, Podgorsak EB, et al. Fractionated stereotactic radiation therapy for intracranial tumors. Cancer 1991;68(10):2101–8.

[59] Ahn YC, Lee KC, Kim DY, et al. Fractionated stereotactic radiation therapy for extracranial head and neck tumors. Int J Radiat Oncol Biol Phys 2000;48(2):501–5.

[60] Laramore GE. Radiotherapy as the primary treatment for malignant salivary gland tumors. In: Johnson J, Didolkar M, editors. Head and neck cancer III. New York: Elsevier Science; 1993. p. 599–617.

[61] Catterall M, Errington RD. The implications of improved treatment of malignant salivary gland tumors by fast neutron radiotherapy. Int J Radiat Oncol Biol Phys 1987;13(9): 1313–8.

[62] Risler R, Eenmaa Y, Jacky J, et al. Installation of the cyclotron based clinical neutron therapy system in Seattle. In: Marti E, editor. Tenth International Conference on Cyclotrons and Their Applications. Piscataway (NJ): IEEE Service Center; 1984. p. 428–30.

[63] Hummel SM, Buchholz TA, Laramore GE. Treatment of adenoid cystic carcinoma of the salivary gland, a three-field technique. Med Dosim 1990;15(3):99–105.

[64] Douglas JG, Laramore GE, Austin-Seymour M, et al. Treatment of locally advanced adenoid cystic carcinoma of the head and neck with neutron radiotherapy. Int J Radiat Oncol Biol Phys 2000;46(3):551–7.

[65] Kudchadker RJ, Hogstrom KR, Garden AS, et al. Electron conformal radiotherapy using bolus and intensity modulation. Int J Radiat Oncol Biol Phys 2002;53(4):1023–37.

[66] Kudchadker RJ, Antolak JA, Morrison WH, et al. Utilization of electron bolus in head and neck radiotherapy. J Appl Clin Med Phys 2003;4(4):321–33.

[67] Ma C-M, Pawlicki T, Lee MC, et al. Energy- and intensity-modulated electron beam radiotherapy for breast cancer. Phys Med Biol 2000;45(8):2293–311.

[68] Hogstrom K, Boyd RA, Antolak JA, et al. Dosimetry of a prototype retractable eMLC for fixed-beam electron therapy. Med Phys 2004;31(3):443–62.

[69] Archambeau JO, Forell B, Doria R, et al. Use of variable thickness bolus to control electron beam penetration in chest wall irradiation. Int J Radiat Oncol Biol Phys 1981;7(6):835–42.

[70] Beach JL, Coffey CW, Wade JS. Individualized chest wall compensating bolus for electron irradiation following mastectomy: an ultrasound approach. Int J Radiat Oncol Biol Phys 1981;7(11):1607–11.

[71] Low DA, Starkschall D, Sherman NE, et al. Computer aided design and fabrication of an electron bolus for treatment of the paraspinal muscles. Int J Radiat Oncol Biol Phys 1995; 33(5):1127–38.

[72] Leavitt DD, Stewart JR, Moeller JH, et al. Optimization of electron arc therapy doses by multi-vane collimator control. Int J Radiat Oncol Biol Phys 1989;16(2):489–96.

[73] Ma C-M, Ding M, Li J, et al. A comparative dosimetric study on tangential photon beams, IMRT and MERT for breast cancer treatment. Phys Med Biol 2003;48(3):909–24.

[74] Moran JM, Martel MK, Bruinvis IAD, et al. Characteristics of scattered electron beams shaped with a multileaf collimator. Med Phys 1997;24(9):1491–8.

[75] Ding M, Li J, Price R, et al. Modulated electron radiation therapy using a conventional multileaf collimator: a feasibility study. Med Phys 2003;30(6):1447.

[76] Brun E, Kjellen E, Tennvall J, et al. FDG PET studies during treatment: prediction of therapy outcome in head and neck squamous cell carcinoma. Head Neck 2002;24(1): 127–35.

[77] Lowe VJ, Dunphy FR, Varvares M, et al. Evaluation of chemotherapy response in patients with advanced head and neck cancer using [F-18] fluorodeoxyglucose position emission tomography. Head Neck 1997;19(4):666–74.

[78] Wong RJ, Lin DT, Schoder H, et al. Diagnostic and prognostic value of [18F] fluorodeoxyglucose position emission tomography for recurrent head and neck squamous cell carcinoma. J Clin Oncol 2002;18(7):4199–208.

[79] Beyer T, Townsend DW, Brun T, et al. A combined PET/CT scanner for clinical oncology. J Nucl Med 2000;41:1369–79.

[80] Schöder H, Yeung HWD, Gonen M, et al. Head and neck cancer: clinical usefulness and accuracy of pet/ct image fusion. Radiology 2004;231:65–72.

[81] Ciernik IF, Dizendorf E, Baumert BG, et al. Radiation treatment planning with an integrated positron emission and computer tomography (PET/CT): a feasibility study. Int J Radiat Oncol Biol Phys 2003;57(3):853–63.

[82] Sobel S, Rubin P, Keller B, et al. Tumor persistence as a predictor of outcome after radiation therapy of head and neck cancers. Int J Radiat Oncol Biol Phys 1976;1(9):873–80.

[83] International Commission on Radiation Units and Measurements. Report 62: prescribing, recording, and reporting photon beam therapy. Bethesda (MD): International Commission on Radiation Units and Measurements; 1999.

[84] Yan D, Wong J, Vicini F, et al. Adaptive modification of treatment planning to minimize the deleterious effects of treatment setup errors. Int J Radiat Oncol Biol Phys 1997;38(1): 197–206.

[85] Yan D, Lockman D. Organ/patient geometric variation in external beam radiotherapy and its effects. Med Phys 2001;28(4):593–602.

[86] Lattanzi J, McNeeley S, Pinover W, et al. A comparison of daily CT localization to a daily ultrasound-based system in prostate cancer. Int J Radiat Oncol Biol Phys 1999;43(4): 719–25.

[87] Morr J, DiPetrillo T, Tsai JS, et al. Implementation and utility of a daily ultrasound-based localization system with intensity-modulated radiotherapy for prostate cancer. Int J Radiat Oncol Biol Phys 2002;53(5):1124–9.

[88] Balter JM, Sandler HM, Lam K, et al. Measurement of prostate movement over the course of routine radiotherapy using implanted markers. Int J Radiat Oncol Biol Phys 1995;31(1): 113–8.

[89] Shimizu S, Shirato H, Ogura S, et al. Detection of lung tumor movement in real-time tumor-tracking radiotherapy. Int J Radiat Oncol Biol Phys 2001;51(2):304–10.

[90] Kitamura K, Shirato H, Seppenwoolde Y, et al. Three-dimensional intrafractional movement of prostate measured during real-time tumor-tracking radiotherapy in supine and prone treatment positions. Int J Radiat Oncol Biol Phys 2002;53(5):1117–23.

[91] Johnson LS, Milliken BD, Hadley SW, et al. Initial clinical experience with a video-based patient positioning system. Int J Radiat Oncol Biol Phys 1999;45(1):205–13.

[92] Yan Y, Song Y, Boyer AL. An investigation of a video-based patient repositioning technique. Int J Radiat Oncol Biol Phys 2002;54(2):606–14.

[93] Jaffray DA, Siewerdsen JH, Wong J, et al. Flat-panel cone-beam computed tomography for image-guided radiation therapy. Int J Radiat Oncol Biol Phys 2002;53(5):1337–49.

[94] Ruchala KJ, Olivera GH, Kapatoes JM, et al. Megavoltage CT image reconstruction during tomotherapy treatments. Phys Med Biol 2000;45(12):3545–62.

[95] Kuriyama K, Onishi H, Sano N, et al. A new irradiation unit constructed of self-moving gantry-CT and LINAC. Int J Radiat Oncol Biol Phys 2003;55(2):428–35.

[96] Mackie TR, Kapatoes J, Ruchala K, et al. Image guidance for precise conformal radiotherapy. Int J Radiat Oncol Biol Phys 2003;56(1):89–105.

[97] Court L, Rosen I, Mohan R, et al. Evaluation of mechanical precision and alignment uncertainties for an integrated CT/LINAC system. Med Phys 2003;30(6):1198–210.

[98] Barker JL, Garden AS, Ang KK, et al. Quantification of volumetric and geometric changes occurring during fractionated radiotherapy for head-and-neck cancer using an integrated CT/linear accelerator system. Int J Radiat Oncol Biol Phys 2004;59(4):960–70.

[99] Buck D, Alber M, Nusslin F. Potential and limitations of the automatic detection of fiducial markers using an amorphous silicon flat-panel imager. Phys Med Biol 2003;48:763–74.

[100] Nederveen AJ, Lagendijk JJW, et al. Feasibility of automatic marker detection with an a-Si flat-panel imager. Phys Med Biol 2001;46(4):219–30.

ELSEVIER
SAUNDERS

Otolaryngol Clin N Am
38 (2005) 397–411

OTOLARYNGOLOGIC
CLINICS
OF NORTH AMERICA

Alternative Surgical Dissection Techniques

Thomas Carroll, MD*, Keith Ladner, BS,
Arlen D. Meyers, MD, MBA

*Department of Otolaryngology, University of Colorado Health Sciences Center,
4200 East Ninth Avenue, B 205, Denver, CO 80262, USA*

The steel blade and monopolar electrocautery have been and remain the mainstay in surgical dissection instruments for the majority of practicing otolaryngologists. Despite advances in technology and bioengineering, these two instruments remain widely used and are often preferred, although newer, emerging technologies have been demonstrated to improve surgical time, decrease postoperative pain, and reduce collateral tissue damage and unwanted side effects for select procedures. This article focuses on four alternative surgical dissection instruments and their applications in select otolaryngologic surgeries. These instruments include the ultrasonically activated scalpel (ie, UltraCision Harmonic Scalpel, Ethicon Endosurgery, Cincinnati, Ohio), bipolar electrosurgical scissors (ie, PowerStar bipolar scissors, Ethicon, Inc., Somerville, New Jersey), temperature-controlled radiofrequency probes (ie, Somnoplasty, Somnus Medical Technologies, Inc., Mountain View, California), and Coblation (ie, Evac 70 Plasma Wand, ArthroCare Corp., Sunnyvale, California).

A basic understanding of conventional monopolar electrocautery is imperative to understand the benefits and shortcomings of the newer dissection tools. Tissue ablation with the Bovie monopolar cautery unit, a conventional electrosurgical tool, is achieved by introducing current across the physical gap between the source electrode and electrically conductive tissue using an electrode pair. Air or water molecules in the gap are dissociated into charge-carrying ions. Kinetic energy transfer between charge-carrying ions and tissue molecules results in heating of intracellular and extracellular fluids and injures localized tissue cells [1]. Compared with a standard scalpel, electrocautery provides an excellent tool for achieving

---

* Corresponding author.
E-mail address: Thomas.carroll@uchsc.edu (T. Carroll).

cutting, ablation, coagulation, desiccation, and rapid surgical hemostasis because the heat generated denatures proteins. It has a larger area of collateral thermal damage than other dissection tools, however, and has been shown to extend postoperative recovery for certain procedures when compared with cold techniques [2–4].

Bipolar scissors

How it works

The PowerStar bipolar scissors is discussed most frequently in the otolaryngolic literature. It is a modified 7-inch Metzenbaum scissors with two normal blades that have been modified to allow bipolar electrocautery without excessive collateral damage. The inner surface of one blade is covered with a ceramic coat. The other blade is coated with a clear surface-hardening material. The handles and part of the outer surface of the blades are covered with plastic [5]. Some have modified the instrument further to bring the outer plastic coating to within 10 mm of the tip of the scissors [6]. A diathermy machine is used to supply the electrical current. Reportedly, after 25 to 40 operations, the scissors become dull and need to be discarded [5,6]. Bipolar scissors, like bipolar forceps, are as effective as monopolar cautery but offer less lateral tissue injury and do not interfere with cardiac pacemakers or joint prostheses. Bipolar scissors and forceps have recently been coupled into one automatic unit that is linked to a computer and turns on when touched to tissue. It stops working automatically once coagulation has taken place and before desiccation or fulguration occurs [7].

Applications

Bipolar scissors have been described for use in multiple otolaryngologic procedures such as tonsillectomy, facial plastic surgery, microvascular free-flap surgery, and parotid surgery. The most frequently reported application for the bipolar scissors in otolaryngologic surgery is tonsillectomy. The technique for tonsillectomy uses the scissors' ability to dissect with and without cautery. The procedure involves slow movements to allow the cautery to work in the surgeon's favor. As blood vessels are identified, the bipolar scissors can maintain hemostasis by allowing current to pass between the tips of the blades until the vessel is sealed. The surgery is usually reported as bloodless with a slight blanching seen at the end of the procedure in the tonsillar bed [6]. If bleeding is seen, the tips of the scissors can cauterize in a manner similar to that of bipolar forceps. As in monopolar blade electrocautery and bipolar forceps electrocautery, the blades of the scissors require periodic cleaning during a procedure for optimal functioning.

Saleh et al [6] reported 40 cases of tonsillectomy using bipolar scissors. They found that operative times for bipolar scissors were shorter than reported for blunt dissection and bipolar forceps and that blood loss was less than reported for laser, bipolar forceps, and blunt dissection. In the amount of blood lost during tonsillectomy, Bovie cautery was comparable to bipolar scissors. Posttonsillectomy hemorrhage with bipolar scissors was comparable to previously reported values using other methods.

A later prospective, randomized study of 183 patients by Raut et al [5] compared bipolar scissors with the cold dissection technique. Statistically significant differences in blood loss and operative time favored the bipolar scissors. A difference in postoperative pain between the two groups was not statistically significant. Postoperative hemorrhage was also similar between the two groups. Isaacson and Szeremeta [8] found low operative time, no blood loss, and no posttonsillectomy hemorrhage using bipolar scissors.

Other applications for bipolar scissors have been reported in the literature. Uchida et al [9] describe a role for bipolar scissors dissection in superficial lobectomy of the parotid gland. Conventional monopolar cautery was used until the facial nerve was identified; then surgery was completed with bipolar scissors in one half of the patients and monopolar cautery was continued in the other patients. Operating time was significantly less, and blood loss was also less, but not significantly so, in the bipolar scissors group. Permanent facial weakness was not observed in either group, although traction was thought to play a role in the few patients with temporary weakness.

Winslow et al [10] report the usefulness of bipolar scissors in an array of plastic surgery and microvascular procedures. They emphasized their use in free-flap harvest and endoscopic brow lift. In the endoscopic brow lift, hemostasis of the sentinel vein can be accomplished without thermal injury to the adjacent temporal branch of the facial nerve. They also found that the tourniquet was no longer needed in harvesting their fibular free flaps because of the ease of hemostasis offered by the bipolar cautery. Wax et al [11] reported significantly improved time under the tourniquet when using bipolar scissors to elevate radial forearm fasciocutaneous free flaps.

Complications and controversies

The only complication mentioned more than once in the literature pertaining to the bipolar scissors is superficial burn. A noninsulated screw on the body of the scissors has reportedly caused two tongue burns during tonsillectomy and a skin burn during a submentoplasty [10,12]. The distal handles are also reported to become hot despite insulation [12]. Winslow et al [10], who describe the problems, state that technique and care when using bipolar scissors can help avoid this complication.

Coblation

How it works

Cold ablation, or coblation, has received much attention in recent medical literature. Coblation technology, first developed by ArthroCare (Sunnyvale, California), was originally designed for cartilage repair during arthroscopic surgery. Since its introduction, however, the applications of coblation in the operating room have drastically expanded. The field of otolaryngology has arguably benefited from this new technology. Coblation is currently being used for such procedures as tonsillectomy, turbinectomy, and palate reduction.

Coblation is a direct extension of standard electrosurgical techniques in that it also employs an oscillating electrical current to disrupt surrounding tissue. Electrodes at the tip of the coblation probe serve as sources of radiofrequency energy. This energy is not conducted directly through the surrounding tissue as in conventional electrosurgery; rather, a conductive medium (either normal saline fluid or gel) is used to deliver the electrical energy. The radiofrequency excites the saline solution, thereby creating a field of electrically active sodium ions that are able to dissociate tissue molecular bonds. (Therefore coblation is commonly referred to as an electro-dissociation procedure.) Because there is a steady flow of saline from the probe, this system generates relatively low tissue temperatures (40°C–70°C) when compared with standard electrosurgery (400°C–600°C) [13,14].

Coblation is also able to operate at a much lower frequency (100 kHz) than conventional electrosurgery generators (350 kHz–2000 kHz). Because impedance is inversely related to the frequency magnitude, the tissue impedance is four to five times greater than in standard electrosurgery [14]. Like the Bovie device, coblation probes also allow for hemostasis through the coagulation option. When the coagulation pedal is pressed, the applied voltage cycles on and off and produces hemostasis.

By operating at lower temperatures and frequencies, coblation has been purported to decrease healthy tissue destruction and result in more rapid wound healing. For example, Chinpairoj et al [14] concluded that incisions created by electro-dissociation resulted in faster wound healing and less collateral tissue injury than those of conventional electrosurgery. Therefore several recent clinical studies, as discussed later, have reported better outcomes with coblation surgery than with traditional methods.

Applications

By far, the most widely explored application of coblation has been in tonsil removal, one of the most common head and neck procedures. Otolaryngologists have experimented with a myriad of different techniques for tonsillectomies in searching for a method that decreases postoperative pain and the frequency of postoperative hemorrhage. Through improved precision in tissue dissection and decreased collateral tissue damage, coblation was hypothesized to minimize these side effects.

Tonsillectomies are thought to cause postoperative pain by disrupting muscle fibers and nerve endings lying beneath the lateral tonsil capsule. With the electro-dissociative method, a subtotal intracapsular tonsil reduction that avoids injury to the constrictor muscles can be performed

[15]. In a double-blind, randomized, controlled study, Timms and Temple [16] compared postoperative pain and healing time in 10 adults receiving tonsil coblation on one side and bipolar dissection on the other. They reported a markedly lower range of pain scores and an earlier fall to very low pain scores on the side of coblation. Similarly, there was a significant difference in the appearance of tonsillar fossae at 9 days after surgery, with the coblation side often fully healed and the bipolar side containing considerable slough. Many studies, including those of Friedman et al [15] and Arya et al [17], have subsequently affirmed the findings of Timms and Temple, reporting reduced postoperative pain, more rapid return to normal diet and activity, and diminished analgesic requirements in both adults and children receiving coblation tonsillectomies [16].

Based on these recent studies, most experts agree that coblation subtotal tonsillectomies significantly reduce postoperative pain and allow quicker recovery. This method is generally accepted as a superior option for patients with obstructive tonsillar hypertrophy who do not require complete tonsil tissue removal and as a suitable alternative for patients with chronic or recurrent tonsillitis. Clearly, postoperative comorbidities need to be evaluated further, but initial results for coblation tonsillectomy are promising.

Inferior turbinate hypertrophy is a common manifestation of chronic rhinitis and leads to significant obstructive symptoms. Definitive treatment requires surgical reduction of the inferior turbinates. Various methods, including coblation, have been used to minimize nasal obstructive symptoms. This technique creates channels within the anterior and posterior aspects of the inferior turbinates by ablating tissue as the probe is inserted into the submucosal plane. One to six passes may be made in the tissue, and each pass requires approximately 10 to 20 seconds [18].

Bhattacharyya and Kepnes [19] conducted a consecutive series of 24 adult patients who were treated for inferior turbinate hypertrophy with the coblation technique. The patients returned to the clinic for follow-up visits at 2 weeks, 3 months, and 6 months. At 3 months and 6 months, 75% and 85% of patients, respectively, reported improvement in nasal breathing. The authors also concluded that the procedure was safe, with only 8% of patients experiencing postoperative epistaxis. Although these results are consistent with those of standard techniques, a controlled trial comparing the safety and effectiveness of coblation with that of conventional methods is necessary.

Still in its experimental stage, soft palate reduction for snoring and obstructive sleep apnea can be achieved with coblation technology. As in inferior turbinate reduction, the probe is passed into the submucosal plane of the palate to form necrotic lesions that shrink with time. Although no studies have been performed to assess the efficacy and safety of this procedure, results from a similar procedure, bipolar radiofrequency thermal ablation, were favorable [20].

Complications and controversies

Opponents have argued that subtotal tonsillectomy using the coblation system leaves a significant remnant of tonsillar tissue that can regrow. Koltai et al [20] reported regrowth of tonsil tissue following partial tonsillectomy with a microdebrider in one child, supporting this suggestion. In a small, randomized, control study of subtotal coblation tonsillectomy versus complete coblation tonsillectomy, Arya et al [17] assert that there is no difference in postoperative pain between the two groups. Based on these findings, these investigators believe that coblation technology can be used to resect the tonsils completely, thus avoiding tissue regrowth.

Two recent conflicting studies have evaluated the incidence of post-operative hemorrhage in coblation tonsillectomy. Using a retrospective analysis of 65 cases, Noon and Hargreaves [21] described a significant increase in the rate of secondary hemorrhage in adult patients treated with coblation tonsillectomy compared with standard dissection (22.2% versus 3.4%). In contrast, in a large, prospective, observational cohort study, Belloso et al [22] found that the rate of secondary hemorrhage in both children and adults was much lower in coblation tonsillectomies than in blunt dissection tonsillectomies (2.25% versus 6.19%). Clearly, further investigation is needed to resolve this debate.

Harmonic scalpel

How it works

Ultrasonic coagulation achieved by the harmonic scalpel is similar to that of electrocautery in that the ultimate result remains a denatured protein coagulum that coapts and tamponades blood vessels. The mechanism by which the proteins become denatured is completely different, however. Both electrocautery and lasers form the coagulum by heating tissue to denature the protein. The harmonic scalpel denatures protein by using ultrasonic vibration to transfer mechanical energy sufficient to break tertiary hydrogen bonds [23]. At least two mechanisms exist by which the harmonic scalpel cuts: cavitational fragmentation and mechanical cutting. The blade vibrates at 55.5 kHz over a distance of 80 μm. This device generates minimal heat, resulting in much lower lateral thermal damage than seen with monopolar or laser cautery. The lateral zone of injury for the harmonic scalpel has been shown in the porcine model to be 0 to 1000 μm, versus the 240-μm to 15-mm range for monopolar electrocautery [24]. In a porcine study comparing vessel-sealing systems using various modalities of energy, including the harmonic scalpel, the LigaSure vessel sealing system (Valleylab, Boulder, Colorado), and two types of bipolar forceps, the harmonic scalpel was found to seal arteries 3.8 mm in diameter on average and veins 9.9 mm in diameter on average. This sealing ability was essentially inferior to that of the other systems. The harmonic scalpel showed the smallest area of lateral thermal damage, however [25].

The harmonic scalpel set-up consists of a generator, a hand piece, and a blade. The hand piece contains an ultrasonic transducer that consists of a stack of piezoelectric crystals sandwiched between two metal cylinders under pressure [23]. The transducer is attached to the blade through a mount. The 110-volt generator is a high-frequency switching power supply controlled by a microprocessor that pulses the transducer in the hand piece with AC current. This current allows the transducer to vibrate at its natural harmonic frequency of 55.5 kHz. The blade used most frequently in otolaryngologic procedures looks like a paddle with a sharp inner beveled side for cutting and a blunt outer radius for coaptive coagulating. The generator can be adjusted from a level of 1 to 5 to increase cutting speed and decrease coagulation by increasing the blade's lateral excursion [23,26]. A descriptive article by Wiatrak and Willging [26] reports the benefits of less charring and smoke, giving the surgeon a more visible surgical field.

Applications

The harmonic scalpel was originally developed for its applications in laparoscopic abdominal surgery but has found its way successfully into the specialty of otolaryngology [27]. The primary applications for the harmonic scalpel in the otolaryngologic literature pertain to its uses for tonsillectomy and thyroidectomy. The use of the harmonic scalpel has also been described in excising cancer of the tongue and soft palate [28], submandibular sialadenectomy [29], parotidectomy [30], treating allergic rhinitis by means of inferior turbinate alteration [31], and surgical treatment of rhinophyma [32]. The advantages and disadvantages of the harmonic scalpel pertaining to tonsillectomy and thyroidectomy are discussed here.

The most noticeable and worrisome complications for tonsillectomy surgeons and patients alike are intraoperative blood loss, postoperative hemorrhage, and postoperative pain and return to daily activities. Operative time and cost are also considerations. In theory the harmonic scalpel is a superlative dissection instrument, when compared with electrocautery, because the decreased lateral tissue damage should lead to decreased postoperative pain and quicker recovery. Because the harmonic scalpel has the ability to coagulate as it dissects, it should be comparable to electrocautery in controlling intraoperative bleeding and in operative times.

Results of the studies pertaining to the use of the harmonic scalpel in tonsillectomy have been mixed. An early observational study by Sood et al [33] reported shorter operation times, a mean operative blood loss of 7 mL, and low levels of early postoperative pain in 59 patients who underwent harmonic scalpel tonsillectomy. Two small, early, prospective studies investigating postoperative pain compared harmonic scalpel with traditional cold dissection tonsillectomy. Both studies included adult subjects who had cold dissection tonsillectomy performed on one side and harmonic scalpel tonsillectomy performed on the other. In the first study, Arena et al [34] reported that in 26 patients there were no differences in pain score during the 14 days postoperatively. They did observe, however, that the need for cauterization was significantly less on the sides treated with harmonic scalpel. On the other hand, a study by Akural et al [35] showed that pain on postoperative day 1 was significantly better in the harmonic scalpel group, but by the second week of recovery pharyngeal pain and otalgia were worse in the harmonic scalpel group.

Intraoperative and postoperative blood loss findings for harmonic scalpel versus electrocautery tonsillectomies are variable. In a 50-patient prospective, randomized trial by Haegner et al [36], intraoperative blood loss was significantly less for the harmonic scalpel group, but the postoperative blood loss was higher (7/25 versus 3/25). Walker and Syed [23] found no differences between the groups for either intraoperative or postoperative bleeding in their prospective study of 316 children. Willging and Wiatrak [37] found intraoperative blood loss to be equivalent for the two methods in their study of 117 patients, as did Morgenstein et al [38] with 156 patients in a community-based practice.

The ability of a patient to return to normal diet and activity has also been studied in many of the studies comparing harmonic scalpel to electrocautery. Walker and Syed [23] reported that at both 24 and 72 hours postoperatively patients from the harmonic scalpel group returned to normal activity and normal diet significantly more often than those in the electrocautery group. This observation was true for all patients combined but especially true for those 7 years old and younger. Only at the 24-hour mark was the subclassified 8-year-and-older group treated by the harmonic scalpel not significantly better in terms of return to normal diet that age-matched patients treated with electrocautery. No significant difference was found between groups in narcotic and non-narcotic analgesic use. Morgenstein et al [38], in their community-based study, revealed no significant difference between the groups for pain at days 1, 3 and 6, for days until soft foods could be eaten, and days until regular diet taken. This study split out a number of harmonic scalpel patients (14/95) who required Bovie cautery for control of hemorrhage and again found no advantages in that group over patients treated using harmonic scalpel alone. On the other hand, Willging and Wiatrak [37] report that on days 1,2,3, and 14, the harmonic scalpel patients reportedly slept more soundly than the electrocautery group reflecting their comfort level. Superior but not statistically significant pain scores on postoperative days 2, 3, and 4 for the harmonic scalpel groups correlated with the sleep findings.

Unlike the variable results described with the use of the harmonic scalpel in tonsillectomy, the literature is consistent concerning the usefulness of the harmonic scalpel in thyroid surgery. Operative times are consistently lower, bleeding is insignificant, and the resulting cost containment is evident. In addition to the shorter operating time (30 minutes less for lobectomy and 40 minutes less for total thyroidectomy), Shemen [39] reports the advantage of a smaller incision (4.5 versus 5.5 cm). Vach et al [40] report that pathologists can more easily evaluate thyroid specimens obtained with the harmonic scalpel. In their work with video-assisted thyroidectomy, Miccoli et al [41] confirmed the significant reduction in operative time and a lack of complications in the harmonic scalpel group. Finally, in a prospective, randomized study of 200 patients, Ortega et al [42] confirmed a 15% to 20% reduction in operative time. Hospital stays were similar to those with traditional thyroidectomy, so the reduced operating time resulted in a lower global charge for the harmonic scalpel group.

Complications and controversies

Certain minor complications from using the harmonic scalpel have been reported in the literature. Haegner et al [36] reported significant uvular swelling and slower wound healing in his prospective study on ultrasonic tonsillectomy. Shemen [39] reports two superficial skin burns that healed uneventfully. The shorter operative time for thyroidectomy using the harmonic scalpel has been shown to reduce overall costs, but for tonsillectomy, in which the operative times for harmonic scalpel and electrocautery techniques are not widely different, the financial benefit is not as obvious. Walker and Syed [23] point out that at their institution (like many others), the general surgeons had already met the initial capital expense of buying the reusable equipment (generator and wand). The net cost of the disposable blade, after figuring in the cost of the previously used cautery and Teflon tip, is approximately $80. They point out that this small cost burden may save the hospital the enormous expense of readmissions for dehydration because of the quicker initial recovery seen by the patients in their study. Also, they suggest a second cost benefit is realized by the parents of the child who recovers quickly, who can return to work sooner. Finally, concern for whether the harmonic scalpel releases viable airborne cancer cells has been addressed in the literature. A study by Nduka et al [43] looked at colon cancer in rats being dissected by the harmonic scalpel. The smoke plume generated by the surgery was aspirated, but no viable tumor cells were isolated or grown in vitro.

Temperature-controlled radiofrequency ablation

How it works

Temperature-controlled radiofrequency ablation (TCRFA) technology is now widely used by otolaryngologists for treatment of sleep-disordered breathing (SDB). The technology behind TCRFA is not new: it has been studied and used extensively by other medical specialties in the treatment of such diseases as atrial fibrillation, trigeminal neuralgia, prostatic hypertrophy, and liver tumors [44]. In otolaryngology, the Somnoplasty system is well described for its use in tissue reduction for the base of tongue, soft palate, inferior turbinates, and palatine tonsils. The Somnoplasty device consists of a radiofrequency control unit that delivers variable energy (power) levels at controlled temperatures. This unit attaches interchangeable hand-held probes for different applications.

TCRFA allows the ear, nose, and throat surgeon to deliver a specific amount of low-temperature, low-voltage energy in the form of radio-frequency (measured in joules) to a specific site. Radiofrequency energy delivered in this fashion agitates tissue ions by the inherent changes in electrical flow with an alternating (AC) current. The tissue then heats because of its inherent resistance but does so only to temperatures of 60° to 90°C. Laser and electrocautery techniques, in contrast, deliver energy at temperatures above 750°C. Because proteins denature at temperatures in excess of 47°C, the Somnoplasty probe causes tissue and vascular coagulation in the area of application. The radiofrequency energy causes an acute inflammatory response within the first 24 hours, leaving the tissue congested and edematous. Within 72 hours, the treated area undergoes tissue necrosis and subsequently, over 10 days, changes to fibrotic tissue [44,45]. The ultimate goal of the TCRFA technique is tissue reduction. This reduction occurs in two stages: contraction and resorbtion. Initially, the area of fibrosis contracts and pulls the adjacent tissue with it. Subsequently, over the next several months the body resorbs this area, causing further volumetric tissue reduction [45]. Stuck et al [46] describe the ideal amount of energy to be applied to the tongue base as 600 J at 85°C. After an initial in vitro porcine model they used 11 human subjects and MRI technology to measure lesion size in vivo. They determined that energy above 600 J resulted only in slight increases in lesion length but not diameter. The final lesion size at this ideal energy and temperature was approximately 8.3 mm in diameter by 10.9 mm in length.

Applications

TCRFA is primarily used with in-office or operating room procedures for the treatment of SDB. The location of the obstruction, lesion placement, and underlying patient diagnosis (ie, simple snoring or nasal obstruction versus obstructive sleep apnea syndrome [OSAS]) normally determine whether TCRFA can be done as an outpatient procedure.

As an outpatient office procedure, TCRFA has been used in the treatment of habitual snoring and nasal obstruction caused by inferior turbinate hypertrophy. For habitual, nonapneic snorers, Boudewyns and Van de Heynig [47] describe their prospective, nonrandomized findings in 45 patients. They made one midline lesion of approximately 700 J in the soft palate in one to three sessions and performed pre- and postsession full-night polysomnography on each patient. Forty-five percent of patients had a posttreatment snoring index of less than 3, and 84% had subjective improvement. Sandhu et al [48] performed a pilot study to obtain objective data on 10 patients, delivering three lesions in each of two sessions (700 J at midline and 350 J on each side at 85°C). They found that 60% of patients reported subjective improvement, but only 30% showed objective improvement based on full polysomnography 3 months after the last treatment. Velopharyngeal function and speech quality are not affected by TCRFA of the soft palate [49].

TCRFA to the inferior turbinates is widely used and has been shown numerous times to be effective for nasal obstruction [50–54]. Most studies exclude patients with septal deformity. TCRFA of the turbinates has also shown benefit to patients who can tolerate continuous positive airway pressure (CPAP) for OSAS, although further, larger studies are needed [55]. Nasal function as measured by ciliary beat frequency and saccharin transit time was preserved after TCRFA to the inferior turbinates [54].

TCRFA is also used in certain procedures for OSAS or obstructive tonsillar hypertrophy that require overnight observation in the hospital. Nelson [44] has evaluated the use of TCRFA for reduction of tonsillar tissue in patients who suffered from obstructive symptoms such as dysphagia and dysphonia but not overt OSAS. He initially performed the reduction in the operating room but has moved his procedure to an office setting after which patients are observed overnight in the hospital. Using a two-needle probe, he makes two to four passes per tonsil with an average dose of 2301 J per tonsil under local anesthesia. Patients reportedly tolerated the procedure well and returned to normal activity in 1 to 2 days. In a later pilot study looking at the long-term effects of this procedure, Nelson [56] found that tonsil somnoplasty maintained its effectiveness up to the 1-year mark.

TCRFA to the base of tongue has also become an effective adjunct to the arsenal of OSAS surgical procedures. The base of tongue is normally entered with a double-tipped probe under direct visualization, and energy is delivered in multiple passes. Studies are variable in the total joules and number of sessions required to complete the procedure. Woodson et al [57] compared outcomes between OSAS patients receiving CPAP versus those who underwent TCRFA to the base of tongue. They found superior outcomes in those patients who had saline injected into the surgical site before TCRFA was performed. The apnea hypopnea index (AHI) did improve in those undergoing TCRFA, and clinical outcomes were similar between TCRFA and CPAP groups. For patients with an AHI less than 20, TCRFA to the base of tongue produced better subjective improvement than seen in the CPAP patients in the same category. Li et al [58] investigated long-term outcomes. They demonstrated that the effect of TCRFA to the base of tongue may reduce objectively over time, but subjective quality-of-life scores remained strong.

Since the addition of TCRFA to the base of tongue as a treatment of OSAS, studies have evaluated its effectiveness when used in tandem with other procedures to improve outcomes in patients with OSAS. Fischer et al [59] demonstrated that after 9750 J in total was delivered to the tongue base, tonsils, and soft palate using TCRFA, 60% of participants were treated successfully or had marked improvement. Friedman et al [60] concluded that uvulopalatopharyngoplasty alone can be successful for patients with stage I OSAS (minimal oropharyngeal obstruction on examination and a body mass index less than 40) based on the Friedman staging system. For those with higher-stage OSAS, TCRFA to the base of tongue in addition to UPPP will be more effective.

Complications and controversies

Many minor complications have been described in the literature pertaining to TCRFA. Superficial ulceration of the soft palate, mucosal breakdown, and tongue base neuralgia have been described and probably represent non–life-threatening complications. TCRFA has been reported to have caused tongue base abscesses, tongue hematoma, floor of mouth edema, and a tonsil abscess, all of which could compromise or have compromised the airway. These instances are rare but necessitate observation and awareness [59,61–64].

Summary

The bipolar scissors, coblator, harmonic scalpel, and somnoplasty techniques are widely available and offer new choices for the operating arena. There are advantages and disadvantages to all four techniques. With time, these dissection methods will prove their lasting power. Otolaryngologists have already begun to expand their applications and will surely play a role in their use and development.

References

[1] Stoker KE, Don DM, Kang DR. Pediatric total tonsillectomy using coblation compared to conventional electrosurgery: a prospective, controlled single-blind study. Otolaryngol Head Neck Surg 2004;130:666–75.
[2] Wexler DB. Recovery after tonsillectomy: electrodissection vs. sharp dissection techniques. Otolaryngol Head Neck Surg 1996;114:576–81.
[3] MacGregor FB, Albert DM, Bhattacharyya AK. Postoperative morbidity following paediatric tonsillectomy; a comparison of bipolar diathermy dissection and blunt dissection. Int J Pediatr Otorhinolaryngol 1995;31:1–6.
[4] Nunez DA, Provan J, Crawford M. Postoperative tonsillectomy pain in pediatric patients: electrocautery (hot) vs. cold dissection and snare tonsillectomy–a randomized trial. Arch Otolaryngol Head Neck Surg 2000;126:837–41.
[5] Raut VV, Bhat N, Sinnathuray AR. Bipolar scissors versus cold dissection tonsillectomy: a prospective, randomized, multi-unit study. Laryngoscope 2001;111:2178–82.

 [6] Saleh HA, Cain AJ, Mountain RE. Bipolar scissor tonsillectomy. Clin Otolaryngol 1999;24: 9–12.

 [7] Stenquist BC, Holt PJ, Motley RJ. Computerized bipolar diathermy with scissors and forceps in cutaneous surgery. Dermatol Surg 2002;28:601–2.

 [8] Isaacson G, Szeremeta W. Pediatric tonsillectomy with bipolar electrosurgical scissors. Am J Otolaryngol 1998;19:291–5.

 [9] Uchida M, Wada Y, Hisa Y. Usefulness of bipolar scissors during superficial lobectomy of the parotid gland. Laryngoscope 2002;112:1119–21.

[10] Winslow CP, Burke A, Bartels S, et al. Bipolar scissors in facial plastic surgery. Arch Facial Plast Surg 2000;2:209–12.

[11] Wax MK, Winslow C, Desyatnikova S, et al. A prospective comparison of scalpel versus bipolar scissors in the elevation of radial forearm fasciocutaneous free flaps. Laryngoscope 2001;111:568–71.

[12] Sood S, Strachan DR. Bipolar scissor tonsillectomy [letter]. Clin Otolaryngol 1999;24:465.

[13] Plant RL. Radiofrequency treatment of tonsillar hypertrophy. Laryngoscope 2002;112: 20–2.

[14] Chinpairoj S, Feldman MD, Saunders JC, et al. A comparison of monopolar electrosurgery to a new multipolar electrosurgical system in a rat model. Laryngoscope 2001;111:213–7.

[15] Friedman M, LoSavio P, Ibrahim H, et al. Radiofrequency tonsil reduction: safety, morbidity, and efficacy. Laryngoscope 2003;113:882–7.

[16] Timms MS, Temple RH. Coblation tonsillectomy: a double blind randomized controlled study. J Laryngol Otol 2002;116:450–2.

[17] Arya A, Donne AJ, Nigam A, et al. Double-blind randomized controlled study of coblation tonsillotomy versus coblation tonsillectomy on postoperative pain. Clin Otolaryngol 2003; 28:503–6.

[18] Bhattacharyya N, Kepnes LJ. Clinical effectiveness of coblation inferior turbinate reduction. Otolaryngol Head Neck Surg 2003;129(4):365–71.

[19] Bhattacharyya N, Kepnes LJ. Bipolar radiofrequency cold ablation turbinate reduction for obstructive inferior turbinate hypertrophy. Operative Techniques in Otolaryngology-Head and Neck Surgery 2002;13(2):170–4.

[20] Koltai PJ, Solares CA, Koempel JA, et al. Intracapsular tonsillar reduction (partial tonsillectomy): reviving a historical procedure for obstructive sleep disordered breathing in children. Otolaryngol Head Neck Surg 2003;129(5):532–8.

[21] Noon AP, Hargreaves S. Increased post-operative haemorrhage seen in adult coblation tonsillectomy. J Laryngol Otol 2003;117:704–6.

[22] Belloso A, Chidambaram A, Morar P, et al. Coblation tonsillectomy versus dissection tonsillectomy: postoperative hemorrhage. Laryngoscope 2003;113:2010–3.

[23] Walker RA, Syed ZA. Harmonic scalpel tonsillectomy versus electrocautery tonsillectomy: a comparative pilot study. Otolaryngol Head Neck Surg 2001;125:449–55.

[24] McCarus SD. Physiologic mechanism of the ultrasonically activated scalpel. J Am Assoc Gynecol Laprosc 1996;3:601–8.

[25] Landman J, Kerbl K, Rehman J, et al. Evaluation of a vessel sealing system, bipolar electrosurgery, harmonic scalpel, titanium clips, endoscopic gastrointestinal anastomosis vascular staples and sutures for arterial and venous ligation in a porcine model. J Urol 2003; 169:697–700.

[26] Wiatrak BJ, Willging JP. Harmonic scalpel for tonsillectomy. Laryngoscope 2002;112:14–6.

[27] Siperstein AE, Berber E, Morkoyun E, et al. The use of the harmonic scalpel vs. conventional knot tying for vessel ligation in thyroid surgery. Arch Surg 2002;137:137–42.

[28] Metternich FU, Wenzel S, Sagowski C, et al. The "Ultracision harmonic scalpel" ultrasound scalpel. Initial results in surgery of the tongue and soft palate. HNO 2002;50(8):733–8.

[29] Komatsuzaki Y, Ochi K, Sugiura N, et al. Video-assisted submandibular sialadenectomy using an ultrasonic scalpel. Auris Nasus Larynx 2003;30(Suppl):S75–8.

[30] Markkanen-Leppanen M, Pitkaranta A. Parotidectomy using the harmonic scalpel. Laryngoscope 2004;114:381–2.

[31] Yamanishi T, Suzuki M, Inoue H, et al. Clinical application of the harmonic scalpel to allergic rhinitis. Auris Nasus Larynx 2003;30(1):53–8.

[32] Metternich FU, Wenzel S, Sagowski C, et al. Surgical treatment of rhinophyma with the ultrasonic scalpel (Ultracision harmonic scalpel). Laryngorhinootologie 2003;82(2):132–7.

[33] Sood S, Corbridge R, Powles J, et al. Effectiveness of the ultrasonic harmonic scalpel for tonsillectomy. Ear Nose Throat J 2001;80(8):514–6, 518.

[34] Arena S, Carney S, Wormald P. The use of the harmonic scalpel and post-operative pain following tonsillectomy: a prospective randomized clinical trial. Aust J Otolaryngol 2000;3: 495–7.

[35] Akural EI, Koivunen PT, Teppo H, et al. Post-tonsillectomy pain: a prospective, randomized and double-blinded study to compare an ultrasonically activated scalpel technique with the blunt dissection technique. Anaesthesia 2001;56(11):1045–50.

[36] Haegner U, Handrock M, Schade H, et al. "Ultrasound tonsillectomy" in comparison to conventional tonsillectomy. HNO 2002;50(9):836–43.

[37] Willging JP, Wiatrak BJ. Harmonic scalpel tonsillectomy in children: a randomized prospective study. Otolaryngol Head Neck Surg 2003;128:318–25.

[38] Morgenstein SA, Jacobs HK, Brusca PA, et al. A comparison of tonsillectomy with the harmonic scalpel versus electrocautery. Otolaryngol Head Neck Surg 2002;127:333–8.

[39] Shemen L. Thyroidectomy using the harmonic scalpel: analysis of 105 consecutive cases. Otolaryngol Head Neck Surg 2002;127:284–8.

[40] Vach B, Fanta J, Velenska Z. The harmonic scalpel and surgery of the thyroid gland. Rozhl Chir 2002;81(Suppl 1):S3–7.

[41] Miccoli P, Berti P, Raffaelli M, et al. Impact of harmonic scalpel on operative time during video-assisted thyroidectomy. Surg Endosc 2002;16(4):663–6.

[42] Ortega J, Sala C, Flor B, et al. Efficacy and cost-effectiveness of the UltraCision harmonic scalpel in thyroid surgery: an analysis of 200 cases in a randomized trial. J Laparoendosc Adv Surg Tech A 2004;14(1):9–12.

[43] Nduka CC, Poland N, Kennedy M, et al. Does the ultrasonically activated scalpel release viable airborne cancer cells? Surg Endosc 1998;12(8):1031–4.

[44] Nelson L. Radiofrequency treatment for obstructive tonsillar hypertrophy. Arch Otolaryngol Head Neck Surg 2000;126:736–40.

[45] Pazos G, Mair E. Complications of radiofrequency ablation in the treatment of sleep-disordered breathing. Otolaryngol Head Neck Surg 2001;125:462–7.

[46] Stuck BA, Kopke J, Maurer JT, et al. Lesion formation in radiofrequency surgery of the tongue base. Laryngoscope 2003;113:1572–6.

[47] Boudewyns A, Vanr de Heynig P. Temperature-controlled radiofrequency tissue volume reduction of the soft palate (somnoplasty) in the treatment of habitual snoring: results of a European multicenter trial. Acta Otolaryngol 2000;120:981–5.

[48] Sandhu GS, Vatts A, Whinney D, et al. Somnoplasty for simple snoring—a pilot study. Clin Otolaryngol 2003;28:425–9.

[49] Haraldsson PO, Karling J, Lysdahl M, et al. Voice quality after radiofrequency volumetric tissue reduction of the soft palate in habitual snorers. Laryngoscope 2002;112:1260–3.

[50] Li K, Powell NB, Riley RW, et al. Radiofrequency volumetric tissue reduction for the treatment of turbinate hypertrophy: a pilot study. Otolaryngol Head Neck Surg 1998;119: 569–73.

[51] Fischer Y, Gosepath J, Amedee RG, et al. Radiofrequency volumetric tissue reduction (RFVTR) of inferior turbinates: a new method in the treatment of chronic nasal obstruction. Am J Rhinol 2000;14(6):355–60.

[52] Coste A, Yona L, Blumen M, et al. Radiofrequency is a safe and effective treatment of turbinate hypertrophy. Laryngoscope 2001;111:894–9.

[53] Nease CJ, Krempl GA. Radiofrequency treatment of turbinate hypertrophy: a randomized, blinded, placebo controlled trial. Otolaryngol Head Neck Surg 2004;130:291–9.

[54] Powell NB, Zonato AI, Weaver EM, et al. Radiofrequency treatment of turbinate hypertrophy in subjects using continuous positive airway pressure: a randomized, double-blind, placebo-controlled clinical pilot trial. Laryngoscope 2001;111:1783–90.

[55] Rhee C-S, Kim DY, Won TB, et al. Changes of nasal function after temperature-controlled radiofrequency tissue volume reduction for the turbinate. Laryngoscope 2001;111(1):153–8.

[56] Nelson LM. Temperature-controlled radiofrequency tonsil reduction: extended follow-up. Otolaryngol Head Neck Surg 2001;125:456–61.

[57] Woodson BT, Nelson L, Mickelson S, et al. A multi-institutional study of radiofrequency volumetric tissue reduction for OSAS. Otolaryngol Head Neck Surg 2001;125:303–11.

[58] Li KK, Powell NB, Riley RW. Temperature-controlled radiofrequency tongue base reduction for sleep-disordered breathing: long-term outcomes. Otolaryngol Head Neck Surg 2002;127:230–4.

[59] Fischer Y, Khan M, Mann WJ. Multilevel temperature-controlled radiofrequency therapy of soft palate, base of tongue, and tonsils in adults with obstructive sleep apnea. Laryngoscope 2003;113:1786–91.

[60] Friedman M, Ibrahim H, Lee G, et al. Combined uvulopalatopharyngoplasty and radiofrequency tongue base reduction for treatment of obstructive sleep apnea/hypoponea syndrome. Otolaryngol Head Neck Surg 2003;129:611–21.

[61] Pazos G, Mair EA. Complications of radiofrequency ablation in the treatment of sleep-disordered breathing. Otolaryngol Head Neck Surg 2001;125:462–7.

[62] Robison S, Lewis R, Norton A, et al. Ultrasound guided radiofrequency submucosal tongue-base excision for sleep apnoea: a preliminary report. Clin Otolaryngol 2003;28:341–5.

[63] Stuck BA, Starzak K, Verse T, et al. Complications of temperature-controlled radio-frequency volumetric tissue reduction for sleep-disordered breathing. Acta Otolaryngol 2003;123(4):532–5.

[64] Back LJ, Tervahartiala PO, Piilonen AK, et al. Bipolar radiofrequency thermal ablation of the soft palate in habitual snorers without significant desaturations assessed by magnetic resonance imaging. Am J Respir Crit Care Med 2002;166:865–71.

ELSEVIER
SAUNDERS

Otolaryngol Clin N Am
38 (2005) 413–417

OTOLARYNGOLOGIC
CLINICS
OF NORTH AMERICA

Index

Note: Page numbers of article titles are in **boldface** type.

A

Adhesives, for wound closure, 296–298

AlloDerm soft tissue implants, 363

Auditory brainstem implants, history of, 262
  technology and outcomes of, 262–263

Auditory nerve, in neurofibromatosis Type 2, 262

Auricular reconstruction, tissue engineering in, 208–209

Autofluorescence, of lesions of oral mucosa, 222

Autologen, as soft tissue filler, 365–366

B

Bioengineering, and classical engineering principles, interaction of, 186
  definition of, 187
  introduction to, **185–197**
  sample projects in, 190–196
  solutions, for hearing loss and related disorders, **255–272**
  subdisciplines of, 187–190

Biofusionary, for wound closure, 301–302

Bioinformatics, in otolaryngology, **321–332**
  future prospects in, 328–329
  microarray technology and, 322–323
  techniques of, for microarray analysis, 323–324

Biomechanics, 189–190

Biomedical imaging science, 188

Biomimetics, 281

Bion microstimulator, in tinnitus, 268

Biophotonics, 215–216

Bipolar scissors, applications of, 398–399
  complications of, 399
  description of, 398

Bone-anchored hearing aids, history of, 264–265
  indications for, 265–266
  outcomes of, 266
  technology of, 265

BoneSource, 367

Bovine collagen, as soft tissue filler, 364

Brachytherapy, interstitial, description of, 372–373
  high-dose-rate, 373–374
  low-dose-rate, 373

Brain functional imaging, portable, using near-infrared light, 190–193

C

Cancer, diagnosis and treatment of, nanomedicine and, 285–286
  of head and neck. See *Head and neck, cancer of.*
  of mouth, 215

Cardiovascular research, bioengineering and, 188

Cell-based therapies, and tissue engineering, **199–214**

Coblation, applications of, 400–402
  complications of, 402
  description of, 399–400

Cochlear implants, electro-acoustic, history of, 261
  technology and outcomes of, 261–262
  external and internal components of, 256–257
  history of, 255–256
  indications for, 257–258
  outcomes of, 258–260
  quality of life and cost effectiveness of, 260
  surgical procedure for, 258
  technology of, 256–257

S

Shoe sole, for prevention of neuropathy in diabetic patients, 193–196

Silastic, for soft tissue implants, 362

Silicone soft tissue implants, 362

Skin tissue, interaction of laser light with, in port-wine stains, 242–243

Sleep apnea syndrome, obstructive, temperature-controlled radiofrequency ablation in, 407–408

Sleep-disordered breathing, temperature-controlled radiofrequency ablation in, 406–407

Soft tissue filler(s), Autologen as, 365–366
    bovine collagen as, 364
    Cymetra as, 366
    Dermalogen as, 366
    hyaluronic acid as, 364–365
    hydroxyapatite as, 367
    Isolagen as, 365

Soft tissue implants, AlloDerm, 363
    and fillers, **361–369**
    approval of, 361
    autologous, 362
    Gore-Tex, 362–363
    ideal, 361
    materials for, 361–362
    silicone, 362

Spectroscopy, diffuse reflectance, of lesions of oral mucosa, 218–220
    infrared, of oral mucosa, 225–226
    near-infrared, 190
    Raman, of oral mucosa, 227
    tri-modal, in lesions of oral mucosa, 222–223

Stereotactic radiosurgery, 381–382

Surgical dissection techniques, alternative, **397–411**

Systems neuroscience, 188–189

T

Temperature-controlled radiofrequency ablation, applications of, 406–408
    complications of, 408
    description of, 405–406

Tinnitus, bion microstimulator in, 268
    pathology of, 266

sensorineural, 267
    transcutaneous electrical stimulation in, 267

Tinnitus suppression devices, 266–268

Tissue engineering, 188
    cell-based therapies and, **199–214**
    cellular aspects of, 201–202
    challenges of, 199–200
    clinical aspects of, 202–203
    concept of, 199, 200
    in auricular reconstruction, 208–209
    in nose and nasal septum reconstruction, 209
    of facial skeleton, 210–211
    of larynx and trachea, 209–210
    polymeric scaffolds for, 203
        bioactive molecules of, 204
        compatibility of, 204
        degradability of, 204
        in situ-forming, 206–208
        prefabricated, 204–206

Tissue fusion, inductive, for wound closure, 301–302
    seamless, for wound closure, **295–305**

Tissue welding, laser, for wound closure, 299–300

Tomography, optical coherence, of oral mucosa, 228

Tonsillectomy, coblation for, 400–401
    harmonic scalpel for, 403–405

Trachea, tissue engineering of, 209–210

Transcutaneous electrical stimulation, in tinnitus, 267

Tumor markers, identification of, microarray analysis in, 327

Turkey test, 195

V

Vascular lesions, of face, advances in treatment of, 242–248

W

Wound closure, energy-based, 298–301
    modern adhesives for, 296–298
    seamless tissue fusion for, **295–305**
    traditional, 295–296

Changing Your Address?

Make sure your subscription changes too! When you notify us of your new address, you can help make our job easier by including an exact copy of your Clinics label number with your old address (see illustration below.) This number identifies you to our computer system and will speed the processing of your address change. Please be sure this label number accompanies your old address and your corrected address—you can send an old Clinics label with your number on it or just copy it exactly and send it to the address listed below.

We appreciate your help in our attempt to give you continuous coverage. Thank you.

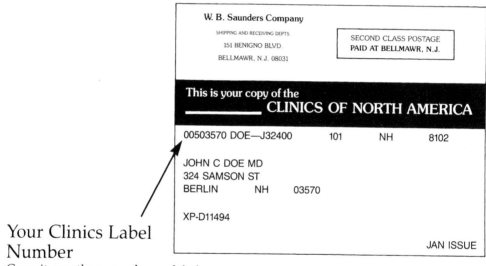

W. B. Saunders Company

SHIPPING AND RECEIVING DEPTS
151 BENIGNO BLVD.
BELLMAWR, N.J. 08031

SECOND CLASS POSTAGE
PAID AT BELLMAWR, N.J.

This is your copy of the
_____ **CLINICS OF NORTH AMERICA**

00503570 DOE—J32400   101   NH   8102

JOHN C DOE MD
324 SAMSON ST
BERLIN   NH   03570

XP-D11494

JAN ISSUE

Your Clinics Label Number

Copy it exactly or send your label
along with your address to:
W.B. Saunders Company, Customer Service
Orlando, FL 32887-4800
Call Toll Free 1-800-654-2452

Please allow four to six weeks for delivery of new subscriptions and for processing address changes.